Implementing Cancer Survivorship Care Planning

Workshop Summary

A National Coalition for Cancer Survivorship and
Institute of Medicine National Cancer Policy Forum Workshop

In Partnership with

The Lance Armstrong Foundation and
The National Cancer Institute

Maria Hewitt and Patricia A. Ganz, *Rapporteurs*

INSTITUTE OF MEDICINE
OF THE NATIONAL ACADEMIES

THE NATIONAL ACADEMIES PRESS
Washington, D.C.
www.nap.edu

THE NATIONAL ACADEMIES PRESS • 500 FIFTH STREET, N.W. • Washington, DC 20001

NOTICE: The project that is the subject of this report was approved by the Governing Board of the National Research Council, whose members are drawn from the councils of the National Academy of Sciences, the National Academy of Engineering, and the Institute of Medicine. The members of the committee responsible for the report were chosen for their special competences and with regard for appropriate balance.

This study was supported by the National Coalition for Cancer Survivorship, in partnership with the Lance Armstrong Foundation and the National Cancer Institute. Any opinions, findings, conclusions, or recommendations expressed in this publication are those of the author(s) and do not necessarily reflect the view of the organizations or agencies that provided support for this project.

International Standard Book Number-10:   0-309-10318-5
International Standard Book Number-13:   978-0-309-10318-3

Additional copies of this report are available from the National Academies Press, 500 Fifth Street, N.W., Lockbox 285, Washington, DC 20055; (800) 624-6242 or (202) 334-3313 (in the Washington metropolitan area); Internet, http://www.nap.edu.

For more information about the Institute of Medicine, visit the IOM home page at: **www.iom.edu.**

The serpent has been a symbol of long life, healing, and knowledge among almost all cultures and religions since the beginning of recorded history. The serpent adopted as a logotype by the Institute of Medicine is a relief carving from ancient Greece, now held by the Staatliche Museen in Berlin.

"Knowing is not enough; we must apply.
Willing is not enough; we must do."
—Goethe

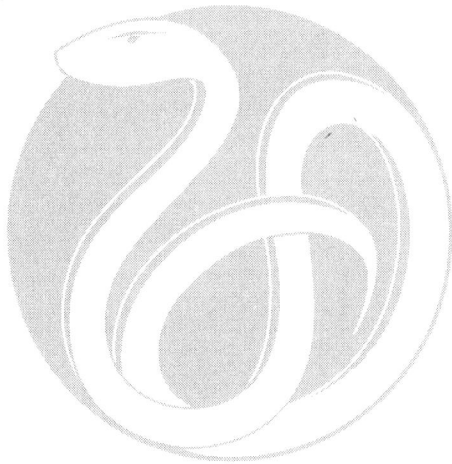

INSTITUTE OF MEDICINE
OF THE NATIONAL ACADEMIES

Advising the Nation. Improving Health.

THE NATIONAL ACADEMIES
Advisers to the Nation on Science, Engineering, and Medicine

The **National Academy of Sciences** is a private, nonprofit, self-perpetuating society of distinguished scholars engaged in scientific and engineering research, dedicated to the furtherance of science and technology and to their use for the general welfare. Upon the authority of the charter granted to it by the Congress in 1863, the Academy has a mandate that requires it to advise the federal government on scientific and technical matters. Dr. Ralph J. Cicerone is president of the National Academy of Sciences.

The **National Academy of Engineering** was established in 1964, under the charter of the National Academy of Sciences, as a parallel organization of outstanding engineers. It is autonomous in its administration and in the selection of its members, sharing with the National Academy of Sciences the responsibility for advising the federal government. The National Academy of Engineering also sponsors engineering programs aimed at meeting national needs, encourages education and research, and recognizes the superior achievements of engineers. Dr. Wm. A. Wulf is president of the National Academy of Engineering.

The **Institute of Medicine** was established in 1970 by the National Academy of Sciences to secure the services of eminent members of appropriate professions in the examination of policy matters pertaining to the health of the public. The Institute acts under the responsibility given to the National Academy of Sciences by its congressional charter to be an adviser to the federal government and, upon its own initiative, to identify issues of medical care, research, and education. Dr. Harvey V. Fineberg is president of the Institute of Medicine.

The **National Research Council** was organized by the National Academy of Sciences in 1916 to associate the broad community of science and technology with the Academy's purposes of furthering knowledge and advising the federal government. Functioning in accordance with general policies determined by the Academy, the Council has become the principal operating agency of both the National Academy of Sciences and the National Academy of Engineering in providing services to the government, the public, and the scientific and engineering communities. The Council is administered jointly by both Academies and the Institute of Medicine. Dr. Ralph J. Cicerone and Dr. Wm. A. Wulf are chair and vice chair, respectively, of the National Research Council.

www.national-academies.org

Staff

MARIA HEWITT, Study Director
ROGER HERDMAN, Director, National Cancer Policy Forum
ALIZA NORWOOD, Research Assistant
MARY ANN PRYOR, Senior Program Assistant

Reviewers

This report has been reviewed in draft form by individuals chosen for their diverse perspectives and technical expertise, in accordance with procedures approved by the NRC's Report Review Committee. The purpose of this independent review is to provide candid and critical comments that will assist the institution in making its published report as sound as possible and to ensure that the report meets institutional standards for objectivity, evidence, and responsiveness to the study charge. The review comments and draft manuscript remain confidential to protect the integrity of the deliberative process. We wish to thank the following individuals for their review of this report:

Betty R. Ferrell, PhD, RN, FAAN, City of Hope National Medical Center
Len Lichtenfeld, MD, FACP, American Cancer Society
Kevin Oeffinger, MD, Memorial Sloan-Kettering Cancer Center
Jerome W. Yates, MD, MPH, American Cancer Society

Although the reviewers listed above have provided many constructive comments and suggestions, they were not asked to endorse the final draft of the report before its release. The review of this report was overseen by **Melvin Worth, MD,** Scholar-in-Residence at the Institute of Medicine. Appointed by the National Research Council and Institute of Medicine, he was responsible for making certain that an independent examination of this report was carried out in accordance with institutional procedures and that all review comments were carefully considered. Responsibility for the final content of this report rests entirely with the rapporteurs and the institution.

Contents

Abstract

T his workshop proceedings was compiled from presentations and discussion during a two-day Institute of Medicine (IOM) National Cancer Policy Forum workshop sponsored by the National Coalition for Cancer Survivorship (NCCS) in partnership with the Lance Armstrong Foundation and the National Cancer Institute. The purpose of the workshop was to discuss a key recommendation of the joint IOM and National Research Council report, *From Cancer Patient to Cancer Survivor: Lost in Transition.* That report recommended that patients completing their primary treatment for cancer be given a summary of their treatment and a comprehensive plan for follow-up. This "Survivorship Care Plan" would also be provided to the patient's primary care providers. Such a plan would inform patients (and their providers) of the long-term effects of cancer and its treatment, identify psychosocial support resources in their communities, and provide guidance on follow-up care, prevention, and health maintenance. The purpose of the IOM workshop was to further inform the National Cancer Policy Forum on the next steps to implementing cancer survivorship care planning. The workshop featured commissioned papers, invited presentations, and discussions on formats for templates for treatment summaries and care plans; implementation issues, such as reimbursement; and potential practice sites for pilot tests of survivorship care planning. The workshop was open to the public and was attended by stakeholders with an interest in survivorship care: cancer survivors, nurses, primary care physicians, oncology specialty physicians, health services researchers, and representatives of government agencies, health insurance companies and managed care organizations.

The first day of the workshop was devoted to (1) an overview of the goals of survivorship care planning, (2) a review of the status of treatment summaries for oncology care, and (3) a general discussion and reaction to a series of qualitative research efforts. Structured one-on-one interviews and focus groups with consumers, nurses, and oncology and primary care physicians were conducted to help the forum better understand opportunities for, and barriers to, survivorship care planning. Reactants with diverse perspectives (consumers, nurses, physicians, insurers) were invited to participate in the discussion of these efforts. Topics for discussion included:

- What are the essential elements of the care plan? Will a single template work?
- Who is responsible for creating the plan and discussing the plan with patients?
- What are the respective roles of oncology/primary care and physicians/nurses?
- What economic strategies could encourage implementation of care planning?
- What barriers exist to creating the care plan? How can they be overcome?

On the second day of the workshop there were presentations and discussion on the following topics:

- Resources for completing the care plan template (survivorship guidelines, psychosocial support resources, recommendations on healthy behaviors/prevention).
- Adapting care plans to electronic record systems and information technologies.
- Statewide and collaborative approaches to implementation.
- Opportunities to pilot test survivorship care planning and assess its impact.
- An evaluation and research agenda for survivorship care planning.

At the end of the second day of the workshop, moderators led a wrap-up discussion of highlights of the two-day workshop.

1

Introduction

Chair, Institute of Medicine Committee on Cancer Survivorship:
Dr. Sheldon Greenfield

This workshop is designed to advance one of the key recommendations of the Institute of Medicine report *From Cancer Patient to Cancer Survivor: Lost in Transition* (see the workshop agenda and list of participants in Appendix A and B, respectively). The recommendation states that patients completing primary treatment should be provided with a comprehensive care summary and follow-up plan that are clearly and effectively explained. This Survivorship Care Plan should be written by the principal provider or providers who coordinated oncology treatment, and it should be reimbursed by third-party payers of health care. Such a plan would inform patients (and their providers) of the long-term effects of cancer and its treatment, identify psychosocial support resources in their communities, and provide guidance on follow-up care, prevention, and health maintenance (see the IOM recommendation in Appendix C).

The charge to workshop participants is to identify barriers to implementing survivorship care planning and then outline concrete steps that can be taken to address the challenges and the opportunities ahead.

Vice-Chair, Institute of Medicine Committee on Cancer Survivorship:
Ms. Ellen Stovall

Twenty-six years ago, when the founders of the National Coalition for Cancer Survivorship (NCCS) got together, they envisioned a world in which cancer research, cancer treatment, and cancer care would be very integrated and almost seamless. They described a model of care in which the psycho-social and spiritual concerns, vocational and financial barriers, and bother-some symptoms that often accompany a cancer diagnosis would be addressed with as much seriousness as the cancer itself. The term "survivor-ship" was the term coined to describe this optimal approach to cancer care. Today, survivorship is in the mainstream lexicon. It is the foresight of the NCCS founders that has brought us together today and closer to realizing this vision.

The Institute of Medicine is to be commended for its compendia of work on cancer survivorship and quality of care. Between 1999 and 2005, it issued a series of reports dealing with quality cancer care writ very large and then with a focus on policy issues specific to survivorship and palliative care for both children and adults with cancer.

We are very grateful to the authors of background papers commis-sioned for the workshop: Tim Byers; Wendy Demark-Wahnefried and Lee Jones; Craig Earle; David Poplack, Marc Horowitz, and Michael Fordis; and Deborah Schrag (see commissioned papers in Appendix D). Qualitative researchers Annette Bamundo, Rebecca Day, Marsha Fountain, Reynolds Kinzey, and Catherine Harvey also contributed an invaluable body of work for discussion today.

NCCS is sponsoring this workshop in partnership with the Lance Armstrong Foundation and the National Cancer Institute, through its Of-fice of Cancer Survivorship.

In closing, I would like to acknowledge the thousands of survivors who every day inform our work. Their day-to-day experiences with survivor-ship are what we are here to address in terms of how to ensure optimal care in clinical practice.

2

Suvivorship Care Planning

IMPLEMENTING THE SURVIVORSHIP CARE PLAN
Presenter: Dr. Patricia Ganz

As the Institute of Medicine (IOM) committee finished its deliberations on recommendations for the report *From Cancer Patient to Cancer Survivor: Lost in Transition*, there was a perception that the benefits of implementing the Survivorship Care Plan would be so obvious that everyone would jump on the bandwagon to make it happen. This rapid adoption may occur, but some effort to facilitate implementation is likely to be necessary. Overcoming some of the challenges and barriers to implementation is critical because survivorship care planning is a sentinel project in the drive for quality cancer care.

A key message of the report is that the needs and concerns of the large and growing number of cancer survivors cannot be ignored. The report also raised awareness of cancer as a chronic condition that requires long-term monitoring for its aftereffects and sequelae. That cancer increasingly involves long-term maintenance therapy is another chronic-care feature of the disease, not too unlike diabetes. Also documented in the IOM report is the problem of poor coordination of care and, as the title of the report indicates, the fact that cancer survivors are often "lost in transition."

Why is cancer different from other chronic diseases? Cancer is a very complex set of diseases, and treatments are often multimodal, involving a multidisciplinary team of providers. The treatments themselves are toxic and expensive, and very often care is poorly coordinated. Cancer treatment is often provided in isolation from other care, even though cancer patients tend to be elderly, with multiple comorbidities and health care needs. Oncology professionals at the onset of treatment provide some initial communication to the primary care physician, but during treatment such contact may decline. Given the demands of cancer treatment, most patients do not have time to see their primary care physician, and consequently cancer treatment may seriously disrupt patients' routine care and distance them from the care system to which they will have to return following their treatment.

The development of evidence-based guidelines has been impeded by the lack of research on the late effects of cancer therapy. The American Society of Clinical Oncology (ASCO) is developing guidelines for many important domains of survivorship care, but it has often had to rely on descriptive cohort studies as an evidence base. Even in the childhood cancer arena, in which survivorship issues have long been recognized, there are few studies on which to base guidelines. Support for research in this area is needed to advance understanding of cancer's late effects.

Follow-up care plans, to the extent that they have been developed and used, do not have a standard format and have focused on surveillance for recurrence. ASCO has developed guidelines for breast and colorectal cancer that include recommendations for follow-up for recurrent disease. These guidelines, however, do not deal with other complex and multidimensional issues facing survivors. Absent from most guidelines, for example, is information on health promotion and disease prevention. As cancer survivors live longer, they will need comprehensive health care that includes preventive services to address their cancer and other chronic conditions. In the area of infertility, which is a concern of many cancer survivors, many patients have been told, "You should be happy just to be alive." In this example, potential late effects need to be addressed during treatment planning to help ensure that individuals make informed choices and have an opportunity to lead full, normal lives to the extent possible.

Why does cancer care present such a challenge? Health services researchers engaged in cancer-related quality of care studies find that they have to request as many as three to five medical charts to examine the content of an episode of care. Cancer treatment is often prolonged and may occur in numerous outpatient and inpatient settings, some of which are specialized treatment facilities. There may be very limited communication among the treating physicians, and each of the multiple medical records may document only a portion of the treatment history. In large urban areas, patients may be operated on at one institution, have their chemotherapy at an oncologist's office, have radiation therapy at another institution, and then see a primary care physician somewhere else. Cancer care can be very complicated, and with no electronic records and limited communication, achieving integrated coordinated care can be very difficult.

How can one address this challenge? There are many solutions on the horizon. Integrated electronic medical records will be helpful if somebody is cared for within one system but, as previously mentioned, many patients are in and out of different care settings, often with incompatible information systems. Patient navigators can help patients with communication and coordination of care to ensure completion of the recommended treatment. Posttreatment consultation planning and counseling may also help, but issues that are salient at the end of treatment may not be fully addressed at the outset. None of these strategies is widely available for patients receiving active treatment today. Transition care planning is needed to address issues of coordination of care and quality of care throughout the care trajectory.

Why is survivorship care planning needed, and why is it so vital now? The Survivorship Care Plan is a vehicle that summarizes and communicates what transpired during cancer treatment. It is, in some respects, similar to a hospital discharge summary. Imagine someone being discharged from the hospital without a discharge summary. Whether it is a short or long hospital stay, it would be very cumbersome and time-consuming for the primary care provider responsible for postdischarge care to review the hospital chart to learn what went on during the stay and to divine the care plan for his or her patient. Providers are not reimbursed for preparing the hospital discharge summary, yet completing them is legally required. This obligation to document is inculcated into students throughout medical training. In an analogous fashion, it makes common sense for treating physicians, at the conclusion of treatment, to summarize and document the episode of cancer care.

The Survivorship Care Plan also needs to be prospective and record the known and potential late effects of cancer treatments with their expected time course. This may be very challenging because, as mentioned, there is a paucity of follow-up data for some treatments. More importantly, though, oncologists need to communicate to the survivor and to the other health care providers not only what has been done, but also what needs to be done in the future. This prospective plan is especially important in light of the mobility of the patient population, as well as the difficulty in retrieving older records. If patients were routinely given a formal document at the end of treatment that explained what went on, both in technical and lay terms, it would help them wherever they went and wherever they sought later care. This record could be updated fairly easily if there were such a foundation document.

As envisioned, the Survivorship Care Plan would also function to promote a healthy lifestyle to prevent recurrence and reduce the risk of other comorbid conditions. A summary document with a recommended follow-up plan completed at the conclusion of treatment gives patients an opportunity to take some responsibility for their care and may help to ensure adherence to follow-up recommendations. If patients move or go to a new primary care physician, the Survivorship Care Plan becomes the blueprint for future care.

The Survivorship Care Plan described in the IOM report incorporates recommendations from other IOM reports. The IOM, in its call for quality care, has promoted the ideal of: (1) continuous healing relationships between patients and providers; (2) customization of care based on patient needs and values; (3) the patient as the source of control; (4) shared knowledge and the free flow of information; (5) use of evidence-based decision making; (6) safety as a system property; (7) the need for transparency, and, thus, communication among all involved; (8) anticipation of needs; (9) a decrease in waste; and (10) cooperation among clinicians.[1] Survivorship care planning helps everyone know what needs to be done and who is going to be in charge of the various aspects of a person's care. Such planning helps to avoid the fragmentation of the surgeon's doing one thing, the radiation therapist's repeating it, and the primary care physician's not knowing if anything was done and doing it again. Having a care plan and a clear sense of assigned responsibility, with the patient or survivor as the custodian of the document, could potentially lead to substantial improvement in care efficiency.

Figure 2-1 illustrates the place of survivorship care in the cancer care trajectory. Patients may cycle out of survivorship care back into treatment again, but the focus is on patients who are being managed either with chronic or intermittent disease or who have long-term cancer-free survival and need a prospective plan of care.

The IOM report identified key elements that should be included in the Survivorship Care Plan:

- Specific tissue diagnosis and stage;
- Initial treatment plan and dates of treatment;
- Toxicities during treatment;
- Expected short- and long-term effects of therapy;
- Late toxicity monitoring needed;
- Surveillance for recurrence or second cancer;
- Who will take responsibility for survivorship care;
- Psychosocial and vocational needs; and
- Recommended preventive behaviors/interventions.

---

[1]IOM (Institute of Medicine) Committee on Quality of Health Care in America, 2001. *Crossing the Quality Chasm: A New Health System for the 21st Century*. Washington, DC: National Academy Press.

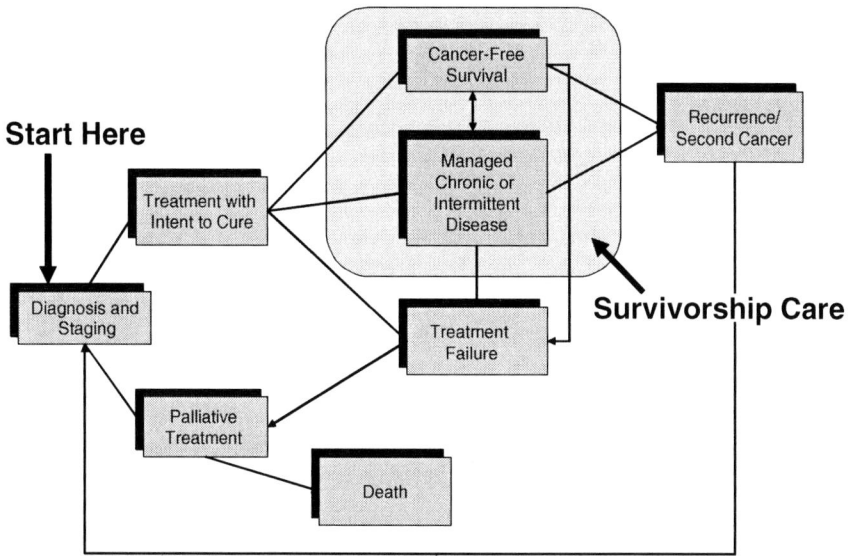

FIGURE 2-1 Cancer care trajectory.
NOTE: Palliative care is provided throughout the cancer care trajectory
SOURCE: Adapted from IOM Committee on Cancer Survivorship, 2006. *From Cancer Patient to Cancer Survivor: Lost in Transition.* Washington, DC: The National Academies Press.

Implementing such comprehensive care planning presents challenges to providers, and some may judge the IOM recommendation premature given the state of the evidence. Evidence is beginning to emerge on the value of this kind of care planning, or guided care, after patients complete their primary treatment.

Eva Grunfeld is a family physician who has conducted a number of randomized controlled trials to test whether primary care or family physicians provide the same quality care as oncologists to patients—in this case, breast cancer patients—after their initial treatment. She performed a randomized controlled trial most recently in Canada in which half of the women who were approached agreed to participate. Family physicians did as good a job as oncologists in terms of detecting recurrences, and women's satisfaction with care and assessment of quality of life did not vary by whether they received follow-up care from their family physician or oncologist.[2] A one-

---

[2]Grunfeld E et al. 2006. Randomized trial of long-term follow-up for early-stage breast cancer: a comparison of family physician versus specialist care. *Journal of Clinical Oncology* 24(6):848-855.

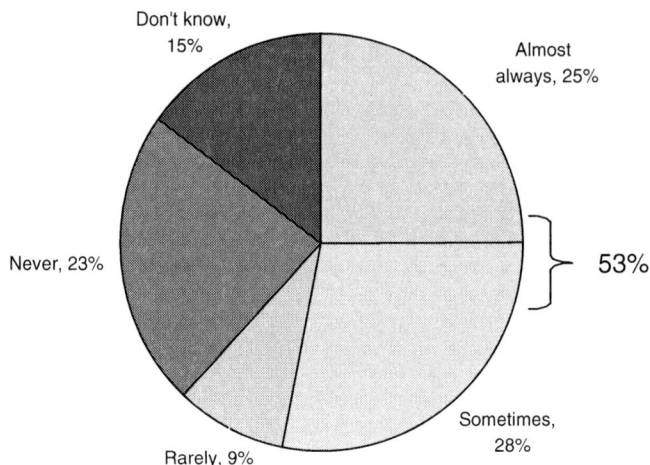

FIGURE 2-2 Primary care physicians receiving end-of-treatment summaries from oncologists.
SOURCE: Ganz presentation of information adapted from BlueCross of California, 2006.

page follow-up guideline was given to the family physician, similar to the Survivorship Care Plan under discussion, telling the physician exactly what to do, and when told, these family physicians performed as well as oncologists. This is a very nice piece of evidence to support survivorship care planning.

Dr. Ganz reported experience working with BlueCross of California to develop a course on the primary care physician's role in the care of cancer survivors. BlueCross of California conducts regular surveys of primary care physicians, and, in anticipation of the course, a few questions about survivorship care planning were added to the survey. The survey was fielded at about the time of the IOM report's release (November 5, 2005). The response rate was very low (5 percent), so the results should be interpreted with caution. Among the 75 respondents, only 25 percent said that they "almost always" received a detailed end-of-treatment summary from the oncologist treating their patients (Figure 2-2). An additional 28 percent said that they "sometimes" received such a summary. Therefore, about half of the primary care physicians reported either not receiving, rarely receiving, or not knowing whether they received care summaries at the end of treatment.

The primary care physicians were also asked two additional questions: "How prepared are you to monitor and manage your patients' late health effects that may arise as a result of the therapeutic exposures used during cancer treatment?" and "How prepared are you to handle transition-of-care issues for your patients after discharge from cancer treatment, including communication with oncology providers?" Only 33 percent of the primary care physicians felt "very prepared" for managing the late health effects, and 41 percent felt "very prepared" about the transition care (Figure 2-3).

Notably, there was an increased perceived ability to manage the late health effects and the handling of transition issues when providers had received end-of-treatment summaries from oncologists (Figure 2-4).

According to this small convenience sample of primary care physicians, confidence in managing cancer survivors' care increased when treatment summaries were available, but oncologists are not routinely sending such summaries to them. The quality of the treatment summaries sent to these primary care physicians was probably somewhat limited, but even so, they did appear to make a difference in how competent primary care physicians felt in terms of following up their survivors. Again, the numbers were small and the physicians participating are not likely to be representative of the population of BlueCross primary care providers in California, but the findings lend some credence to the value of survivorship care plans.

An example of a Survivorship Care Plan is shown in Box 2-1. This care plan was drafted for use in IOM's qualitative research (Chapter 3) and should be considered a work in progress. It is likely to be modified for use on

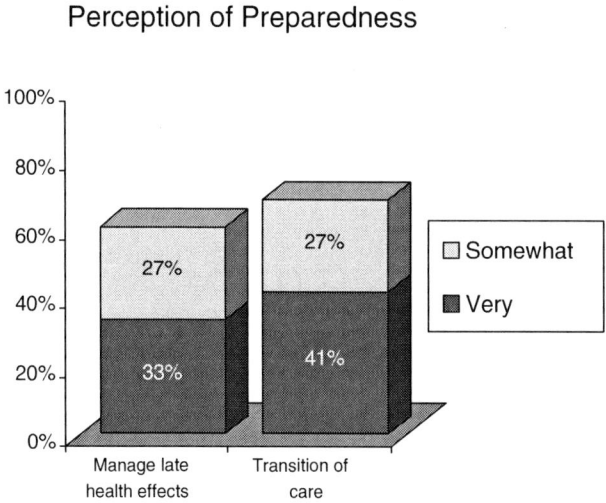

Perception of Preparedness

FIGURE 2-3 Primary care providers' confidence in managing cancer patients' late health effects.
SOURCE: Ganz presentation of information adapted from BlueCross of California, 2006.

% of physicians reporting they are prepared to . . .

Manage late health effects

Handle transition issues

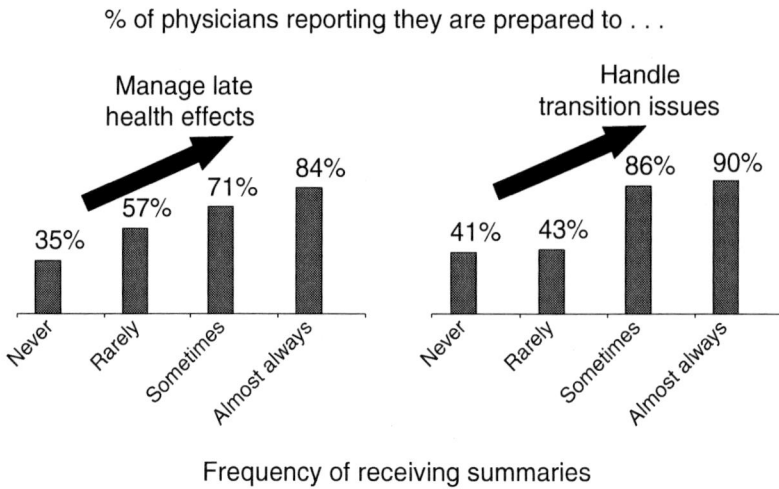

Frequency of receiving summaries

FIGURE 2-4 Relationship between confidence of the primary care physicians in managing cancer patients' late effects and receipt of an end-of-treatment summary. SOURCE: Ganz presentation of information adapted from BlueCross of California, 2006.

the basis of the results of the qualitative research and the experience of others who are testing these templates. The plan describes treatment and follow-up for a relatively young man with stage III colon cancer with lymph node involvement. The treatment summary portion of the plan documents the treatment he had, his surgery, the kind of staging studies that were performed, and the results of recent tumor marker tests. The summary lacks some details of treatment, but it is felt to provide appropriate general information for a primary care physician. Essential to communicate to primary care providers is information on what they need to be looking for and what management issues need to be addressed. To foster communication, the Survivorship Care Plan would be maintained in the oncologist's medical record, sent to the primary care physician, and shared with the patient.

As described in the sample care plan, the patient has high-stage cancer with increased risk of recurrence, which puts providers on alert that this individual has to be under good surveillance. The care plan also outlines what symptoms the patient should report if he experiences them (e.g., blood in the stool, abdominal pain, changing bowel habits). In terms of necessary medical assessments, he needs to be seen every 3 to 6 months for the first 3 years after primary treatment and then every 6 months for years 4 and 5. This schedule and the specification of recommended tests and imaging studies are based on the ASCO guideline. The care plan recommends genetic counseling due to his

BOX 2-1
Sample Cancer Survivorship Care Plan

Date of note: 4/3/06

Provider	**Affiliation:**	**Telephone number:**
Name: Mary Jones, M.D.	State Univ	000-000-0000

Survivor
Name: John Smith   Date of birth: 5-25-59

CANCER TREATMENT SUMMARY

Colorectal Cancer Diagnosis:
Date of tissue diagnosis of cancer: 7-15-05
Stage of cancer: III Lymph node involvement
Pathologic findings: high grade cancer arising in a large polyp, 3 of 10 nodes positive

Diagnostic tests done: dates and results
  Colonoscopy: 7-1-05, obstructing lesion at hepatic flexure
  CT scan Chest: no mets
  CT scan Abdomen: enlarged mass in right colon, no liver mets
  CT scan Pelvis; no abnormalities

Pre-operative and Post-operative serum CEA levels (dates and results): 7/5/05 10; 8/15/05 3.9
  Last CEA 2.0 on 3-10-06

Treatment history (attach relevant treatment summaries):

Date(s)	Surgery 7-15-05	Chemotherapy 9-05 to 3-06	Radiation none	Other
Location(s)	State Univ.	State Univ		
Provider name(s)	John Woods	Mary Jones		
Procedures	Right hemi-colectomy	Systemic chemo: 5 FU + Leuco-vorin +/- Ox-aliplatin (FLOX)		

Risk of cancer recurrence and second cancer: Patient has high-stage cancer with increased risk of recurrence.

continued

BOX 2-1 Continued

Patient should report these signs and symptoms if persistent:
Blood in stool, abdominal pain, change in bowel habits, cough that doesn't go away, bone pain, new lumps, nausea, vomiting, loss of appetite, weight loss, fatigue

Recommended surveillance to detect recurrence/second cancer (specify frequency):
- Clinical assessments:
    Every 3-6 months for the first 3 years after primary treatment, then every 6 months for years 4 and 5, and subsequently to be determined (ASCO, 2005)
- Tests:
    Serum CEA every 3 months for at least 3 years after diagnosis, if the patient is a candidate for surgery or systemic therapy (ASCO, 2005); data not sufficient to recommend other tests such as CBC, LFTs, and stool for occult blood (ASCO, 2005)
- Imaging:
    Annual CT of the chest and abdomen for 3 years after primary therapy (for patients who are at higher risk of recurrence and who could be candidates for surgery with curative intent).

- Other: Colonoscopy at 3 years after operative treatment; if results normal, every 5 years thereafter (ASCO, 2005);
    Genetic counseling for those who are high risk (colorectal cancer or polyps in a parent, sibling, or child younger than 60 or in two such relatives of any age or colorectal cancer syndromes in family)
    This patient needs genetic testing due to young age and family history.

Potential late effects of treatment (e.g., cardiovascular, skeletal):
Surgery: Bowel problems, such as diarrhea, fecal leakage/incontinence, constipation, bowel obstruction, hernia, pain, psychological distress

Chemo/Biotherapy: fatigue, peripheral neuropathy

Patient should report these signs and symptoms if persistent:
Diarrhea, constipation, pain with urination, erectile dysfunction, painful intercourse, infertility, numbness or tingling in hands or feet

Recommended surveillance for late effects of treatment(s): monitor for recovery of peripheral neuropathy

Preventive care recommendations (e.g., osteoporosis prevention, weight management, smoking cessation, diet): **This patient needs counseling about smoking cessation and weight loss.**

BOX 2-1 Continued

Physician(s) who will monitor recurrence/second cancer, late effects, and preventive care:

Dr. Adams will monitor for late effects and preventive care recommendations. Dr. Jones will monitor CEA and do endoscopy and imaging studies at prescribed intervals.

Identified concerns:	Referrals:
x Depression/anxiety:	o Psychiatry
o Fertility:	x Psychology/social work
o Marital/partner/family relationships:	o Fertility/endocrinology
o Sexuality:	x Genetic counseling
x Genetic risk:	x Smoking cessation
x Wellness (e.g., diet, exercise, smoking cessation)	x Dietician/weight control
	o Exercise program
o Employment, health insurance, finances:	o Physical therapy/rehabilitation
o Other:	o Counseling regarding employment, health insurance, finances
	o Other:

---

young age and family history. Under the section on late effects, the care plan specifies potential surgical and chemotherapy complications and, in addition, any other signs or symptoms that could be related to treatment, including sexual dysfunction and peripheral neuropathy. The care plan also addresses lifestyle issues. This particular patient was a smoker and is overweight, and so health promotion and disease prevention action items are included, along with a delineation of who should take charge of monitoring these interventions. As indicated on this care plan, the oncologist assumes responsibility for some of the cancer-related surveillance issues, while the primary care physician takes care of monitoring for late effects and prevention counseling and interventions.

What are the barriers to routine generation of treatment summary and survivorship care plans? There are some specialties, for example surgery and radiation oncology, that routinely create an operative note or radiation treatment summary note. That has not been the case in medical oncology, perhaps because as recently as the early 1970s, oncologists did not have as much to offer patients. With current treatment modalities, many more cancer patients are surviving, but the treatments have become very complex. In addition, most medical oncology care occurs in the outpatient arena.

Oncologists report that they have very busy practices, lack time, and do not get reimbursed for this type of service. This may be a perception rather than a reality, and there may be ways to overcome these impediments by designing efficient mechanisms for preparation of treatment summaries and survivorship care plans. Efficiency will be essential, given the number of cancer survivors that are cared for in oncology practices. Completing the care in real time when people are finishing their treatment should make the task less burdensome.

Another potential barrier to survivorship care planning is a lack of awareness on the part of oncologists that cancer survivors are lost in transition, that survivors want this service, and that care planning may help patients take charge of their care. Oncologists also need to appreciate that primary care physicians can be actively involved in providing follow-up care.

How can the Survivorship Care Plan be used in practice? The care plan should facilitate an end-of-treatment consultation with the patient, including a discussion of specific follow-up recommendations. Even if the patient does not want to hear everything about late effects at that point in time, the information will be available in this document. Patients face many issues at the end of treatment, and they may not be able to hear or digest all of the information in the care plan, but having the information in one place will be helpful as questions arise later. Setting out who is to be responsible for what aspects of survivorship care and who is to take responsibility for implementing the plan can lead to efficiencies in health care delivery and potential cost savings. Survivorship care plans also represent a standardized way of communicating to all involved in the patient's care about what went on and essential next steps.

What is needed to implement the Survivorship Care Plan? Five elements are key to implementation: (1) acceptance of cancer as a chronic disease; (2) adequate reimbursement; (3) time, either time for the oncology specialist or a physician extender working collaboratively, to create and deliver care plans in a systematic way; (4) more research to expand the evidence base, so that survivorship recommendations have a solid basis; and (5) training for all health professionals in the needs of the growing number of survivors and how to act on the care plan recommendations.

THE STATUS OF TREATMENT SUMMARIES FOR ONCOLOGY CARE

Presenter: Dr. Deborah Schrag

An ASCO initiative, "Treatment Plan/Treatment Summary" that is under way is integral to survivorship care planning. The purpose of this

---

BOX 2-2
Motivations for the ASCO
"Treatment Plan/Treatment Summary" Initiative

- IOM cancer survivorship report
- National Initiative on Cancer Care Quality (NICCQ)
- Quality Oncology Practice Initiative (QOPI)
- Burden of documentation reported by oncologists
- Patient demand as expressed by the advocacy community
- Pay for performance initiatives
- Electronic medical record vendor requests
- Lessons on fragmentation of care from 2005 hurricanes

---

initiative is to standardize a format for medical oncologists to prepare a treatment plan when patients embark on a new course of therapy. This treatment plan summary would document the diagnosis, purpose of treatment, agent, schedule, anticipated toxicities, and the plan for reevaluation. The need for this summary has emerged from decades of quality-of-care research documenting how much information patients do not hear or retain during initial oncology consultations.[3]

The other part of the ASCO initiative is to standardize a format for medical oncologists to complete a treatment summary when patients complete a chemotherapy regimen. The purpose of this summary is to describe treatment tolerance, response, outcomes, and planned next steps. The preparation of this summary is of particular importance to patients who have completed curative or potentially curative regimens and subsequently transition all or some of their care to other providers.

The IOM cancer survivorship report and several other influential reports and initiatives have motivated this effort (Box 2-2).

The recognition of poor oncology documentation practices came into sharp focus with the National Initiative on Cancer Care Quality (NICCQ), a study that examined the quality of care for patients with breast and colon cancer diagnosed in 1998 in five U.S. cities. This study, which was supported by ASCO and the Susan G. Komen Foundation, determined that the quality of care for study patients was quite good, but that it was incredibly difficult for researchers to retrieve treatment information from medical charts to assess cancer care.

---

[3]For more information, a background paper by Dr. Schrag, "The Cancer Treatment Plan and Summary," is included in Appendix D.1.

Volunteers from the ASCO membership are piloting the use of templates for treatment plans and treatment summaries. Oncologists involved in this initiative are motivated by a desire to streamline the burden of documentation and to be responsive to the advocacy community, which has identified such summaries as key to providing much-needed information to survivors and their families. A move toward "pay for performance" on the part of Medicare and other insurers is another factor driving this initiative. There is an acknowledgment that clinical audits and evaluations of performance depend on good documentation. Electronic medical record systems hold great promise for improving documentation, and vendors who are developing these systems are eager to accommodate oncologists on what they want in terms of content and format. Finally, the events surrounding recent hurricanes tragically illustrated the consequences of not having portable health records. Patients in the midst of their cancer treatment were dislocated without any documentation of their diagnosis and treatment.

Treatment Summaries

The treatment summary is responsive to evidence of problems in three important interrelated domains of quality:

1. *Care coordination:* physician-to-physician communication has become more difficult as more subspecialists have become involved in care. A cancer patient may have a pain doctor, two kinds of endocrinologists, and two gynecology specialists.
2. *Patient-physician communication:* patients' information and psychosocial needs are not being adequately addressed, and the process of shared decision making may not be documented when multiple treatment options are available.
3. *Efficiency:* providing information to insurance companies and to other physicians involved in the patient's care is time-consuming, and mechanisms are needed to streamline the burden of record review, document creation, transmittal, and flow management.

Preparation of treatment summaries can also facilitate quality improvement by aiding providers' self-scrutiny, as is the case for Quality Oncology Practice Initiative (QOPI) participants, as well as external review for quality assurance. Public health tracking, for example for cancer registries, could also be expedited. Cancer registrars currently find it difficult to extract information from medical records.

Some physicians routinely prepare treatment summaries. Surgeons document their care through operative reports. Radiation oncologists have standardized treatment summaries. More generally, all physicians are responsible for completing a summary for patients discharged from the hospital. Pediatricians have agreed on a standard format for the pediatric health record, which is not necessarily comprehensive but does include the basic growth curve and immunization record. Obstetricians have an agreed-on standard obstetrical summary.

Medical oncologists have not yet taken this approach to documentation, perhaps because oncology care is often complex, variable, and prolonged, making it difficult to summarize. It is these very traits that make it a necessity to have good documentation of care. Other medical specialties that are involved with the management of complex chronic disease have also recognized and tried to address their documentation shortcomings. Psychiatrists must contend with chronically mentally ill individuals, who over the years may be cared for in health care, social services, or criminal justice institutions. Documentation is also problematic in the case of diabetes, renal dialysis, transplantation, and HIV/AIDS. In all of these areas, in which it is common for patients to transition between providers and care settings, a treatment summary can provide valuable information to caregivers.

In an attempt to promote the use of treatment summaries, ASCO will develop a sample template that will be:

• Synoptic, not a comprehensive, detailed review of the medical record (and not a replacement for informed consent or flow sheets);
• Available as "open source" and modifiable by its users (templates could be downloaded from the ASCO website);
• Adaptable in its formatting;
• Minimally burdensome; and
• Multipurpose.

Treatment Plans

As a complement to the treatment summary that is prepared at the conclusion of treatment, ASCO is also working on a template for a treatment plan that would be prepared at the onset of chemotherapy and reviewed with patients. This plan would include:

• Summary information, such as regimen name and administration plan (e.g., FOLFOX with Bevacizumab every 2 weeks as an outpatient), numbers of cycles until reevaluation, reevaluation plan (e.g., CT scan in 10 weeks);
• Contact information for cancer care team members (e.g., patient support, medical oncologist, oncology nursing, radiation oncologist, primary care);

II. Important Background Information About My Cancer	
Date of Initial Cancer Diagnosis	01/10/ 2003
Primary Cancer Site	Right colon (Cecum)
Primary Cancer Type (Histology)	Adenocarcinoma
Stage of Initial Cancer Diagnosis	Stage II
Current Disease Status	Metastatic
Current Sites of Disease	Liver, lung, lymph nodes, intestines
Disease Evident on Physical Exam	No
Symptoms at Start of this Treatment	Mild Back pain
Overall Function at Start of this Treatment (Functional Status)	No Limitations (ECOG 0)
Previous Surgery for this Cancer	1. Right hemicolectomy : 1/2003, 2. Ileostomy for intestinal obstruction 8/2005
Previous Radiation for this Cancer	None
Previous Chemotherapy for this Cancer	Adjuvant 5Fu and Leucovorin 03 -11/2003
Baseline Radiologic Study	CT scan of Chest/abdomen and pelvis with contrast and PET
Date of Baseline Radiologic Study	CT: 9/1/05 PET: 9/10/05

FIGURE 2-5 Example of a portion of the medical oncology treatment plan template that provides background information.
SOURCE: Schrag, 2006.

- Disease status at the start of treatment;
- Rationale for treatment; and
- Basic ingredients of the regimen.

Figure 2-5 is an example of the part of the treatment plan template showing important background information.

One of the advantages of the treatment plan is that, once it is completed, it can be used repeatedly for notes and it can also be used to formulate the preamble for the treatment summary.

Status of Treatment Plans/Treatment Summaries

The ASCO group working on the design of the treatment plan and summary recognized the importance of both documents, but in discussing the concept with practicing medical oncologists, realized that it would be difficult to have both documents adopted simultaneously. The ASCO group

---

BOX 2-3
Potential Audience for Treatment Summaries

- Patients
- Other medical oncologists
- Surgeons, radiation oncologists
- Other physicians
- Nurses
- Non MD/RN providers (psychologists, physical therapists)
- Insurers
- Researchers

---

had to decide where to put their initial efforts and focus. Was it more important to first encourage medical oncologists to adopt treatment planning to help ensure patients' informed decision making, or should the completion of treatment summaries be the first priority to improve the survivorship care transition? The ASCO planning group decided to initially focus on the treatment summary with the ultimate goal of having two integrated documents that would span the care trajectory.

Identifying the key audience for the care summary has implications for its design. There are many potential audiences for the care summary (Box 2-3). The ASCO designers are focusing on other "nononcology" physicians and will encourage those completing the summary to avoid overly technical oncology jargon.

Another challenge is defining the end of treatment, the time when a treatment summary needs to be prepared. The ASCO planning group developed some ground rules:

- Do not prepare a treatment summary if a component of a regimen is discontinued;
- Do not prepare a summary if the patient has a brief (e.g., less than 2 month) break or "holiday" from treatment (e.g., during hospitalization or a comorbid event);
- Do prepare a summary if the patient proceeds to surgery, radiation, or a new chemotherapy regimen;
- Completion of adjuvant/neoadjuvant treatment or of primary curative therapy is a logical time to prepare a summary; and
- Transition to full-fledged survivorship presents another opportunity to prepare a summary.

It may not be easy to define when the treatment summary should be

---

BOX 2-4
Why Physicians Document

Greater emphasis:
- Medicolegal requirement to create a record
- Justify reimbursement
- Jog memory
- Communicate with support staff

Less emphasis:
- Communicate with colleagues
- Communicate with patients
- Create a record for public health reporting
- Create a record for research

---

created, and practicing oncologists will have to use their judgment in determining when the summary has value. There are, however, some logical points for its creation—at the completion of adjuvant or neoadjuvant treatment regimes or completion of primary curative therapy. It is at these times that having the treatment summary dovetails with survivorship care planning. In oncology, these transitions probably account for nearly 50 percent of all chemotherapy treatment.

The incentives and disincentives that shape physicians' documentation practices are important to understand when planning for implementation of treatment summaries. Why do physicians document, and what factors could bring about a change in the documentation culture? Some of the key motivators include medicolegal requirements, reimbursement, and a simple jog to providers' memories during subsequent visits (Box 2-4). There is less emphasis in terms of documentation on communicating with colleagues. Oncologists generally formally communicate with colleagues through letters. Chart documenting is for nuts-and-bolts business and workaday inner office communication. Communicating with a primary care physician or a colleague is an entirely separate endeavor. There has been little emphasis on written communications with patients or creating a record for either public health reporting, research, or quality monitoring. There are some deep-seated cultural patterns in terms of how and why physicians document that need to be overcome in order to get treatment summaries into routine practice.

What are some strategies for implementation? Many have suggested that reimbursement will be key to implementation, but it is unclear if existing reimbursement codes for complex coordination of care are sufficient for both the creation of the treatment summary and the end-of-treatment consultation. The level 5 code for a highly complex visit and coordination of care may suffice.

Patients are also key to implementation. There is a new Joint Commission on the Accreditation of Healthcare Organizations (JCAHO) initiative that requires providers to wear buttons that say, "Ask me if I have washed my hands." Advocacy organizations have promoted the idea of survivorship care plans, and as patients become informed and start asking for these documents, physicians will be in a position to meet their expectations. Adoption would rapidly occur if health care payers asked for treatment summaries and linked their receipt to reimbursement.

The various groups that are involved with quality-of-care measurement (e.g., the National Committee on Quality Assurance, the American Board of Internal Medicine) can also help drive this process. When surgeons, on whom oncologists depend for referrals, start anticipating and requesting these documents, oncologists will be motivated to change.

Working with the electronic medical record vendors will help with implementation, but evidence will be needed that creating the summary can be efficient and that this documentation will be acceptable in lieu of other forms of documentation. At the present time, because of reimbursement requirements, the medical records include many repeat reviews of systems and physical exams that do not inform other providers. This redundant information is provided to meet reimbursement requirements. ASCO's new vision of documentation will have to replace the current system, but the dialogue with payers has not yet commenced.

At the time of the workshop, ASCO's development strategy was being led by Dr. Molla Donaldson, the head of Quality Policy Initiatives within ASCO.[4] The goal of the development strategy thus far has been to identify critical content and to get feedback from oncologists, other cancer and noncancer providers, and patients. ASCO aims to develop templates and sample formats that have flexible formatting, including a two-dimensional, fill-in-the-blank paper form that can be completed by hand, as well as a dictatable version. Eventually, the goal is to have three-dimensional versions with drop-down menus. Dissemination strategies ultimately are going to include simply making the software and downloadable forms available. Evaluations will help determine the extent and value of the use of the templates.

A prototype of the treatment summary (see end of Appendix D.1) was designed to answer very basic questions:

---

[4]Dr. Donaldson has since left her position at ASCO.

- When was the treatment given and over what time period?
- Why was this treatment given and what was the context of treatment?
- What was the treatment? What are the basic details of the regimen?
- How was the treatment tolerated?
- What are the planned next steps?
- Who will perform follow-up?

The form looks deceptively easy to complete, but according to the experience of pilot testers, it is actually somewhat time-consuming to complete.

There is some preliminary feedback from some pilot tests in select oncology practices and from National Comprehensive Cancer Network (NCCN) facilities. Every physician who has participated in the pilot testing has said that the ASCO initiative is valuable, but it has implications for maintaining the volume of patients in their practices given the time necessary to complete the forms. There are also some concerns about liability. Oncologists worry that if a plan is written down and then is not implemented, there may be legal ramifications. These are some of the issues that need to be examined further and resolved. Although this initiative remains in its very early phases, there is widespread interest and support for this endeavor from providers and patients alike. All recognize that there are considerable obstacles to implementation and that changing entrenched habits will be a challenge.

DISCUSSION

Dr. John Rainey, a medical oncologist in private practice who participated in some of the pilot testing, reported that it took about 20 minutes to complete the treatment summary template. He felt that it would have been easier to complete if a treatment plan had been available. Summarizing the treatment is time-consuming, and there is a tendency to give insufficient attention to psychosocial and long-term aspects of care. Having a treatment plan would make it relatively easy to prepare the summary in about 10 minutes at the end of treatment. The focus then could be on toxicity and the long-term plan. He indicated that it might have been better to start initially with the treatment plan and then work on the summary.

Dr. Lee Newcomer, of the UnitedHealth Group, suggested that the treatment summary and care plan have great potential to save time. When on weekend call and picking up a case, for example, an oncologist could look at one page, rather than flip through the chart, saving a good 20 minutes per case. In terms of reimbursement, Dr. Newcomer indicated that the treatment plan would likely be reimbursed as part of a new patient consultation, that the plan would definitely be considered part of that new patient consultation. If radiation oncologists have a distinct ICD-9 code for their treatment summary, this is perhaps a model to examine. There may need to be some rethinking about how to compensate medical oncologists for the extra time involved in its preparation.

Dr. Lawrence Shulman of Dana-Farber Cancer Institute mentioned that private insurers are concerned about haphazard follow-up and the potential under- or overordering of tests. They are beginning to realize that good care can be less expensive care. In his opinion, if treatment plans and summaries are ultimately cost saving, there will be opportunities for reimbursement. Writing the summary itself may not be reimbursed, according to Dr. Ganz, but oncologists do get paid for counseling visits. If the treatment plan facilitates an additional 20 minutes of discussion with the patient, this time spent counseling could be reimbursed. She suggested that the summary could replace the often fragmentary documentation of the content of those visits.

Dr. William Kraybill, a surgeon from Roswell Park Cancer Institute, indicated that the multidisciplinary conference may provide an opportunity to create the treatment plan summary. Dr. Schrag added that radiation and surgical oncologists have developed treatment summaries, and informal discussions with representatives of these specialties suggest that medical oncology needs to develop a treatment summary for its specialty. She thought that one specialist will have to assume the responsibility of preparing the document after the multidisciplinary team meeting. The patient does not usually attend the multidisciplinary conference, so the posttreatment consultation would need to be held separately.

Dr. Betty Ferrell, a nurse and researcher from City of Hope National Medical Center, described how, over the past 25 years, there has been an interdisciplinary effort to document that cancer survivorship is more than just physiological effects, late effects, and drug treatments. She pointed out that the IOM report recognized that survivorship is also about serious psychosocial issues, including family disruption, economic concerns, and fertility. Dr. Ferrell expressed some concern that the ASCO plans for a treatment plan and summary appeared to be reducing survivorship care planning to physical issues and drugs and to also be focused on reimbursement issues. Critical at this junction is to establish what patients need and then design documents to meet those needs. Ultimately, the Survivorship Care Plan should capture psychosocial issues and be designed to be interdisciplinary in nature. It is crucial to have nursing and social work involved, in addition to medical and radiation oncologists. Survivorship care plans without an interdisciplinary focus would represent a step backward, not forward.

Dr. Michael Fordis from Bayor College of Medicine thought that, to minimize the burden of documentation, it is very important for the ASCO planning group to define clearly the purpose of the summary documents. There appear to be different expectations and potential multiple uses. It is also important to consider the level of evidence and research that is available to support the various applications.

The oncology care and survivorship issues under discussion represent a domain in health care that is a "poster child" for why interoperability within health care is needed, according to Dr. Ross Martin of Pfizer Human Health. He added that electronic medical records and the associated communication between electronic medical records and personal health records are vital to success in this area. The multimodal delivery, the multiple domains involved in care, the long duration of care, and the high costs of care all point to the need to deliver this complex care efficiently. The American Health Information Community was formed last year, with the express purpose, according to Secretary Leavitt of the U.S. Department of Health and Human Services, to look at these "breakthrough-use" cases for how one can accelerate interoperability among and within health care through electronic medical records. Continuity of care was one of the identified breakthrough-use cases. Many of the applications will be dependent on paper first, because that is the reality of many practices. Progress must accelerate, however, to reach the next stage of development. There are many ongoing initiatives to produce electronic formats for continuity-of-care records, but the templates for treatment plans and summaries can easily be integrated into these formats.

Dr. Schrag reiterated that the goal of the ASCO initiative is to have the treatment plans and summaries available electronically with drop-down menus, so that in a limited amount of space a lot more detail can be captured, whether it is a follow-up referral to a fertility specialist or to a psychologist or a therapist. Starting with a two-dimensional paper template is necessary because the majority of medical oncology practices remain paper based. Estimates are that 30 to 40 percent of medical oncologists do not use a computer for their medical records. The goal is to proceed on multiple fronts simultaneously, at the same time reaching consensus on the documents' audience and content. It has been a challenge to meet the range of needs that have been identified. A document that satisfies a patient is not the same as a document that will satisfy a fellow oncologist, a future oncologist, a surgeon, and a primary care physician. In trying to create documents that meet some of everyone's needs, they may meet all of no one's needs. Achieving a balance is a challenge.

Dr. Martin pointed out how critical it is during the early stages of development to have in mind the end optimal model, which in this case is a template with an electronic format. There is a need to accommodate existing paper processes, but it is difficult to adapt a paper process later if an electronic model is not conceived of in the beginning. Dr. Sheldon Greenfield agreed on the importance of clarity of purpose at the outset. He raised the point Dr. Ferrell made earlier that there may have to be a different focus, a separate but equal track for patients and providers. He added that it is sometimes difficult for professional societies to champion these activities because the rank-and-file members may thwart the progressive leadership and refuse to adopt the new recommendations for documentation. The right people need to be assembled, particularly payers and quality assurance groups, such as the National Committee for Quality Assurance. They are taking the initiative on similar issues. It is important to establish the composition of the group that is needed to make decisions about the purpose and scope of the initiative.

Dr. Schrag mentioned that the practicing community of oncologists who have been consulted on the ASCO initiative acknowledge that the innovations in documentation envisioned are important. Although they are recognized as a good idea, there is resistance. She added that, as described in the book by Malcolm Gladwell, there may need to be a "tipping point," a cultural shift to an expectation that everyone creates and uses these documents. There will have to be simultaneous effort from multiple directions, including from survivor groups. Aggressive strategies, such has having providers wear buttons that say, "Ask me if I gave you a treatment summary" would probably not be appreciated by the provider community.

Ms. Stovall described how many patients are very intimidated by their physicians and have the perception that if they asked about hand-washing they would be labeled as a bad patient. In her opinion, the JCAHO hand-washing initiative gives patients permission to ask the question. From the patient perspective, it relieves a burden and may not be such a bad thing. From the physician perspective, it may be viewed as a "stick"; however, it may be preferable to prevent an infection than to have the question asked.

In terms of the content of the treatment plan and summary, it is essential for psychosocial issues to be addressed. It must be understood that relieving the anxiety and depression that almost every person with cancer faces when he or she is diagnosed will improve the patient's experience and make cancer care more manageable. Dr. Schrag agreed and suggested that providers will probably need to have both carrots and sticks to implement survivorship care planning.

From the perspective of primary care, Dr. Jean Kutner of the University of Colorado Health Sciences Center thought that providers of diabetes care are probably at the forefront of shared care across specialties. Oncology, when the treatment plan and summary are adopted, would be lauded as a shining example in terms of specialist to primary care communications. She felt that primary care providers would appreciate enormously having oncologists take the lead in establishing who is responsible for what elements of follow-up care and documenting succinctly the status of care and the presence of clinical and psychosocial concerns. Having a comprehensive but short treatment summary and follow-up plan would make primary care visits more efficient.

Ms. Susan Leigh, a cancer survivorship consultant, indicated that, from an advocacy perspective, survivorship care planning must be viewed as a team effort not limited to doctors. Nurses and social workers are critical members of this team. Attention needs to be paid to how to communicate this kind of information to survivors. It involves a lot more than simply giving them a paper and talking about all the specifics of their treatment. Sharing such information can be very traumatizing and anxiety-producing. Communication research is needed to better understand how to deliver this type of information effectively and compassionately. Mr. Richard Boyajian, a nurse practitioner from Dana-Farber Cancer Institute, added that it is important to keep in mind that the treatment plan and summary should be considered a starting point from which the various disciplines—nursing, social work, and others—will be involved to address the entire array of patient needs. The focus on the needs of the patient must be maintained. Patients are entitled to the information that these documents provide.

Health care payers could be integral to the adoption of the treatment plan and summary, according to Dr. Newcomer of the UnitedHealth Group. He suggested that interest may initially be greater in the initial treatment plan because the plan could serve as a document that counselors could use to help patients address questions about coverage or find appropriate support groups. If it could be used as a precertification tool, it would generate payer interest very quickly. When payers get involved, things can happen quickly. For example, despite having a standard for colon cancer surgery established for 10 years, it has not been adhered to for half the patients in the country. This year, in less than 3 months, UnitedHealthcare told surgeons in four cities that if they could not demonstrate adherence to the standard regarding node resection, then they would not be eligible to see patients with UnitedHealthcare coverage. Change in practice occurred very quickly. Some providers dropped out, but most are adhering to the standard. This example illustrates how payers can initiate a tipping point in physician practice.

Dr. Newcomer thought that one central purpose needs to be identified for the treatment plan and summary. The plan should clarify what is anticipated and also include both medical and psychosocial aspects of care. Many oncologists will need tools to assist them in making psychosocial assessments. The development of comprehensive treatment plans will illustrate how little is known about follow-up.

For some aspects of the care plan, such as symptom management and psychosocial issues, the particular treatment that a person has may not be that important, according to Dr. Greenfield. It is important to keep in mind that the summaries are only a starting point for sets of discussions. Dr. Peter Raich of Denver Health Medical Center added that an interdisciplinary approach is needed to develop the treatment plan and summary, and these tools need to be aimed at the patient. Perhaps two instruments are needed, one for physician communication and the other for patient communication. These documents would provide a proactive way to educate and guide patients into the survivorship phase of their treatment. This phase of care provides a teachable moment, and it should be used to help patients with lifestyle changes that will be very important as they continue in their survivorship.

Dr. Greenfield concluded that however the treatment plan and summary evolve, with perhaps two tracks, a physician track and a patient track, it would put oncology at the forefront of many other medical specialties. There have been many quality-related activities in other disciplines, but the focus is usually entirely on the medical and not on the psychosocial aspects of care. If there were a way to put the two together, it would represent a huge national step forward, and, as has been pointed out, payers may be able to use the documentation and facilitate adoption.

Dr. Donaldson congratulated Dr. Schrag for the enormous amount of work she has undertaken on the treatment plan and summary, and pointed out that, although the effort has been led within ASCO, there is an understanding that additional members of the survivorship community will have to be involved in further development. Development will move ahead to accommodate practices with and without an electronic health record, but, regardless of the platform, some agreement is needed on content. A question was raised regarding dissemination and the role of specialty societies. A group called the Cancer Quality Alliance has recently been formed, cochaired by Ellen Stovall and Patricia Ganz, which includes representatives from insurance companies, the federal government, social work, nursing, and so on, across the board. The Cancer Quality Alliance is therefore a logical place for both development and dissemination activities relating to treatment plans and summaries.

Ms. Carol Curtiss raised the concern that the draft templates under discussion would appear to be very useful to health care providers in understanding what is happening to patients, but they may not be very useful to patients in learning to live well through diet and exercise and getting back to wellness. Not enough is known in these areas to provide very specific advice; however, she thought that it could be frightening for patients to simply receive a list of potential late effects without some guidance on what they themselves can do to maintain or improve their health.

Ms. Wendy Landier described how the Children's Oncology Group (COG) has developed evidence-based, long-term follow-up guidelines and treatment summary forms (see Appendix F). A lesson learned over years of development is that it is very important to establish what will be done with the summary information. The pediatric oncology community has honed the summary down to key elements that are needed to generate patient-specific guidelines. It is through the COG guidelines and not through the treatment summary that psychosocial issues are addressed. Appropriate guidelines are generated on the basis of the treatment summary that documents the patient's treatment-related risk factors.

Dr. Loria Pollack of the Centers for Disease Control and Prevention concluded the discussion by pointing out that one of the potential uses of a treatment plan is to assist patients in treatment following a disaster. She described how there were an estimated 24,000 people diagnosed with cancer in the past year in the areas affected by Hurricane Katrina. Many of these individuals were displaced during their treatment, and when they sought care in another setting, some could not tell the oncology providers what type of cancer they had. In discussions of whether to start with plans or summaries, it would be helpful to keep these experiences in mind.

3

Perspectives on Suvivorship Care Planning

INTRODUCTION

Moderator: Ms. Caroline Huffman

To further understand the opportunities and challenges associated with cancer survivorship care planning, the Institute of Medicine (IOM) commissioned work from three qualitative research groups:

1. Rebecca Day and Reynolds Kinzey of Kinzey & Day Market Research conducted focus groups among cancer survivors.
2. Catherine Harvey and Marsha Fountain of The Oncology Group conducted interviews and focus groups among nurses.
3. Annette Bamundo of Bamundo Qualitative Research conducted interviews with oncology physicians and focus groups with primary care providers.

This section of the report summarizes the results of the qualitative research conducted by the individuals listed above and presented at the workshop. When interpreting the findings described below, it is important to consider the limitations of qualitative research. Insights and hypotheses, rather than firm conclusions, have been generated from these research efforts. In addition, the behavior, attitudes, and perceptions expressed in the interviews and focus groups are not necessarily representative of those of the general population or of particular population subgroups.

PERSPECTIVES OF CANCER SURVIVORS

Presenters: Ms. Rebecca Day and Mr. Reynolds Kinzey

Three focus groups were conducted among cancer survivors to learn more about follow-up care that is currently being provided, levels of satisfaction with posttreatment care, receptivity to the concept of a Survivorship Care Plan, and reactions to a specific draft care plan template that would summarize a particular patient's cancer treatment and specify a plan for follow-up care (see draft template in Appendix E). The composition of the three groups was as follows:[1]

1. Older cancer survivors (age 56 to 70), both men and women,
2. Younger women survivors only (age 25 to 55), and
3. Younger men only (age 25 to 55).

Participants had completed their primary treatment for various types of cancer (excluding superficial skin cancer) and their initial follow-up care within the past 5 years. All groups were held in Fairfax, Virginia, on April 5, 2006.[2]

Views on Follow-Up Care

In general, participants reported that they were satisfied with their follow-up care, most rating it 7 or above on a 10-point scale on which 10 means "completely satisfied." Only a few expressed open dissatisfaction initially. In describing their follow-up care, it became evident that satisfaction was high for the medical or clinical aspects of their care; however, many expressed dissatisfaction with their physician's lack of attention to their psychological needs. One man said, "They are very good clinically, but there wasn't much attention paid to the psychological aspect, just very clinical." And an older person said, "They also did nothing in terms of follow-up, in terms of the psychological follow-up, nutrition, exercise, support groups, none of that, and I know some of the hospitals and doctors do things that way, but even a sheet of paper would have been nice, so I was not struggling on the Internet."

Older patients, more of whom have survived past the 1-year mark, and

---

[1]The first (older) group was led by Ms. Day, the all-women group was led by Ms. Day, and the all-men group was led by Mr. Kinzey.

[2]Fairfax is a fairly affluent community and group membership reflected this. For example, all group members were well educated and had searched the Internet for information on their cancer. Responses to survivorship care planning would probably have been different if the groups had been held in a rural area or among individuals of low socioeconomic status.

younger women were the most likely to vividly describe feeling somewhat "abandoned" after active care, and they even described the difference in using the word "plan." They said that during active treatment, they felt that there was a plan in place, and they knew what to do and what to expect. Once active care was over, however, they did not know what to do or what to expect, and some felt that they were not being cared for. One woman, for example, said that she felt, during active care, that she was in the front seat of the car. Somebody was driving, they were going along, and she could see where they were going. As soon as she finished her active care, she had to get into the backseat, and then she did not know and could not see what was going on. Some men also agreed and said that they felt their follow-up care was "sporadic."

At least some participants in all three groups complained that they found their specialist (oncologists, urologists) "uncommunicative" and even "uncompassionate" or "uncaring" during follow-up. Younger women were not only the most vocal about this, but also they were much more likely to report switching oncologists because of the problem. Men were more reticent about complaining about any aspect of their care, but they said very directly that their physicians had not done a good job of meeting their psychological needs. They agreed that counseling should be part of follow-up care. One also pointed out that physicians need to be more active in this area with men, precisely because men are so reluctant to seek out psychological help. Men particularly said that physicians had not even warned them about the possible sexual consequences of their treatment. One man said, "I think they treated everything that was physical, but if I wanted any support—mental health, anything like that—I would have to seek it out. It was available, but it wasn't like I was offered it or it was talked about at all." One woman pointed out in a similar way that she had not even considered that she might need spiritual counseling, but if a plan had suggested it, she might have understood her need better. Relatively few participants seemed to have been directed to support groups, but those who had used such groups seemed to have benefited tremendously. One of the participants said, "I don't feel cared for. The treatment ended, and then you are out the door of the hospital, and you don't know what happens next. I don't have any information about what the effect might be on the rest of my life." Another group member said, "Posttreatment is really important for your peace of mind, if nothing else. I was terribly fearful. I woke up in the middle of the night. I felt like I was just dropped."

Reactions to Survivorship Care Plans

Participants in all three groups expressed a great desire for a written follow-up plan. Only one or two members in the three groups had received anything in writing. Most received information orally, but some were told only when their first follow-up appointment was scheduled. One participant said, "At least in my situation, when I was being discharged, the doctor came in and sat down and talked to me, and you are going through a fire hose of a lot of stuff. You are happy, but there is a lot of stuff. There is just so much going on. I nodded and smiled a lot, and I am not sure how much I took in. If I had had something that I could have carried home and then read over, maybe later, you know, it would have put things in perspective a little more. Walking out of there, probably the only thing I remember is that I got an appointment in three months. That was it."

Most participants said that a written follow-up plan would have given them greater "peace of mind" and would have made them feel better psychologically (one said that having a plan would reassure him that the doctors were confident that he "would be around to follow the plan" and that he had survived). Given what the participants said they felt about the failures of their doctors to provide for their psychological needs, this seems very significant. One or two of the younger women suggested that they might have had significantly better clinical outcomes if they had been given better supervision during follow-up care. Participants also said that having a follow-up plan "in front of them" would have been very helpful. Many said that they had been overwhelmed at the end of active treatment, and they were given so much information about follow-up care orally that they "couldn't take it all in." The younger women, in particular, said that a written plan would have been very helpful in explaining to their families what they still needed to do.

Participants were very clear in demanding that everything be written in lay terms. Generally, group members said, the plan needed to be given in both paper and digital formats. They liked the idea of a paper copy in a binder form so that information could be added, and they were very receptive to a Web-based personalized site, which their physicians could update with the latest information, including ongoing research.

There was an expectation that the specialist (oncologist or urologist) would complete the plan with necessary information. Most participants said that their primary care physicians were not very involved with their follow-up care, and virtually none was using oncology nurses or social workers for follow-up care (some said that oncology nurses had been extremely helpful during their active treatment, but not with follow-up).

Receiving a written plan at the final session of their active care was viewed favorably by most participants, although some suggested that a written plan, including follow-up care, should have been given to them when they began active treatment (they commented that the plan could always be changed, according to how treatment went).

Participants were generally very receptive to the template they were shown.[3] They did not, however, like the use of the term "cancer survivor" in the title (even though most, if not all, generally found the term acceptable in general). They suggested that the plan should be titled something "more descriptive," such as "Cancer Patient Follow-Up Care Plan."

Participants generally liked the format and the content of the draft template they were shown, but participants in all groups stressed that the more personalized and tailored the treatment plan was for the individual, the more helpful it would be. Men particularly seemed to want something very specific to them to avoid "information overload." Some of the specific content areas that were recommended by group members included contact information for providers (including e-mail); the location where tests were done; normal ranges for test results; risk of recurrence or second cancer; specific information related to worrisome signs and symptoms; a follow-up schedule; and recommendations for diet and good health. Finally, participants in all groups strongly agreed that they would have wanted this kind of plan in writing.

Summary of Key Observations from Qualitative Research

There appears to be strong patient demand for a written follow-up plan for cancer patients, and a template should be developed and distributed to cancer specialists for their use. The proposed template appears to be on target both in terms of organization and format, although it should use a more descriptive title, such as Follow-Up Care Plan for Cancer Patients. The more individualized and personalized the care plan is for the patient, the more helpful it will be. Obtaining full participation among health care providers will be key to the development and implementation of these plans. The plans could be given in both paper and digital formats. The paper copy may be most useful if kept in a loose-leaf binder so that information can be added. For the digital format, the possibility of Web-based formats could be considered, although a CD or even a file that can be sent through e-mail may be sufficient.

---

[3]A copy of the draft template that was tested in this qualitative research is included in Appendix E. Two versions of the template were available: one was blank and the other was filled out for a "typical" patient with colorectal cancer. Survivors were shown the blank version and were told that the template would be personalized to reflect their clinical situation and needs. Providers were shown both the blank and completed versions and were told that they could complete the template electronically.

PERSPECTIVES OF NURSES

Presenter: Dr. Catherine Harvey

Three focus groups were held with nurses during the Oncology Nursing Society (ONS) annual meeting in Boston, Massachusetts (May 4-7, 2006). Nurses were asked about their current and potential roles in providing posttreatment survivorship care, reactions to the draft templates, and suggested approaches to adoption of survivorship care planning. The focus groups also addressed perceptions that nurses have of patient and family needs at the juncture between active treatment and the transition to extended follow-up.

Special efforts were made to identify nurses in community-based physician practice settings and, in addition, advanced nurse practitioners who currently function in expanded roles in outpatient and/or physician practices. There were 34 nurses representing various practice settings: academic centers (13), hospital-based (6), and private practice (15). Of them, 16 were certified as oncology nurses, and a number of others were certified through organizations representing nurse practitioners. More than half (19) of the nurses were employed and paid by a third party, not the physician in their practice. The remaining nurses (15) were dependent on a physician for their salary as part of their office-based responsibilities. If nurses are to be compensated for some aspects of survivorship care planning, there will have to be acceptance of such involvement on the part of hospital administrators and office-based physicians. About half of the nurses worked in environments in which electronic medical records were in use.

In terms of the potential nursing workforce that might be available to provide survivorship care, about 3,000 certified nurses have an advanced oncology certification. In the past year, the ONS split the certification exam between advanced nurse practitioners, who are considered clinical nurse specialists, and nurse practitioners. ONS reports that it has about 1,600 nurse practitioner members. These Advance Practice Nurses could play an important role in creating and implementing survivorship care plans.

The focus groups explored existing clinical practices and survivorship programs and examined:

- Current development and use of care plans and transition from active treatment to surveillance;
- Perceived (and observed) needs of patients and families as they complete active therapy and transition to extended follow-up;
- Reaction to the proposed content of care plans and treatment summaries;

- The role of nurses in the survivorship care planning process, including levels of participation and needed skill sets; and
- Barriers to implementation of care planning.

Current Practice

In describing current survivorship care practices, nurses acknowledged that there is not a formalized approach to the posttreatment transition period. Most of the nurses agreed that patient education and treatment planning at the initiation of treatment had improved markedly over the past 15 years. Chemotherapy teaching has been institutionalized so that most practices now have packets of materials reviewing what chemotherapy is, the treatment side effects, signs and symptoms to watch for, and guidance on when to call for assistance. If this model were applied to the posttreatment transition, there would be some synergy at the beginning and end of primary treatment.

Most nurses reported that some informal activities are in place, for example, routine conversations after treatment about the critical importance of follow-up, plans for surveillance, and the schedule for visits. A distinction was often made between what happened in the short term (within 2 years) and the longer term surveillance period.

When they were asked whether there was any kind of "handoff" of patients following treatment, variations in practice emerged. Some nurses indicated that patients returned to their primary care physician at about 5 years, while other nurses reported that handoff practices were inconsistent and could vary by practitioner or by disease. Nurses in academic programs were more likely to have a formalized handoff to some kind of a survivorship or long-term follow-up program. The handoff process was usually not well defined. In some cases, the volume of survivors in their active treatment clinics necessitated the development of survivorship programs because the medical staff could not handle both survivors and their patients in active treatment.

Nurses Perceptions of Survivors' Needs

Nurses observed that patients often felt abandoned or "cut loose" following their treatment and were often uncertain and anxious about what was going to happen next and who should be seen for various aspects of their care. It used to be common practice to have end-of-treatment celebrations for patients, but this has been largely discontinued because of the adverse psychological consequences for those who, 2 or 3 months later, have a recurrence. There is now a recognition that it is important to acknowledge this new survivorship phase of the cancer experience and to let patients know how nurses can help.

During the active treatment phase, medical oncologists often manage comorbid medical conditions, but at the end of active treatment, there is an expectation for patients to return to their usual provider for hypertension or diabetes management. This handoff causes some confusion among patients. Concerns about finances and time arise when patients realize that they are scheduled to see their radiation therapist, surgeon, and oncologist for follow-up. So while patients report being anxious about being cut loose, they are also concerned about the number of visits they have scheduled with so many different practitioners.

Nurses reported a common set of questions asked by patients at the conclusion of treatment: What is going to happen to me now? How long are my side effects going to last? When am I going to feel normal again? What can I do? How am I going to feel about returning to work? What level of physical activity should I have? What about my sexual feelings and function? Nurses pointed out the importance of managing patient expectations in the first 6 months after treatment. Helping patients deal with the fear of recurrence was identified as a key nursing role. Some patients really look forward to their last treatment but then feel anxious because they sense that the treatment has been "keeping them going." These anxieties relate to not being able to do something active at that point.

Nursing Roles in Survivorship

Nurses in the groups believed that they could develop and deliver survivorship care plans from the materials they had available to them and the experiences they had with their patients. The nurse practitioners, as a group, noted that this role was consistent with their training, skills, and experience. They stated "We ought to do it. We can do it. We want to do it, and we will try to do it." The evolving nature of surveillance guidelines and the rapidity with which cancer treatment is advancing were felt to pose major challenges to implementing care planning. They recognized the need to keep the care plan updated and, in some instances, change recommendations for the patient.

All participants felt strongly that in order for nurses to assume a key role in survivorship care planning, attending physicians would need to reinforce the importance of the nursing role with patients. This could be accomplished by having the physician say to a patient, "We have asked this person to assume this role for you. They have the skills, the competence and the referral base to help you with this." Physicians would also need to approve of nurses allotting time in their schedules for this role.

In terms of billing, the 99211 Evaluation and Management (E&M)

code is available for patient education when another code is not billed on the same day. For chemotherapy counseling, a number of practices have the physician provide some information regarding treatment on the first visit, and then schedule time with the nurse the next day for additional education and counseling. Because the patient is not seeing the physician that day, the 99211 billing code can be used. The 99211 code is associated with very low payments, and it does not actually cover the nurse's time spent counseling. When patients come in for a separate counseling visit, they can avoid having to absorb too much information at once. However, scheduling multiple visits may not work well for those with transportation problems or who live in rural areas.

In terms of referrals, although nurses reported knowing who to call for social work or nutritionist support, most acknowledged that they do not have formalized referral mechanisms. If patients were routinely screened to assess their need for support services, there were concerns expressed by nurses regarding the adequacy of local resources. Many office-based practices depend on the hospital-based social worker. A few office-based nurses had a system in place for social workers and/or dieticians to work with them, but this arrangement was not common.

Components of the Care Plan

Participants in the focus groups were asked to itemize important elements of survivorship care plans before they were shown an example of a care plan template. Their suggestions, summarized in Box 3-1, included a plan for surveillance, the postrecovery treatment period, and the long term. They recommended that the treatment summary be included at the end of the plan.

Language and how information is presented was viewed as critical. Nurses pointed out that many patients have difficulty understanding written materials and that any information provided had to be in lay terms and at a sixth grade reading level. There were concerns about raising anxiety and a need to craft the language so as to not raise fear. Important also is the need to be culturally sensitive. The care plan should be viewed as being delivered to someone, not necessarily handed to them, so attention must be paid to the quality of the interaction with patients at this juncture. The nurses felt strongly that the treatment summary should go at the very end of the plan. This "future first, history last" approach was viewed as addressing immediate concerns and focusing on the positive and hopeful aspects of survivorship. The focus group participants did not like the title "Survivorship Care Plan" for this document and suggested alternatives: Cancer Recovery Plan; Cancer Wellness Plan; End-of-Treatment Care Plan, Prescription for Living; and Cancer Rehabilitation Plan.

BOX 3-1
Elements of the Survivorship Care Plan Suggested by Nursing Focus Group Participants

- Surveillance plan
  — Immediate
  — Longer-term
- Posttreatment recovery period
  — Expectations of next few months
  — Port removal
  — Side effects management
  — Rehabilitation
  — Psychosocial issues
- Longer term issues and risks
  — Importance of ongoing evaluation for long-term effects/recurrence/second malignancy
- Treatment summary
  — Care/treatment to date
  — Pathology report

A suggestion to facilitate nursing involvement in care planning was the establishment of a website for current surveillance guidelines. Without such a resource, it would be difficult for nurses to keep up with the issuance of new guidelines or changes in existing guidelines. Alternatively, having the guidelines embedded in an online survivorship plan template would ease access to the latest guidelines.

Nurses suggested that the care plan be viewed as an active and not a static document and felt that, given the rapid pace of advancement in oncology, the plan would need to be updated at least annually or when the patient's disease status changed.

One subgroup of patients may require special attention: those who never get off therapy. Nurses report that they have many patients in their practices who are stable and receiving maintenance therapy, but they need surveillance education and some of the same transition education as those who have completed their treatment.

Nurses indicated that how the care plan is packaged is important. They said it should "look important, feel important, and be important." The value of the document needs to be emphasized as it is given to patients in a good binder, and the materials need to be organized in such a way that when other providers are consulted, the binder will provide easy access to all necessary information.

Legal issues and the need for a disclaimer were discussed. Nurses were concerned that as surveillance guidelines change and as information about late effects becomes available, the care plan should indicate that the recommendations reflect the best current thinking and that the plan may need updating as recommendations change. Nurses felt that, like hospital discharge summaries, care plans should be required by the Joint Commission on Accreditation of Healthcare Organizations. After a hospital-based nurse discusses discharge plans with a patient, he or she signs and the patient signs the plan. Nurses thought this formal agreement following the interaction would be appropriate in the context of care planning following cancer treatment.

Several concerns were raised about the interface between specialty and primary care. Nurses felt that the roles of oncology and primary care physicians needed to be clearly delineated and that it is the responsibility of the oncology community to educate referring physicians about posttreatment surveillance and late effects. The handoff from oncology to primary care also needs to be more actively managed to avoid duplication of effort or having patients fall between the cracks and not receive needed follow-up care and services.

Barriers to Care Planning

Nurses identified three main barriers to their involvement in care planning: staffing, the recognition of a nursing role in care planning, and reimbursement. Nurses report being very busy with their current patient loads and responsibilities and indicated that current staffing levels would not permit them to incorporate care planning into their practices. The creation of the treatment summary was viewed as especially time-consuming, given the lack of electronic medical records in most offices. Many nurses are, however, skilled chart abstractors, because they have experience in data collection for clinical trials. It is not only nursing time that needs to be factored in. The ability to implement survivorship care planning into practice will also depend heavily on having access to support services for patients, for example, social workers, nutritionists, and financial counselors. Nurses concluded that they could assume an active role in care planning only if additional resources are allocated and practice patterns change to accommodate survivorship visits. In terms of adapting practice patterns, private office-based practices, because of their size, may have more flexibility than academic medical centers to innovate to meet the needs of survivors. In the nurses' view, innovation will be predicated on physicians "blessing" their role in survivorship planning and committing the necessary resources.

The adequacy of reimbursement to cover a survivorship visit was also a concern expressed by nurses. An office-based nurse could use a 99211 code for billing purposes, but the associated reimbursement would be inadequate for the time needed to both develop and administer the care plan. It is not clear what code could be used in hospital-based programs for reimbursement (99211 codes cannot be used in hospital-based settings).

In summary, the nurses recognized the importance of the transition plan and indicated that such planning can be incorporated into their clinical practice. Key to implementation is physician partners making this a priority. Nurses can and want to take a key role, but they cannot assume these new responsibilities unless there is agreement on collaboration and innovation.

PERSPECTIVES OF PRIMARY CARE PHYSICIANS AND ONCOLOGISTS

Presenter: Ms. Annette Bamundo

To gain the perspectives of physicians on survivorship care planning, 20 in-depth interviews were conducted among oncologists[4] and two focus group sessions were conducted among primary care physicians.[5] In-depth interviews were conducted with oncology providers because it was felt that they would probably have the primary responsibility of creating and administering the care plan. The purpose of the one-on-one interviews was to obtain the unique perspectives of different oncology providers (e.g., medical oncologists, urologists) practicing in varied settings. Focus groups were held with primary care physicians because they would be likely to reap the benefits of care planning along with the cancer survivors. It was productive to have them in a group, because they had an opportunity to react to and build on the template.

This qualitative research was conducted the week of April 10, 2006, in Bethesda, Maryland, and St. Louis, Missouri. Physicians were asked about their current practices, their levels of satisfaction with the status of post-treatment care, and their reactions to the draft care plan templates. Also discussed were the roles of oncology/primary care providers in the post-treatment phase of care, methods of communication among physicians and with patients, and practical issues related to the completion and communication of the care plan.

---

[4]Oncology providers included 12 medical oncologists, 4 radiation oncologists, 3 urologists, and 1 gynecologic oncologist.

[5]Nearly equal numbers of family practitioners and internists participated at each focus group session.

The Status of Physician Follow-Up Practices

Cancer patients often feel abandoned after acute care, according to the survivor focus groups presented by Ms. Day and Mr. Kinzey. Members of the medical oncology community interviewed believe that they are making every effort possible to stay in clear communication with all other physicians involved to provide patients the very best of care. Interestingly, all of this appears to be happening in the background, with the patient completely unaware that their oncology providers are in constant communication with their primary care physician, their primary care physician is getting updates following each oncology visit, and their primary care physician feels very intimately involved in their follow-up care.

According to the practice patterns described by oncology and primary care physicians, there appears to be a duplication of effort, rather than a breakdown in effort, to ensure that cancer patients remain cancer free. Contrary to previously held assumptions, oncology providers report rarely discharging their cancer patients to their primary care physicians for follow-up after active treatment. Instead, the primary oncology provider monitors the patient for as long he or she lives. Oncology providers indicate that this long-term commitment provides patients with a level of assurance that any potential problems will be detected as soon as possible. Oncology providers consider themselves to be better able than any other physician to detect a recurrence or the onset of a negative long-term effect of the cancer or the treatment. Consequently, they feel that monitoring patients, at least annually, is prudent.

Cancer patients' primary care physicians report that they also closely monitor their patients who have a history of cancer. They do so by continually reminding them of the tests that oncology providers recommend, reminding them to report on any unusual symptoms, especially those that are long-lasting, and asking them pertinent questions designed to assess their overall health and well-being. Though oncology providers believe that they are the "quarterbacks" of their patients' care, in actuality it seems as if patients' primary care physicians are the true quarterbacks and coordinators of their care. It is the primary care physician:

• who typically suspects the cancer and then refers the patient to a surgeon and/or oncology provider.
• who monitors the patient's overall health and well-being throughout his or her acute and follow-up treatment and beyond.
• who often has a long-standing relationship with the patient and the patient's family and whose counsel is sought:
  — before patients begin the recommended acute or follow-up treatment to ensure that they are in agreement with the recommendations;

— while being treated, patients or their families often visit primary care physicians to discuss their overall state of health as well as their psychological and emotional state of mind.

• who knows the patient well enough to detect if he or she is suffering from unusual emotional or psychological symptoms (or both).

• who is relied on to explain, in a way that is comprehensible, what is going on and the treatment path that is recommended.

According to the interviews and focus groups, the goals of oncology providers and those of primary care physicians differ in one significant way. Oncology providers appear to be focused on one thing only—that is, treating the cancer and ensuring against a recurrence. It was the rare oncology provider who actually talked to his or her cancer patients about their psychosocial needs during their acute or their follow-up treatment. The very few oncology providers who address these critical issues acknowledge that they typically learn about their patients' psychosocial problems from their nurses. They report that cancer patients who acknowledge that they are experiencing psychosocial problems seem to feel more comfortable discussing them with nurses than with oncology physicians.

The focus and concern of primary care physicians is quite different. Primary care physicians focus on the patient's achieving the same quality of life that he or she enjoyed prior to the cancer diagnosis. Consequently, as a general rule, it is primary care physicians, rather than oncology providers, who assess and counsel their patients on their overall health, as well as their psychological state of mind and their social and emotional well-being. While primary care physicians recognize the psychological stress of dealing with cancer and try to broach this subject, they are inundated with work and may not have sufficient time to address their patients' concerns.

Oncology providers report that they do not broach the subject of follow-up until the patient has come back after the last acute treatment. This approach is taken to avoid overburdening patients with too much information when they are often overwhelmed, depressed, and fearful. After the acute treatment, patients are relieved and can then address issues related to follow-up care.

Oncology providers keep all other physicians involved in the patient's care informed about the patient's progress. This is achieved by sending letters to all involved physicians each and every time that a patient is seen. The net result of these constant updates is that primary care physicians' files, and those of oncology providers, are overloaded. Although the letters are well intentioned, primary care physicians acknowledge that:

• the sheer volume of correspondence makes it difficult to assess the patient's status at a glance;

• their limited knowledge and their workload prevent them from studying all that is contained in each of the letters received. Some just look to the last page, because it typically provides them with information about the tests that the oncology providers are recommending.

As a general rule, when discussing follow-up treatment, oncology providers inform patients about the frequency of follow-up office visits, the tests and the medications that they will be taking, and that it is critical for patients to contact them if they notice any medical condition that is persistent or unusual. They do not address psychosocial issues, recurrence possibilities, or the specific symptoms that patients should be cognizant of. Oncology providers typically do not write down the follow-up treatment plan. This is done only when requested by the patient.

Reactions to the Concept of a Survivorship Care Plan

The oncology providers and primary care physicians generally agreed that cancer patients and their primary care physicians would benefit greatly if a summary of the patient's diagnosis, acute treatment, and follow-up plan was provided. However, oncology providers were not inclined to provide such a summary.

Patients would benefit because they change physicians as a result of relocating, changing their health care plan, or because their health care plan is no longer accepted by their current physicians. Their new physicians and any emergency department physician who is treating them would be in an excellent position to provide beneficial care if the patient had this document in his or her possession. Patients who have gone through a traumatic experience, such as cancer, are often unable to provide new physicians with useful and accurate information about their diagnosis and their treatment.

Primary care physicians would also benefit. When treating a patient who has a history of cancer, they need not wade through multiple letters from oncology providers or surgeons just to recall their patient's diagnosis, acute treatment, or follow-up treatment plan. Consequently, the summary would make it easier for them to:

• address the questions that patients often raise, even years after treatment;
• be fully aware of their patient's follow-up plan of treatment, so that they can remind them of tests that must be taken;
• be fully aware of the signs that signal a possible recurrence or a problem that may be due to a long-term effect of the cancer or the treatment.

The primary care physicians were so intrigued by the concept of this template being made available to them that many suggested that, all other things being equal, they would refer patients to oncology providers who distributed this plan over those who did not.

In general, the oncology providers were disinclined to provide such a summary because they would receive no time-saving or monetary benefit as a result of doing so.

• Oncology providers would benefit only if the document created could replace that which is sent to insurance companies, Medicaid, Medicare, and the other physicians who are treating the patient. The templates presented for review would not be acceptable to insurance companies, Medicaid, or Medicare, and they were not considered to be personalized enough to send to the other physicians who are treating the patient.

• Of seemingly lesser importance to oncology providers is the belief that they would not be compensated for filling out the template. There is no reimbursement code for doing so.

Although oncology providers acknowledged that possession of a care plan could be beneficial to cancer patients, some said that they would not give it to all of their patients. There was a concern that certain cancer patients, who are exceedingly anxious or fearful, could become more so if they were given a document that spells out the possibility of recurrence, the long-term effects of the cancer or treatment, and symptoms that they should be aware of. Consequently, if a care plan were available, it would not necessarily be given to all patients.

A few oncology providers believed that their "undereducated" patients would not benefit from the template. Consequently, they suggested that they would give the template only to patients who were well educated.

It was typically suggested that, for oncology providers to even consider filling out the template, it must take no longer than 20 minutes. Even if the template could be completed in an acceptable time frame, the vast majority doubted that the oncology community will embrace it. Older oncology providers do not appear to be inclined to change their recordkeeping methods or their reporting habits and practices. This was confirmed by a young oncology provider in St. Louis: even though she had demonstrated to the older oncology providers in the practice she joined that her summary document could ultimately save them time, they refused to use it.

The Content of the Follow-Up Care Plan

The prudence of developing templates that include the recommended follow-up guidelines for specific types and stages of cancers does not seem warranted. Including this information will not make it any easier or faster for oncology providers to fill out the form. The recommended follow-up guidelines are viewed, by oncology providers, as merely a guide that is designed for the general population. Oncology providers view it as their prerogative, in fact their responsibility, to alter recommended guidelines for cancer patients' acute and follow-up treatment. Therefore, embedding the recommended guidelines into the care plan template (for example, as drop-down options) would not make it any easier for oncology providers to complete the form. In fact, it might complicate the process.

The oncology physicians indicated that the templates did not provide as complete a picture of the patient's diagnosis and history of treatment as desired. Although no consensus was sought, it was suggested that the template could be improved:

• For many, if the number of cycles of each chemotherapy medication that was administered is included.
• For many, if the document provides space to record a recurrence, should it occur.
• For some, if the total amount of milligrams of each chemotherapy medication that was administered is included.
• For some, if significant side effects for each medication or treatment (such as allergic reaction, effect of toxicity, and insight into how long this effect may last—e.g., "numbness in fingers and toes that may last 1 to 2 years or longer," significant weight loss, effect on teeth) are included.
• For some, if information on current and prior medications and any allergic reactions are included. In addition, space should be left so that new medications can be added.
• For a few, if laboratory tests and radiology tests are separated and if the date and the results of each test are included.
• For one, if the document contains a family history section.
• For one, if the document includes diet and exercise recommendations.
• For one, if the document provides space to record insurance coverage information.

In order for the template to capture all of these elements, the care plan has to be designed as a dynamic tool and not one that presents a static picture. Such a dynamic template increases the burden on the oncology community because it means continually updating and maintaining an accurate real-time document.

The draft template contains two sections that are not needed. Primary care physicians believe and oncology providers' practices confirm that it is rare for oncology providers to address cancer patients' psychosocial problems. Consequently, the section that requires oncology providers to identify these problems and their referrals is not needed and, in the opinion of most, should not be included. If this section is to be retained, then it should be designed so that it:

- can be personalized. This would best be achieved by eliminating the check box and allowing the oncology provider to show the areas of concern.
- includes a space to record the name and phone number of the professional they are referring the patient to.
- includes space to record if the patient has followed their recommendation and, if so, the outcome of the visit.

Primary care physicians and oncology providers believe that the three-page section that provides patients with information on services that are available to them and useful websites to access for information should not be a part of the document. Although this information is extremely useful, it was not considered critical. Instead, it was recommended that this information be included in a booklet that could be made available to cancer patients in their doctors' offices.

Overcoming Oncology Providers' Resistance

Several factors may have to work in tandem to overcome oncology providers' reluctance to create a document that summarizes a patient's diagnosis and the acute and follow-up plan of treatment. Oncology providers' reluctance to provide this summary may be overcome if:

- primary care physicians encourage them to do so. Primary care physicians' referrals are essential to the success of oncology providers' practices.
- patient advocate groups encourage patients to insist that they receive this summary.
- medical schools that educate oncology providers and the institutions in which they train encourage this practice.
- insurance providers are encouraged to reimburse oncology providers for the time spent creating the summary.
- insurance providers and Medicare/Medicaid are encouraged to accept the initial summary and updates as proof of service for reimbursement purposes.
- steps are taken by medical professional associations, hospitals, medical teaching facilities, and consumer advocacy groups to encourage lawmakers, Medicare/Medicaid, and insurance companies to mandate physicians to embrace electronic medical records. The creation of the summary and care plan will be much easier when medical records are electronic. Virtually all participants felt that, for the document to be of value, it could

not be a static snapshot of the patient's diagnosis, acute treatment, and the initial plan for follow-up treatment. Only when electronic medical records are in place will it be easy for oncology providers to update the summary.

• steps are taken to encourage designers of electronic medical records software to develop packages that allow for the creation of the document with minimal effort.

On the basis of the above criteria, both short-term and long-term strategies are needed to move toward implementing survivorship care planning. In the short term, the oncology community can be encouraged to be engaged through other physician groups, advocacy groups, and insurers. In the long term, investments in electronic medical records technology are needed to develop a dynamic care plan that can be completed throughout a patient's care.

DISCUSSION

Moderator: Ms. Caroline Huffman

Dr. Kevin Oeffinger of Memorial Sloan-Kettering Cancer Center mentioned that, as a primary care physician working with survivors of pediatric cancer, the results of the focus groups reflect what he hears almost daily from patients, physicians, and nurses around the country. One-page summaries or summaries in general can get so complicated and have so much added that their real value is lost. Survivors of pediatric cancer benefit from a one-page summary that, when reviewed, tells them: "This is your cancer. This is your therapy. These are the key things that we are looking for. This is our surveillance plan. This is contact information."

Dr. Oeffinger described how such a summary was tested through the Childhood Cancer Survivor Study as part of a Lance Armstrong–funded feasibility study. The study involved 60 women and men who were at high risk for either breast cancer or cardiovascular disease and were not being followed at the cancer center or by a health care professional who was aware of their risk status. An advance letter was sent, and later a one-page summary letter was mailed that included a 1-800 number and an e-mail address to contact to get questions answered. When the recommendations of the Children's Oncology Group were shared with survivors, they went to their health care professionals and discussed with them the one-page summary. Most of them had the appropriate testing done within a 6- to 12-month period of time. Dr. Oeffinger emphasized the importance of not letting things get too complicated and remembering that even simple things can fill a cognitive void in the patient population.

Ms. Martha Gaines of the University of Wisconsin Law School shared her perspectives as a cancer survivor, a patient advocate, and a supervisor of students from law, medicine, nursing, social work, counseling, and psychology who do advocacy work for people diagnosed with life-threatening and serious chronic illnesses. She stated that if there is no patient acceptance and involvement in survivorship care planning, then it will not happen. Barriers that have been mentioned are provider time and reimbursement, but the importance of buy-in from patients is critical. She noted that the absence of good-quality care for most cancer survivors needs to be acknowledged and that this was not surprising because there is virtually no one trained to provide good long-term survivor care. Survivorship is not a discipline in medical schools, and it is not recognized as a separate body of medicine. Ms. Gaines shared her personal experience with her primary care practitioner and oncologist not communicating very frequently or effectively. She found herself saying, "So, is it time for me to have a colonoscopy or perhaps a bone-density test?" Each one of them responded, "Well, sure, I guess so." That is the general level of planning that goes on. She emphasized the importance of recognizing survivor care as important and necessary from a medical quality-of-care point of view.

Ms. Gaines also described how a consumer focus is needed, given the devastating consequences that cancer can have on an individual and his or her family. For example, a survivor may lose his or her job because he or she cannot work and therefore lose insurance and access to follow-up care, and along the way separate from a spouse or partner and lose custody of children. Whether this survivor should be seen for follow-up every 6 months or every year is not going to make any difference, because he or she will not be able to access care.

Ms. Gaines described how a new wave of activated, empowered consumers will soon emerge as baby boomers enter the higher cancer risk age cohorts. Baby boomers will demand good information in order to be effective consumers. Although the option of having a personalized website mentioned earlier was viewed as far-fetched, Ms. Gaines thought that investments should be made to develop such high-quality, individualized, electronic services. She urged the group "to dream high, listen to what patients feel is important, and collaborate to achieve these goals."

Dr. Wendy Demark-Wahnefried of Duke University Medical Center emphasized the importance of getting important messages to patients in writing, so they can take them home to truly digest them and become partners in care. Home-based interventions have worked very well in the context of lifestyle inventions for cancer survivors, and some of the lessons learned from health behavior and education can be applied to survivorship. Home-based interventions can overcome barriers related to distance and transportation, and they are also effective because individuals can better attend to information when they are in their own homes. Physicians sometimes spend a lot of time with their patients trying to get difficult messages across; if these are put into writing, patients may be better able to understand their care and options.

Dr. James Talcott expressed a concern that many issues have been presented as conflicts, such as conflicts between documentation and care of patients and conflicts between stakeholders, providers, and others. He suggested that this perspective may not be helpful and instead proposed a focus on inclusiveness. In terms of the care plan, essentially the same information should be used initially, when the patients are trying to understand their diagnosis and their options, and later, at the conclusion of treatment, so that patients understand what is going on and can participate knowledgeably in their care. Chart documentation is also needed to chronicle care transitions, changes in the objectives of care, and debriefing points, so that other physicians can be aware of significant events.

In response to Dr. Betty Ferrell's concern that psychosocial aspects of care are being neglected (see Chapter 2), Dr. Talcott again mentioned the need to focus on teamwork, because one person cannot do everything. Nurses in focus group sessions seemed to feel confident that they could provide the posttreatment counseling that is being called for. He doubted whether physicians would want nurses to be describing the reasoning behind their decisions. He also questioned whether nurses would want physicians to be speaking for them in terms of psychosocial issues. Implementing the plan will require input from all the providers. Finally, Dr. Talcott mentioned a stakeholder group that had been left out of the conversation thus far: that is, partners, family members, and friends. In his experience in treating patients with prostate cancer, he has usually found partners to be involved in decision making and care.

Dr. Lari Wenzel, from her perspective as a psychologist at the University of California, Irvine, commented on the apparent disconnect observed in the qualitative research between the survivors indicating that their psychological concerns were paramount and the oncology physicians, who, while recognizing these concerns as important, generally wanted to eliminate psychosocial content from the summary care plan template. There may be a need to reduce the oncologist's burden, or the perceived burden, associated with psychological evaluation and treatment. She pointed out that meeting the psychosocial needs of oncology patients has been an issue for 25 or 30 years in the literature, with little progress having been made. Creative methods for evaluation and intervention should be employed, she noted. These methods could involve social work colleagues or could employ telephone services such as the Cancer Information Counseling Line of Dr. Al Marcus, readily available to survivors around the country. Ms. Bamundo responded to this point by clarifying that physicians who were interviewed as part of the commissioned qualitative research reported that they did not broach these issues with their patients, and therefore they did not feel that content in this area needed to be represented on the care plan template. Ms. Bamundo stated that physicians need training to recognize that this is a critical component to care.

Mr. Richard Boyajian of Dana-Farber Cancer Institute suggested that there will have to be compromise in order to move forward with care planning. Physicians, nurses, and advocates may not all get what they want. Some consensus will need to be achieved on a middle ground. He felt that it would be helpful to have more evidence on which to make decisions; however, as both a survivor and a nurse practitioner, he urged that steps be taken immediately with guidance from the assembled experts, and then people should learn from that experience.

Dr. Sherry Kaplan of the University of California, Irvine shared her perspective from work in the area of diabetes and other chronic diseases. She pointed out that when cancer management is successful, patients go on to survive to get something else. Perhaps for this reason, planning should be considered for a variety of chronic diseases, not just cancer. She also described the concept of "patienthood." In her work with Dr. Sheldon Greenfield, she has evaluated the effects of sharing with patients their medical records, treatment plans, or algorithms for disease management. They have tested showing patients their records before their visit and have audiotaped those visits to look at the effects on the doctor-patient interaction and, more importantly, on physiological and quality-of-life health outcomes. The results of this work indicate that patients want to be involved in their care; patients in this study represented a spectrum, from Mexican American patients with a third grade education to the equivalent of the well-educated Fairfax patients who participated in the IOM focus groups. The study demonstrated that when patients are involved, they get better health care and they experience better health outcomes.

Dr. Kaplan pointed out that information cannot just be dumped on patients. Planned patienthood is needed, so that patients know how to use the information provided. The average male patient in the 15-minute office visit asks no questions. The average woman asks six questions. There is still a perception in the medical culture that, if a patient asks questions, he or she is considered a bad or a difficult patient. Dr. Kaplan suggested that a patient training system is needed that transcends cancer. Such training needs to start in childhood and needs to extend across the health care spectrum.

Dr. Ross Martin of Pfizer Human Health reminded the audience that Dr. Greenfield had asked them at the outset to prioritize problems that need solutions. The problem discussed in the morning related to continuity of the care record and shortcomings of communication between clinicians. In the afternoon there has been a shift to engaging patients and empowering them with their own care plan. In terms of using evaluation and monitoring codes for billing purposes, he pointed out that there are two distinct activities that need to be coded. First is the preparation of the plan, whether it is a patient-centered plan or a provider-to-provider continuity-of-care plan. Second is the actual delivery of that plan and the patient education process that goes along with it. Billing for the delivery of the plan seems straightforward, but billing for the time that goes into preparing the plan is a much more involved process that requires a lot of input from many different sources. He suggested that if the current codes do not capture this activity, then it should be a very high priority to make sure that it can be captured, regardless of whoever puts it together, whether a nurse, the oncologist, or the primary care physician.

As a general internist and as a person living with chronic recurring cancer, Dr. Wendy Harpham suggested that the purpose of the workshop is to figure out how to help each individual patient get good comprehensive care over the cancer trajectory. She described an image that might be helpful in deciding who the care plan should be addressed to and who should carry this record. On group trips involving many people in several cars that caravan to a destination, she insists that each patient's luggage be in the car with that person, because whatever happens along the way, that person will be with the belongings that that person needs. Cancer survivors represent a huge group of widely divergent people trying to get to the same destination, which is good care. If the individual patient is the holder of this magnificent record, then wherever that patient is, that patient can help the doctors, the nurses, the social workers, the rehabilitation therapists, the psychologists, and the psychiatrists provide good care.

Ms. Patricia Buchsel, a representative of the Oncology Nursing Society, described how advanced nurse practitioners have contributed a great deal to survivorship research and have provided leadership in a number of survivorship clinics. She pointed out that most oncology nurses do not have this level of advanced training and yet can assume many of the follow-up responsibilities that have been outlined.

Ms. Kathryn Smolinski, representing the Association of Oncology Social Work (AOSW), emphasized how important a team approach is to the success of survivorship care planning. Social workers are professionally trained, skilled in counseling, and familiar with available community resources. Social workers have been at the helm of psychosocial care in oncology for over 100 years. However, she pointed out, much needs to be done to better connect patients to the many available community resources. When budget cuts hit a health care facility, oncology social workers are often one of the first professions to be cut. Ms. Smolinski and others at AOSW are working hard to overcome these staffing issues. She described physicians as a critical entry point for patients into the health care system.

If a physician says psychosocial care is important, and if it is on the survivorship plan, then patients will follow through and request it. This will reinforce a team approach and facilitate a comprehensive care plan.

Ms. Wendy Landier of City of Hope National Medical Center reported that, from the pediatric perspective, oncologist providers see the value of care plans but feel that they do not have time to prepare one and, second, that nurses are eager to assume a key role in care planning. She noted that the Children's Oncology Group (COG) model uses nurses extensively in survivorship care planning. In pediatrics and in the COG, advanced practice nurses have specialized in long-term follow-up. The majority of long-term follow-up clinics are led by nurse practitioners with active physician involvement. Nurse practitioners prepare the treatment summary, sometimes with specially trained clinical research associates.

Dr. Lawrence Shulman of Dana-Farber Cancer Institute observed in concluding the discussion session that, while there appeared to be some divergence in the perspectives of survivors, nurses, and physicians, there is also a tremendous amount of synergy and concrete ways to move forward to fill the gaps identified from all points of view.

SMALL GROUP DISCUSSION
Moderator: Dr. Sheldon Greenfield

For this portion of the workshop, participants broke into small work groups of 8 to 10 members. Group members were asked to discuss the following questions, to focus on an assigned question, and then report back to the entire group:

• What are the essential elements of the care plan? Will a single template work?
• Who is responsible for creating the plan and discussing the plan with patients?
• What are the respective roles of oncology/primary care and physicians/nurses?
• What economic strategies could encourage implementation of care planning?
• What barriers exist to creating the care plan? How can they be overcome?

Group 1: What Are the Essential Elements of the Care Plan?

Ms. Sarah Davis of the University of Wisconsin Law School summarized the discussion of Group 1 and identified three purposes of care planning. First, the care plan must have a "survivorship perspective" and address patients' feelings of abandonment, maximize recovery, be based on good evidence for surveillance, and attend to the late effects of cancer treatment. Second, the care plan must be mobile. Patients need a care plan that they can take to their various providers, whether that is locally or across country because they move or are displaced because of natural or other disasters. Third, people must know whom to call to address specific issues that come up over time.

She went on to state that the essential elements of the care plan should include diagnostic information, a treatment summary, a risk assessment, and the prospective plan to include both medical and psychosocial issues. Members of the group indicated that it was extremely important to clearly identify roles and responsibilities and to affirm acceptance of these roles. Having local and national resources as part of the plan was felt to be vital. A patient-friendly disclaimer was also felt to be necessary. This disclaimer should be easy to read and acknowledge the responsibility that patients have as they move forward with the plan. Finally, several group members viewed the care plan as a living document that is taken to all appointments and actively used.

During the discussion period, Dr. Greenfield raised the question, "If there is a team assembled, who takes responsibility for the team? He wondered if a virtual team needs to be created, with formal sign-on. One suggestion raised was to have payers require that a team be designated before any reimbursement is provided. Others pointed out that how teams are created and work will depend on location, for example, whether care is provided in a rural or an urban setting, or in a community-based office or an academic center. A physician practicing in a five-person oncology practice suggested that dedicated triage nurses can provide case management, counseling, and referrals. Being able to provide such nursing support was viewed as being a function of the size of the practice. One practitioner estimated that a full-time nurse is needed to provide "navigational" support for every three medical oncologists.

Group 2: Would a Single Template Work?

Members of Group 2 thought that a single template could meet the needs of cancer survivors if there were sufficient adjunctive and supportive materials that would make the plan appropriate and meaningful to the patients and the primary care providers who would use it. Several group members felt strongly that the care plan template should be used at the onset of care, starting with diagnosis and leading up to the handoff at the end of cancer treatment. Individuals without a care plan at the outset of treatment could be given one as they end treatment. Group participants noted that the care plan should also be dynamic and amended as the cancer journey progresses and as issues arise, such as discontinuation of therapy or the onset of a psychosocial issue. Finally, some group members indicated that research is needed to evaluate the success of the care plan in improving follow-up care and outcomes.

During the discussion period, some skepticism was expressed regarding the ability to rely on a single template, given the wide variation in therapies and the long-term effects associated with different types of cancers. Dr. Neil Schlackman pointed out that a single template can accommodate a range of diagnoses and treatments because, ideally, drop-down menus would be available to identify commonly used drugs and their toxicities. A single template provides a standard for common elements for inclusion. With several diverse templates already available, Dr. Greenfield recommended that a minimum standard be set that individual providers could embellish to suit particular needs. Dr. Lee Newcomer raised the possibility of insurers being able to assist in providing information to "populate" the record if the template were standardized. Insurers can easily list hospitalizations, medications, and physicians involved in the care of a patient using claims information. Standardization of the template would be critical to making these data available. Dr. Patricia Ganz and Dr. John Rainey, both involved in the efforts of the American Society of Clinical Oncology (ASCO) to develop a template, agreed that a minimum standard would facilitate implementation, especially in the context of an electronic medical record system. With general agreement on the merits of a standardized template, Dr. Greenfield cautioned that, in order for implementation of survivorship care planning to proceed, there will have to be some compromise on this standard. He cited the example of the development of quality-of-care measures in which reductionist approaches are often taken. Group members agreed that there are empirical questions related to the care plan template. How much detail is needed, and what formats work best to stimulate patient-provider interaction? What level of community-based resources are needed? Dr. Peter Raich, from the Denver Health Medical Center, suggested that, in developing care plans, patient diversity must be addressed in terms of language, culture, and literacy.

Dr. Deborah Schrag described the balance that needs to be achieved between a focus on a document and on documentation standards and changing interactions between patients and physicians. Under discussion is an attempt to use the document to leverage changes in interactions. Dr. Schrag questioned whether it would be more advantageous to start with interventions to change the nature of interactions, for example, requiring psychosocial issues to be adequately addressed and then expecting the related documentation to improve. Alternatively, one could begin by requiring better basic documentation and then expecting communication to improve. Developing a standardized document is easier to accomplish than changing the culture of oncology practice and communication. Dr. Schrag characterized the document as a wedge that can be used to leverage fundamental change in practice.

The inclusion of psychosocial content in the care plan template is very important, according to one group member. It can provide a prompt for the busy clinician to raise these issues and foster interaction. It was pointed out that physicians are gatekeepers and that they themselves do not have to provide psychosocial services. Sometimes it is sufficient to say, "I find it is often helpful for my patients to go to support groups. Let me give you names and references." Having a list of services available opens the door for their use. Dr. Ferrell raised a concern that, in addition to psychosocial issues, symptom management has not received sufficient attention in developing survivorship care plans. Pain management, fatigue, and weight loss are major concerns when people are leaving cancer treatment. Symptom management will become even more significant as therapies become more toxic and as treatment becomes more prolonged. Good symptom management is a necessary component of survivorship care plans.

Dr. Ganz pointed out the challenges ahead in meeting the care planning needs of 10 million prevalent cancer cases and recommended implementation of a standardized template soon with incident cases. Dr. Charles Catcher, a community-based oncologist in New Hampshire, stated that it would be difficult to implement a standardized care plan in his practice of nine physicians and six mid-level practitioners. Clinicians are very busy and involved in both day-to-day practice and research activities. Community-based practitioners will need clear guidance on how to make this concept work in practice. The realities facing many patients also need to be acknowledged. Many patients lack health insurance, making it difficult for them to get all of the clinical and social support services they need. One participant pointed out that the template is a teaching document, providing a systematic way to educate the patient. If adapted to an electronic medical record, it could potentially make patient counseling more comprehensive and efficient. Dr. Greenfield suggested that adoption of care planning could well be incorporated as a quality indicator into plans for pay for performance systems.

Group 3: Who Is Responsible for Creating the Plan and Discussing It with Patients?

Members of Group 3 recognized that more than 90 percent of cancer patients are cared for in the community (and not at academic medical centers) and determined that for care planning to be implemented widely, it must be practical for clinicians in office-based practices. Oncology practices vary in structure and staffing, and who will carry out care planning in any particular practice will vary. The responsibility for completing the plan will probably rest with some combination of the physician and the nursing staff. The group did not think that primary care physicians or other individuals involved in the patient's care could complete the care plan because of their more limited access to diagnostic and treatment information. Group members noted that, ideally, clinicians would start to write the care plan at the first visit. Not knowing the entire treatment plan at the onset of treatment would make it more difficult to fill out prospectively. Increasingly, treatment plans change. For example, a patient may start with neoadjuvant therapy, but, after 8 weeks, another plan may emerge based on the results of further scans. In the short term, several group members stated that the emphasis should be placed on a posttreatment plan. In the long term, technology will permit having a prospective, adaptable document.

Group members anticipated that care planning, in 5 to 10 years, will improve the standard of care and ease care delivery, but they recognized barriers to implementation. Key to implementation will be expectations set by patient and advocacy groups. Peer pressure and demands from referring primary care doctors and surgeons may also prompt adoption. Financial incentives, for example, pay for performance or better reimbursement for care planning, would help. Regulatory requirements may be forthcoming. Just as there is a Joint Commission for the Accreditation of Healthcare Organizations (JCAHCO) requirement for a timely operative note after surgery, there could be a JCACHO requirement for a cancer care plan. A combination of these pressures will help move the field forward, asserted group members. Any one of these pressures alone, however, will not be enough.

During the discussion, Dr. Newcomer described ASCO's voluntary Quality Oncology Practice Initiative (QOPI) as an example of oncologists engaging in quality improvement activities to learn and adapt their practices to better patient outcomes. Initially there were just a few practices involved, and now there are 73. Dr. Greenfield described a provider recognition program, in which doctors submit practice data and the American Diabetes Association puts summary data online by geographic area. As many as 300,000 to 400,000 patients access this information. There are relatively few practitioners involved thus far, but this activity is having a big ripple effect on practice.

While there are some physicians who are voluntarily engaged in such quality initiatives as QOPI, other providers will need to be motivated through incentives. One selling point might be the potential for time saving if the care plan is completed prospectively and an up-to-date record is available at each visit, obviating the need to wade through a thick chart.

Group 4: What Are the Respective Roles of Oncology/Primary Care and Physicians/Nurses?

In responding to the question, "Who is responsible for discussing the plan?" members of Group 4 focused on the quality of care of survivors in community-based oncology or primary care practices. There was a recognition that as patients transition out of cancer treatment, the availability of resources can vary greatly from setting to setting. Group members suggested that the treatment plan portion of the care plan could be written and discussed by the primary oncology physician or by a nurse on the oncology team, but preferably the oncologist. Once the patient has transitioned back into primary care, the discussion of the treatment summary could be extended by the primary care physician.

The group recognized that not all patients are transitioned back to primary care for their follow-up care. Those patients with comorbid conditions would be expected to have these conditions managed by primary care. Group participants suggested that a stratified approach could be adopted in which high-risk patients, such as stem cell transplant patients or patients at high risk for recurrence, continue their primary follow-up care with the oncologist. Members of the group believe that it is as important for a relatively low-risk patient, for example, one treated by surgical resection for a low-grade liposarcoma, to have a treatment summary as a higher risk patient. For the lower risk patient, the summary would help physicians understand that the cancer was not invasive or aggressive and that this surgical therapy was all that had to be dealt with in terms of late effects.

Group members noted that to achieve buy-in on the concept of care planning on the part of primary care physicians, general internists, pediatricians, and obstetricians and gynecologists, involvement is needed from the respective professional societies at the ground level. These providers also need to be involved in the development of follow-up guidelines. Complexities arise in the context of survivorship care, and a multidisciplinary approach is needed as guidelines are developed, refined, and disseminated. In addition to medical and radiation oncology, it may be necessary to involve urologists and surgeons, as they may be the primary provider of oncology care. It was pointed out in discussion that surgeons vary in their facility with the multidisciplinary approach to cancer. As medical oncologists develop care plan templates and survivorship guidelines, it will be important to reach out to different societies that deal with surgical patients, for example, the American Society of Colon and Rectal Surgeons.

Ms. Mary McCabe reported on experience with survivorship care planning at Memorial Sloan-Kettering Cancer Center in New York City. In pilot studies of long-term follow-up care of adult patients, communication with primary care physicians was not as extensive as expected, and investigators concluded that they needed to learn more about the information needs of primary care providers. Not all of the cancer patients had primary care physicians, and so making sure that all survivors have a primary care physician has been incorporated into their follow-up plan. As part of the survivorship program, a one-page care plan has been developed, and focus groups are being held with primary care providers to see how useful it is to them (see Appendix G). These groups will help the oncology providers assess how best to involve primary care in follow-up care.

During the discussion it was pointed out that there are some areas of sensitivity between oncologists and primary care providers, and they should be discussed so that follow-up care can be collaborative and not duplicative. One issue that emerged from the IOM-sponsored focus groups is that oncologists do not like to "let go" of their patients. There may be uncertainty regarding primary care providers' training and experience with cancer surveillance. Workshop participants stressed that the tension between the roles of oncology and primary care physicians in cancer care follow-up must be addressed.

Dr. Greenfield asked the group to consider some options for coordinating physician response to the care plan. He asked, "If the care plan is developed by the physician responsible for oncology care, should the primary care physician be required to respond in some kind of formal way to indicate his or her agreement with the plan and commitment to implement its recommendations?" Dr. Greenfield pointed out that, if there were a requirement for a response from the primary care physician, this would ensure that communication had been established between the providers responsible for implementation. Dr. Talcott felt that it was important to not only specify on the care plan who has responsibilities for follow-up, but also to have all the people charged with some aspect of follow-up to sign off on their obligations. He likened this approach to the person who takes your order at Starbucks saying "a double tall latte," and then having the barista repeat the order. This verification system makes sure that the order is filled and it also provides an opportunity for feedback. Members of Group 4 thought that such a system in the context of survivorship care is crucial.

Dr. Greenfield also asked workshop participants to consider whether nurses could take a lead role in communicating with patients once the plan was created. He reasoned that with their expertise in patient counseling, nurses could ensure that psychosocial issues are addressed and might be able to implement the plans in a more cost-effective manner than physicians. Ms. Buchsel of the University of Washington School of Nursing reiterated the important role that nurses can play in summarizing what went on during treatment and coordinating the many aspects of follow-up care.

Dr. Oeffinger distinguished the responsibility for the creation of the plan with responsibility for its implementation. Members of Group 4 envisioned a future in which the care template could be housed in a central database so that different physicians participating in the patient's care could log in and complete sections of the form. In such an environment, the care plan could also be accessible to the patient. In the absence of information technology that would allow broad accessibility, one office would have to have the primary responsibility for completing the form, which would then be shared with other practices.

Dr. Ross Martin of Pfizer Human Health advised workshop participants to focus on electronic health records as an endpoint solution to survivorship care planning. Although many health care providers do not have electronic communications, any template that is developed must be created with online applications in mind. When President George Bush appointed a National Coordinator for Health Information Technology in 2004, he announced that he wanted to see every American with an electronic health record by the year 2014. Reaching this goal will be very challenging, but any template development must proceed with the prospect of innovation in mind.

In the short term, it may be possible to have secretaries or others properly trained to do a chart review to fill in some portions of the care plan. More highly skilled labor could then be responsible for verifying the information. Dr. Molla Donaldson reported that, as part of the QOPI program, there is a training program for the office staff to pull records and summarize and track information. Highly trained cancer registrars are already collecting data from medical records. They work in every state and could be considered as a potential resource for beginning the treatment summary. In pediatric oncology, clinical research associates often fill out the treatment summaries. They are verified by clinicians, whether a nurse practitioner or a physician, but they do create the summaries, and quality checks can be incorporated.

Group members suggested that the individual who completed the care plan template was not necessarily the provider who would discuss it with the patient. There is some benefit to having more than one person interact with a patient over a particular issue. One group member illustrated this point by his practice of explaining a course of chemotherapy to a patient and then leaving the room to allow the team nurse to go over the treatment plan again in greater detail. His experience has been that the retention of information is better when information comes from both himself and a nurse practitioner, who has a different way of explaining things and responding to the patient. Resources will vary by practice, but group members agreed that having patients hear information more than once is helpful. Dr. Greenfield noted that how the care plan is discussed with patients, and by whom, can be tested by health services researchers.

Group 5: What Economic Strategies Could Encourage Implementation of Care Planning?

Ms. Buchsel, in summarizing the discussion on this topic, highlighted economic strategies to encourage care planning. She stated that reimbursement for completing the care plan template is likely to be insufficient for physician time spent on this activity. Having nurses, clinical research associates, or other trained nonphysicians complete some portions of the care plan would make it feasible from a cost standpoint. Having others involved in its completion may actually result in higher quality data, she noted. Another group member mentioned that oncologists cannot reliably report tumor-node-metastasis (TNM) staging.

According to Ms. Buchsel, incentives to adopt care planning could include: (1) ASCO endorsement of care planning as an expected standard of care; and (2) adoption of care planning as a quality indicator that could be used as part of report card-type quality improvement programs or pay for performance initiatives. Patients and referring physicians may start choosing practices in which care planning is offered.

Insurers have started to ask for preauthorization for chemotherapy, and this practice is going to become common as the cost of cancer drugs escalates. If the treatment plan could be used to fulfill the preauthorization documentation, then providers might be very interested in completing the treatment summary. The prospective plan for follow-up could also be considered for preauthorization. Oncology providers could, for example, list the imaging procedures and tests recommended for the next 3 years and, if approved, could meet the preauthorization requirements prospectively. This could save significant office time and resources. If the template were standardized and confined to one page, all insurers would be likely to want to use it.

Group 6: What Barriers Exist to Creating the Care Plan? How Can They Be Overcome?

Members of Group 6 discussed barriers to care planning, focusing on how they might be overcome. In terms of solutions, the notion of keeping it simple was reiterated by several group members. A minimum standard, not the best that there could be, should be designated for the treatment summary and the prospective care plan. To expedite care planning, group members thought that starting with a few cancers, for example, breast and colon cancer, would be advisable because surveillance and risk guidelines are already available. Advisable also is learning from the pediatric experience with survivorship guidelines and innovative strategies to communicate with survivors and their providers (see the discussion of the Passport for

Care in Chapter 4). Group participants noted that demonstration projects are needed to evaluate alternate strategies for care planning. Ms. Pamela Haylock mentioned the American College of Surgeons' Commission on Cancer surveys as an opportunity to assess care planning in hospital-based cancer programs. As an overarching goal, reeducation of both oncology and primary care physicians is needed for cancer to be considered a chronic illness.

From a pediatric perspective, Dr. Jackie Casillas, from the University of California, Los Angeles, pointed out that survivors of childhood cancer face an additional barrier posed by the transition from pediatric to adult health care. A care plan may be given to the parent in the pediatric setting. An adolescent or young adult may, however, lose touch with their pediatric oncology providers as they age into adult care settings. They also need to have received a copy of the cancer care records from their parents, as they may not be able to recall any of the specifics related to their diagnosis and treatment.

4

Resources for Completing the Care Plan

INTRODUCTION

Moderator: Ms. Ellen Stovall

This second day of the workshop is devoted to implementation issues. Kevin Oeffinger and Charles Shapiro will provide an overview of the status of survivorship guidelines. Diane Blum will then discuss appropriate use of available psychosocial support services. Recommendations for healthy lifestyle behaviors will be reviewed by Wendy Demark-Wahnefried. Information technology is critical to the success of survivorship care planning, and David Poplack, Mark Horowitz, and Michael Fordis will demonstrate its promise with an introduction to the Passport for Health program for survivors of childhood cancer. Lawrence Shulman will then reflect on the state of information technology as it pertains to survivorship care planning. Finally, Tim Byers will discuss regional approaches to cancer survivorship planning.

SURVIVORSHIP GUIDELINES

Two Perspectives

Presenter: Dr. Kevin Oeffinger

I would like to share some guideline-related lessons learned from two perspectives: (1) from working with the Children's Oncology Group's Late

Effects Steering Committee to disseminate and implement follow-up guidelines, and (2) from sitting on the American Academy of Family Physicians' Commission on Clinical Policy and Research, the body that reviews and collaboratively develops guidelines that are adopted by members of the American Academy of Family Physicians.

Evidence-based guidelines are useful in promoting high-quality care, standardizing and facilitating the care of complex patients, and providing a rubric or a set of accepted measures for process evaluation. While they are valuable, there are some pitfalls associated with the use of guidelines. First, the large number of published guidelines may overwhelm and confuse practicing physicians. Second, some physicians reject guidelines because they may not take into consideration the complexities facing their patients. Guidelines may also be perceived to be dictating clinical decisions.

The Children's Oncology Group (COG) long-term follow-up guidelines were developed by a late effects committee cochaired by Melissa Hudson and Wendy Landier over the course of several years. COG is a 244-institution clinical trial consortium. The pediatric community has over the past 15 years wrestled with the issues under discussion at this workshop. Much has been learned from the pediatric experience, and it would be unfortunate if this experience were not applied productively to the challenges ahead in the adult survivor arena.

The goal of the COG guideline effort was to standardize and enhance follow-up care throughout the life span of the survivor. The focus has been on screening for late effects rather than screening for relapse or recurrence, as these were already embedded in ongoing protocols. The COG guidelines start to apply at 2 years following the completion of cancer therapy. The intended users of the guidelines are clinicians who provide health care for pediatric cancer survivors regardless of their age and their care setting.

To develop the guidelines, more than a year was spent conducting in-depth literature reviews, synthesizing the literature, achieving multidisciplinary group consensus, and submitting the guidelines to external review. Some refinements have been made following their initial dissemination in September 2003.

A hybrid approach was used in guideline development. The large body of evidence linking therapeutic exposures and late effects was reviewed and scored according to quality. There are very few studies that examine how surveillance affects outcomes, in part because of the relatively small numbers of pediatric cancer survivors. Consequently, expert clinical experience and principles of screening in the general population and other high-risk groups was relied on for the aspects of care considered as part of the guideline development process.

Version 2.0 of the long-term follow-up guidelines is available online at www.survivorshipguidelines.org. The guidelines are based on therapeutic exposures rather than on cancer type. Shown in Figure 4-1 are some of the late effects of alkylating agents, associated risk factors, recommendations for follow-up and health counseling, and references to the literature.

Throughout the guideline development process, dissemination efforts have been a priority. A methods paper was published in the *Journal of Clinical Oncology* in 2004[1] and general review articles have subsequently been published. Presentations have been made at specialty and primary care conferences. Having the guidelines posted online permits wide accessibility. A computer-based Passport for Care has been developed to tailor the guidelines to individual patients. This effort will be described by David Poplack and colleagues later in this session.

Maintenance of the guidelines depends on 18 multidisciplinary task forces that include pediatric oncologists, radiation oncologists, surgeons, cardiologists, organ-specific specialists, primary care physicians, nurse practitioners, social workers, and psychologists. These groups review the literature, develop and recommend revisions to the guidelines, and engage in dissemination activities.

A publications committee was established through the COG late effects committee to review all concept proposals for literature that would reflect on the COG guidelines. Two types of publications are highlighted: (1) detailed and in-depth systematic reviews on focused topics such as chest radiation and its relationship with breast cancer development; and (2) general reviews that are geared more toward the practicing primary physician and the community-based pediatric oncologist.

Relationships with professional societies have been developed and endorsements, or what one might call "seals of approval" of the guidelines, have been sought. The guidelines are included in the National Guideline Clearinghouse™ (http://www.guideline.gov/).

The backbone of dissemination efforts is through long-term follow-up programs. These programs are generally based at children's hospitals or cancer centers at which a team approach is taken, with physicians working with survivors, nurse practitioners, social workers, and psychologists. There is also a multidisciplinary network of adult and pediatric-based subspecialists. The three core components of the long-term follow-up programs are: (1) a cancer summary and treatment plan that are discussed with the patient; (2) the COG long-term follow-up guidelines; and (3) delivery of risk-based survivorship care.

Long-term follow-up is not uniformly available across the 244 COG institutions. Although more than half of these institutions have a mechanism for long-term follow-up care, only one-quarter of them have a pro-

---

[1]Landier W et al., 2004. *Journal of Clinical Oncology* 24:4979-4990.

CHEMOTHERAPY · ALKYLATING AGENTS

Sec #	Therapeutic Agent(s)	Potential Late Effects	Risk Factors	High Risk Factors	Periodic Evaluation	Health Counseling / Further Considerations
7 (Male)	**ALKYLATING AGENTS** Busulfan Carmustine (BCNU) Chlorambucil Cyclophosphamide Ifosfamide Lomustine (CCNU) Mechlorethamine Melphalan Procarbazine Thiotepa **HEAVY METALS** Carboplatin Cisplatin **NON-CLASSICAL ALKYLATORS** Dacarbazine (DTIC) Temozolomide	Gonadal dysfunction (testicular) Hypogonadism Infertility	**Treatment Factors** Higher cumulative doses of alkylators or combinations of alkylators Combined with radiation to: - Abdomen/pelvis - Testes - Brain, cranium (neuroendocrine axis) **Health Behaviors** Smoking **Info Link** Doses that cause gonadal dysfunction show individual variation. Germ cell function (spermatogenesis) is impaired at lower doses compared to Leydig cell (testosterone production) function. Prepubertal status does not protect from gonadal injury in males.	**Host Factors** Male gender **Treatment Factors** MOPP > 3 cycles Busulfan > 600 mg/m² Cyclophosphamide cumulative dose > 7.5 gm/m² or as conditioning for HCT Any alkylators combined with: - Testicular radiation - Pelvic radiation - TBI	**HISTORY** Pubertal (onset, tempo) Sexual function (erections, nocturnal emissions, libido) Medication use impacting sexual function (Yearly) **PHYSICAL** Tanner stage Testicular volume by Prader orchidometry (Yearly) **SCREENING** FSH LH Testosterone (Baseline at age 14 and as clinically indicated in patients with delayed puberty and/or clinical signs and symptoms of testosterone deficiency) Semen analysis (As requested by patient and for evaluation of infertility. Periodic evaluation over time is recommended as resumption of spermatogenesis can occur up to 10 years post therapy)	**Health Links** Male Health issues **Resources** Extensive information regarding infertility for patients and healthcare professionals is available on the following websites: American Society for Reproductive Medicine (www.asrm.org) Fertile Hope (www.fertilehope.org) **Counseling** Counsel regarding the need for contraception, since there is tremendous individual variability in gonadal toxicity after exposure to alkylating agents. Recovery of fertility may occur years after therapy. **Considerations for further testing and intervention** Bone density evaluation for osteopenia/osteoporosis in hypogonadal patients. Refer to endocrinologist for delayed puberty or persistently abnormal hormone levels. Hormonal replacement therapy for hypogonadal patients. Reproductive endocrinology/urology referral for infertility evaluation and consultation regarding assisted reproductive technologies. **SYSTEM = Male reproductive** **SCORE =** Alkylating Agents: 1 Heavy Metals: 2A Non-Classical Alkylators: 2A

SECTION 7 REFERENCES

da Cunha MF, Meistrich ML, Fuller LM, et al. Recovery of spermatogenesis after treatment for Hodgkin's disease: limiting dose of MOPP chemotherapy. J Clin Oncol. Jun 1984;2(6):571-577.

Gerl A, Mühlbayer D, Hansmann G, Mraz W, Hiddemann W. The impact of chemotherapy on Leydig cell function in long term survivors of germ cell tumors. Cancer. Apr 1 2001;91(7):1297-1303.

Kenney LB, Laufer MR, Grant FD, Grier H, Diller L. High risk of infertility and long term gonadal damage in males treated with high dose cyclophosphamide for sarcoma during childhood. Cancer. Feb 1 2001;91(3):613-621.

Muller J. Disturbance of pubertal development after cancer treatment. Best Pract Res Clin Endocrinol Metab. Mar 2002;16(1):91-103.

Sklar C. Reproductive physiology and treatment-related loss of sex hormone production. Med Pediatr Oncol. Jul 1999;33(1):2-8.

Somali M, Mpatakoias V, Avramides A, et al. Function of the hypothalamic-pituitary-gonadal axis in long-term survivors of hematopoietic stem cell transplantation for hematological diseases. Gynecol Endocrinol. Jul 2005;21(1):18-26.

FIGURE 4-1 Example of COG guidelines related to chemotherapy late effects.
SOURCE: Oeffinger, 2006.

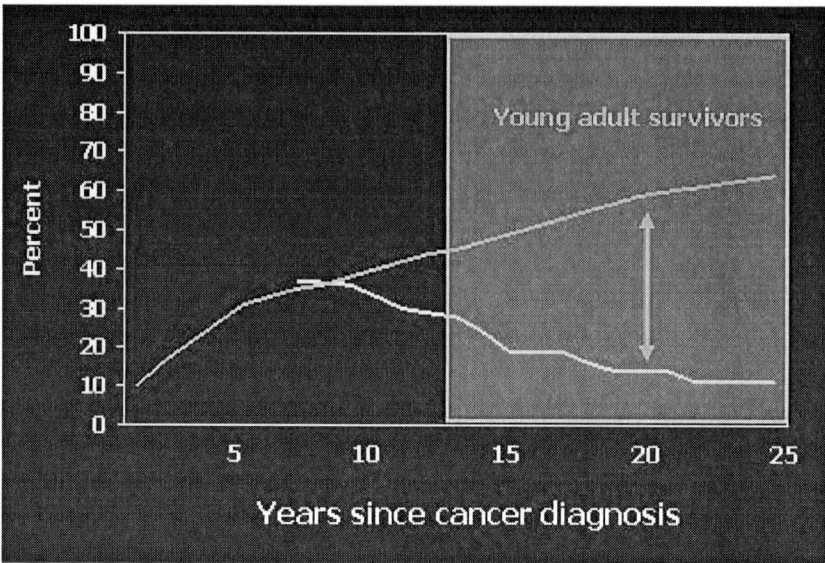

FIGURE 4-2 Cancer center visits and late effects: Results from the Childhood Cancer Survivor Study.
NOTE: Top line represents percent of survivors with incidences of late effects; bottom line represents percent of survivors seen during cancer center visits.
SOURCE: Oeffinger, 2006.

gram that provides comprehensive long-term follow-up care, and only one-tenth of these institutions can follow adult survivors of pediatric cancer.

The proportion of survivors of childhood cancer with a cancer center visit within the past 2 years is about 35 percent at 7 years after cancer therapy or from the cancer diagnosis, according to results from the Child-hood Cancer Survivor Study published a few years ago.[2] As the bottom line on Figure 4-2 illustrates, the further survivors are from their cancer diagno-sis, the less likely they are to have been seen at a cancer center. These results are based on patients who were treated from 1970 to 1986. When the cumulative incidence of late effects is superimposed, as shown in the top line on Figure 4-2, a very significant gap becomes evident as they are 15, 20,

---

[2]See Oeffinger KC, Mertens AC, Hudson MM, Gurney JG, Casillas J, Chen H, Whitton J, Yeazel M, Yasui Y, Robison LL. 2004. Health care of young adult survivors of childhood cancer: a report from the Childhood Cancer Survivor Study. *Annals of Family Medicine* 2(1):61-70.

and 25 years from their cancer therapy. By this time, they are experiencing their highest rate of morbidity but are not being seen at a cancer center.

Some barriers to comprehensive survivorship care extend beyond the reach of long-term follow-up programs. Primary care physicians are not familiar with pediatric cancer survivors, which is not unexpected because, on average, a general internist or a family physician has three to five pediatric cancer survivors in their practice. One of these patients might be a leukemia survivor, one a Hodgkin's disease survivor, and one a brain tumor survivor. Primary care physicians cannot be expected to keep up with this complex and rapidly evolving area of medicine, when it so rarely relates to their practices.

Insurance-related barriers are very significant for survivors of childhood cancer. Many are uninsured, and if insured, their coverage may not adequately cover components of follow-up care, or it may exclude specialized care entirely if the long-term follow-up program is not a designated part of their health care network. There are no survivor-based delivery models in health maintenance organizations or U.S.-based single-payer systems.

Efforts to improve survivor health care have focused on increasing the number and the quality of long-term follow-up programs in COG. Innovative tools, such as the Passport for Care to be demonstrated at the workshop, will facilitate improvements in care not only at cancer centers but also in community-based oncology practices. Work is also under way with insurance companies to develop cost-effective models of survivorship care. Other efforts are aimed at bridging the gap as patients age and transition from pediatric to adult care and transition from specialty to primary care. Engaging primary care physicians in survivorship care is key to improved care. If current practice is to change, efforts must extend beyond the dissemination efforts described.

It is important to note some key differences between pediatric and adult cancer survivors. First, pediatric cancer is rare and, as mentioned, it is not a commonly encountered problem in primary care. In contrast, primary care physicians in the adult arena are engaged in cancer prevention efforts as well as care for the over 10 million survivors of adult cancer. Pediatric cancer survivors, especially as they age, do not maintain strong ties with oncologists, whereas adults survivors, as we learned from the Institute of Medicine (IOM) focus groups, tend to be "followed for life" by their oncologist.

These features of pediatric and adult survivorship suggest different approaches to knowledge transfer. Primary care physicians encountering a pediatric cancer survivor in their practice need a single national site or source of information. In contrast, primary care providers caring for adult cancer survivors usually have a local source of information, the community-based oncologist. In both cases, translating knowledge goes well beyond simply providing follow-up guidelines. Primary care providers need contact with expertise and avenues for continued communication.

Disseminating clinical practice guidelines through journals, continuing medical education opportunities, and postings on websites is insufficient to change practice behavior. What will change practice behaviors? Some recent research conducted at the University of Toronto has provided some clues to effective knowledge translation and subsequent transfer of that knowledge.[3] These investigators have defined knowledge translation as the "exchange, synthesis, and ethically sound application of researcher findings within a complex system of relationships among researchers and knowledge users." To improve knowledge translation and transfer, mechanisms must be developed to "strengthen relationships among health researchers and users of health knowledge, enhance capacity for knowledge uptake, and accelerate the flow of knowledge into beneficial health applications."

In the context of survivorship care, components needed for knowledge transfer include:

- a user-friendly version of survivorship guidelines;
- a patient version of the treatment summary and care plan;
- training to prepare practices for guideline adoption (both the office staff and the clinicians);
- facilitated communication (e.g., between nurse managers, oncologists, and primary care physicians); and
- innovative technology (e.g., cross-platform electronic health records or tools such as the Passport for Care).

In terms of models of care, Eva Grunfeld's series of randomized clinical trials illustrates how follow-up care for breast cancer survivors can be accomplished in the primary care community.[4] The shared care model can be stratified by risk. Some high-risk survivors will need continued follow-up with their oncologist. Lower-risk patients may not need the resources of

---

[3]Information about this program is available at http://www.ktp.utoronto.ca/index.htm.

[4]Grunfeld E. et al., 2006. Randomized trial of long-term follow-up for early-stage breast cancer: a comparison of family physician versus specialist care. *Journal of Clinical Oncology* 24(6):848-55. Grunfeld E. et al., 1999. Comparison of breast cancer patient satisfaction with follow-up in primary care versus 2specialist care: Results from a randomized controlled trial. *British Journal of General Practice* 49(446):705-710. Grunfeld E. et al., 1999. Follow-up of breast cancer in primary care vs specialist care: Results of an ecomonic evaluation. *British Journal of General Practice* 79(7-8):1227-1233. Grunfeld E. et al., 1995. Evaluating primary care follow-up of breast cancer: Methods and preliminary results of three studies. *Annals of Oncology* 6(Suppl 2):47-52.

a cancer center or an oncologist and may be best seen by a primary care physician. There is a unique opportunity to develop and test models of care through partnerships of cancer centers, Community Clinical Oncology Practices (CCOPs), and practice-based research networks supported by the federal Agency for Healthcare Research and Quality (AHRQ). An example of such a network is the Federation of Practice-Based Research Networks, which was established in 1997. There are 50 different networks involving over 6,000 primary care clinicians, over 5 million patients, and 24 million patient encounters a year. There are over 100 active research studies through these networks. There are opportunities for cancer centers and CCOPs to collaborate with these practice-based research networks to develop and test survivorship care models and then disseminate successful models for adoption.

In engaging primary care providers in survivorship care, it is important to remember that effective strategies tend to work from the bottom up, not from the top down. Involving primary care physicians in the process at the outset is critical. The American Academy of Family Physicians, the American College of Physicians, and the American Academy of Pediatrics have been integrally involved in developing and disseminating guidelines for many years and have an established process and experience working with other professional societies. Some guideline strategies fail if: (1) there is a "top-down" mentality; (2) guidelines are based on consensus rather than good evidence; and (3) the focus is on who should do it, rather than what should be done. To bring primary care providers and other constituencies into the dialogue, a summit meeting could be held on collaborative approaches to survivorship care.

Survivorship researchers have examined issues related to quality of life, late effects, and health outcomes, but what is needed now are research initiatives to test models of care. A program announcement that established a common set of outcomes, including measures for adherence to guidelines, would allow the research community to test stratified risk models of care and alternative methods to collaborate with primary care providers. A funding mechanism is needed to encourage the development and testing of innovative technology. Support could be used to explore the potential for exciting technologies, like the Passport for Care and electronic health records to further survivorship health care.

Additional research is also needed to better understand the survivorship care paradigm. Cancer survivors are being characterized as having a chronic condition, but cancer is quite distinct from cardiovascular disease and diabetes. Cancer survivors may have a late effect that becomes a chronic health problem, but often it is their risk for developing new problems that presents a different paradigm.

ASCO INITIATIVE

Presenter: Dr. Charles Shapiro

The American Society of Clinical Oncology's (ASCO) initiative is to develop long-term medical care guidelines for adult cancer survivors. The effort began in 2005, and its purpose is to provide health care professionals with the knowledge and expertise to decrease morbidity and to improve the quality of life for adult cancer survivors. The initial audience for the guidelines is health care providers, but the effort could be expanded to include companion patient-friendly survivorship guidelines. The ASCO guidelines will address issues arising during the posttreatment phase of the cancer trajectory.

In contrast to pediatrics, there are few guidelines for adult survivorship care. A limited evidence base has impeded guideline development. The ASCO initiative will be key to highlighting what is known and not known for this phase of cancer care and suggesting critical areas for future survivorship research.

In contrast to the treatment modality approach taken in pediatrics, the ASCO guidelines will be developed using a symptom or organ site paradigm. For many aspects of survivorship care there is limited clinical trial-based evidence, and generalizations about care from cancer registries are difficult because registries do not capture complete information on treatment and late effects. Furthermore, adult cancer survivors often have comorbid conditions that can confound interpretation of outcomes by researchers as they attempt to establish relationships among treatments, late effects, and health outcomes. It has been difficult, for example, to clearly establish the link between doxorubicin and cardiac problems because heart disease increases naturally as patients age. There is also a dependence on surrogate endpoints, for example, using bone mineral density in research on the effects of various treatments on fractures. The more clinically relevant endpoint, fractures, has not been well studied because follow-up periods have not been long enough.

Another challenge facing clinicians as they attempt to use evidence to guide their practice is that data from long-term follow-up studies may reflect outmoded treatment techniques. For example, 30 years ago, radiation techniques were very different from what they are today. These older techniques were associated with an increased incidence of cardiovascular effects that presented in the second decade. With more modern techniques, the latest data show a markedly reduced incidence of cardiac effects. With treatments advancing rapidly, evaluation of late effects of treatments becomes a moving target. It is axiomatic that new therapies will be adopted into standard practice based on short-term improvements in efficacy. For

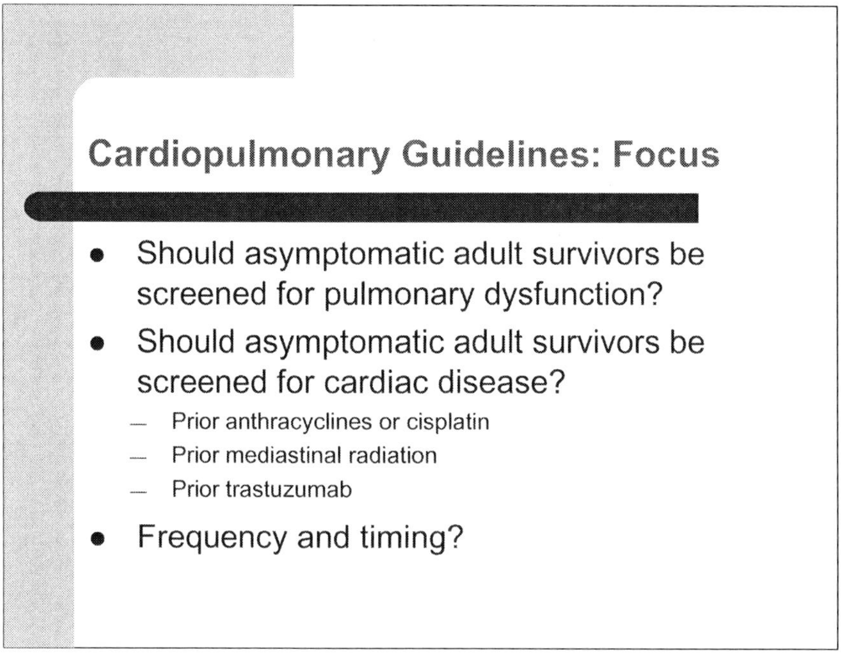

Cardiopulmonary Guidelines: Focus

- Should asymptomatic adult survivors be screened for pulmonary dysfunction?
- Should asymptomatic adult survivors be screened for cardiac disease?
  - Prior anthracyclines or cisplatin
  - Prior mediastinal radiation
  - Prior trastuzumab
- Frequency and timing?

FIGURE 4-3 ASCO's cardiopulmonary guidelines.
SOURCE: Shapiro, 2006.

example, trastuzumab (Herceptin) is markedly beneficial in the early stage of breast cancer according to clinical trials, but the median follow-up period in these trials is 2 to 3 years. It has become the standard of care for women with breast cancer who overexpress the growth factor protein HER2. What is known of trastuzumab cardiotoxicity is reassuring, but absent are long-term follow-up studies and information on interactions between radiation and trastuzumab or anthracyclines and trastuzumab. This represents another kind of moving target that necessitates a continuous reexamination of guidelines after they are created.

The ASCO guidelines will focus on five areas in the following order: cardiopulmonary late effects; bone health; second cancers; hormone deficiency; and anxiety and depression. The guideline development process is moving forward very quickly, and the first guideline is already being reviewed by the ASCO board. Many people have volunteered to expedite the guidelines process.

The focus of the guidelines is on screening questions, for example, whether asymptomatic adult survivors should be screened for pulmonary dysfunction or cardiac disease (Figure 4-3), and if so, when should such screening begin, and at what interval should it be repeated?

One of the recommendations included in the ASCO cardiopulmonary guideline was based on consensus and may be considered controversial. The ASCO guideline suggests screening of asymptomatic high-risk survivors every 5 years and treatment for asymptomatic left ventricular (LV) systolic or diastolic dysfunction based on recommendations of the American College of Cardiology, the American Heart Association, and the Heart Failure Society. Survivors are considered to be at high risk if they have one of the following: age less than 18 years at exposure; prior cardiac disease; greater than 300 mg/m^2 of doxorubicin; or mediastinal radiation. This consensus-based recommendation seems to be reasonable, at least as a starting point.

In terms of challenges and implementation barriers, the first is the paradigm shift to thinking of cancer as a chronic condition. It will be important to raise awareness that people live a long time with cancer and that there are long-term consequences of treatment. A second issue relates to the major legal and financial implications of guidelines. ASCO's consensus guideline states that it is reasonable to screen for cardiac dysfunction in women who have had greater than 300 mg/m^2 doxorubicin or who had breast radiation that involved the chest wall. Such screening is not now part of standard breast cancer follow-up. Physicians are being asked to consider screening for cardiac dysfunction when they have not routinely done so and when there is only consensus among experts to back up the recommendation.

Another challenge in issuing guidelines is establishing who is to accept responsibility for providing guideline-recommended care. ASCO originally viewed this as a responsibility of the oncology community, but more recently, and certainly at this meeting, primary care providers and survivors themselves should be considered as potential constituents for taking action based on the guidelines.

Publishing the guidelines is a starting point, and it may ultimately have the most value in identifying gaps in knowledge and setting the research agenda. The ASCO guideline effort is also an opportunity to link academic and community centers to collaborate on research interventions, education, and information dissemination. The Lance Armstrong Foundation Centers of Excellence, to be described later today, are a model that needs to be developed to fulfill its potential of driving the agenda for research and improvements in survivorship care. The Quality Oncology Practice Initiative (QOPI) is a potential mechanism to assess compliance with the ASCO guidelines. The ASCO guideline initiative will attempt to learn from the experiences of other clinical practice guideline efforts, such as those of the National Comprehensive Cancer Network (NCCN). We need to understand what worked and what did not work, so as not to duplicate effort but rather to learn from the experience of existing programs that are similar to ASCO's in scope and purpose.

Engaging survivors in efforts to improve care is also extremely important. One recent example of a successful engagement is a survey on fertility conducted by a coalition of young cancer survivors. The Internet survey of the members of this coalition resulted in a peer-reviewed publication in the *Journal of Clinical Oncology*. Fertility guidelines issued by ASCO in May 2006 were in part completed as a result of this effort. Directly asking survivors about what they need and want, as well as what is lacking in their care, can inform development of practice guidelines. This experience with the coalition of young survivors represents a good model to emulate. There need to be more opportunities for survivors to be empowered to participate in their own path to wellness and health maintenance. Survivorship care planning, including the development of guidelines, provides such an opportunity.

Discussion

Dr. Sheldon Greenfield asked the speakers whether the timing is right for oncologists to meet with generalists to discuss survivorship care. He suggested that a standing meeting be held, perhaps on a yearly or biennial basis, to discuss advances in clinical practice guidelines and psychosocial issues. Both Dr. Oeffinger and Dr. Shapiro agreed that such a meeting was a very good idea. It would bring together relevant stakeholders and provide an opportunity to collaborate and learn what each other wants and needs. The reality is that the oncology community does not have the resources or capacity to provide care for survivors, and until a partnership is established with primary care providers, quality survivorship care will not be achieved. There are some good precedents for collaboration. The American College of Cardiology has worked with the American Academy of Family Physicians and the American College of Physicians through the Society of General Internal Medicine to develop collaborative guidelines on myocardial infarction posttreatment that have been widely adopted.

Dr. Lawrence Shulman of the Dana-Farber Cancer Institute made the distinction between areas of survivorship care for which there is no or little evidence and areas where there is incomplete evidence. For example, while not all of the evidence is in, it is well established that premature menopause after chemotherapy rapidly affects bone health. In this case, there are interventions to improve bone health. In Dr. Shulman's opinion, the evidence is weaker for the recommendation to screen asymptomatic survivors for cardiac disease after doxorubicin therapy. Dr. Oeffinger reiterated that guideline development will highlight what is known and unknown and help to set a research agenda to fill in the identified gaps. Experience with the pediatric guidelines illustrates the dynamic nature of guideline development in terms of identifying gaps in knowledge, trying to fill those gaps with current research, and then updating the guidelines as new findings are made available.

Ms. Martha Gaines of the University of Wisconsin Law School pointed out that there were many opportunities for survivors to be involved in their own care from its very beginning. An analogy can be made between patients and the captain of a ship. The captain is not always at the helm, but the ship neither leaves the shore nor heads for any destination without the captain's approval. Dr. Oeffinger agreed with this focus on patient empowerment and described how the pediatric survivorship guidelines include over 50 health links that are written on specific topics that can be downloaded, read, and shared by survivors with their physicians. The Passport for Care empowers survivors with information, clinical recommendations, and guidance on improving their own health. Dr. Shapiro suggested that the culture of oncologist practice will have to change to accommodate broader survivor involvement in care.

PSYCHOSOCIAL SUPPORT RESOURCES

Presenter: Ms. Diane Blum

The IOM recommended that the Survivorship Care Plan include information on the availability of community-based psychosocial services. That information and a list of resources be provided to cancer patients at the conclusion of treatment was also called for 3 years ago in the President's Cancer Panel report.[5] It is imperative for an informed cancer survivor in 2006 to be able to use community-based resources. People are increasingly on their own while they are being treated for cancer and in the posttreatment phase of care. They are expected to make decisions, manage treatment, and integrate the cancer experience into their lives as best they can without resources that might have been provided in a hospital. Twenty years ago, being a cancer patient was very much a full-time job. People spent much of their time in a hospital and had access there to education and support. Progress in treatment has shifted care to the outpatient setting. In this environment, patients are seeing nurses less often and are rarely encountering social workers. While there has been a decline in onsite sources

---

[5]President's Cancer Panel, 2004. *Living Beyond Cancer: Finding a New Balance*. Bethesda, MD: National Cancer Institute.

of education, counseling, and support, there has been tremendous growth in Internet-based resources.

The problem for cancer survivors is not that there are too few resources. There are many national and local resources. The American Cancer Society (ACS), for example, has 3,300 offices and thousands of people a day telephone their call center. ACS also has an online searchable database to find local resources by zip code. Cancer*Care*, the National Coalition for Cancer Survivorship (NCCS), the Lance Armstrong Foundation (LAF), the Wellness Community, and numerous disease-specific organizations are among the many other national organizations that provide services. There are also many regional and local resources, particularly for women with breast cancer. Excellent fact sheets and printed guides to resources are also available. The National Cancer Institute (NCI) booklet *Facing Forward: A Guide for Cancer Survivors,* for example, describes the roles of and access to social workers, nutritionists, and physical therapists. Cancer*Care* will issue the fifth edition of its national guide to resources, *A Helping Hand,* that includes tips on evaluating them.[6] "People Living with Cancer" is ASCO's patient website that includes a wealth of information.[7] NCCS, in collaboration with the Oncology Nursing Society and the Association of Oncology Social Work, has produced the Cancer Survivor Toolbox in CD format and online. The toolbox addresses many survivorship issues, including those related to employment and insurance.[8] These sorts of materials should be distributed to every person with cancer in the country, especially those who have finished treatment. The bountiful resources available in print, by telephone, and online are very underutilized.

According to a fairly recent survey of 2,000 oncology professionals, fewer than 60 percent recommended support services or thought such services were helpful. This survey, published in *Cancer Practice* in 2002, included responses from members of professional organizations representing oncologists, oncology nurses, and social workers.[9] Professionals who thought that support services were not helpful were least likely to make referrals and least likely to know about them. These results are alarming, given that the respondents were oncology professionals who belong to their professional organizations. The lack of attention to the psychosocial needs

---

[6]Information on the guide can be found at http://www.cancercare.org/get_help/assistance/helping_hand.php.

[7]ASCO's People Living With Cancer website is at http://www.plwc.org/portal/site/PLWC.

[8]The toolbox can be found at http://www.cancersurvivaltoolbox.org/default.aspx.

[9]This study, "Healthcare Professionals' Awareness of Cancer Support Services," by B. Alex Matthews, Frank Baker, and Rachel Spillers was published in *Cancer Practice*, Vol. 10, No. 1, January/February 2002 (pages 36-44).

of cancer patients was also prominent in the findings from the IOM focus groups (see Chapter 3).

The 2004 IOM report, *Meeting Psychosocial Needs of Women with Breast Cancer*, found psychosocial interventions to be effective but underused for many reasons, including stigma, inadequate insurance coverage, and, very importantly, lack of knowledge on the part of health care professionals.[10]

How can problems related to lack of knowledge and underutilization be addressed? How can one ensure that available materials and services reach the people they are intended to help? The problem lies in the absence of a systematic distribution system and no clear-cut allocation of responsibility. Pharmaceutical companies reach into every place where people with cancer are treated, and they might be enjoined to hand resource materials to a physician or a nurse, but experience suggests that such materials often do not reach the patient. Social workers could assume some responsibilities, but they rarely work in the community settings in which most people with cancer are treated. An additional challenge is keeping resource guides and materials up-to-date. Online guides are somewhat easier to update, but this is time-consuming and has to be assumed as an ongoing responsibility.

Assessing individuals for their psychosocial needs allows providers to refer survivors to a program that is more likely to be individually tailored to their circumstances. Some survivors will require psychological support, while others will need financial or insurance counseling. Making these assessments, however, takes time and should be undertaken only when appropriate resources are available to meet identified needs. Assessments and referrals may be complicated in the case of special populations and the "hard-to-reach." Making resources available across differences in culture, age, and literacy can be a major challenge. These challenges must be overcome, because it is often the economically disadvantaged and individuals with other limitations who are most in need of resources.

Examples of programs that offer resources and resource information to survivors are CancerCare; www.plwc.org, the patient website of the American Society of Clinical Oncology; and the American Cancer Society. CancerCare is a nonprofit organization that provides free professional support services to 90,000 individuals a year. Clients include people with all cancers and their families and friends throughout the country. The services offered include counseling, education, and financial assistance provided by 120 staff, 75 of whom are either trained social workers or health educators. The social work staff works hard to offer quality service to the nearly 1,000 callers each week. CancerCare provides a number of special survivorship

---

[10]Information on this report can be found at: http://www.nap.edu/catalog/10909.html.

programs. A three-part telephone education workshop on survivorship is conducted annually. This program, supported by LAF and NCI, reaches thousands of people with good survivorship educational material. The program is archived on CancerCare's website.[11] CancerCare is part of the LAF LIVESTRONG™ initiative and responds to calls to the foundation from people who need psychosocial services. The potential demand for assistance is very high, and with additional resources, many more individuals could be helped.

ASCO's website, People Living with Cancer, was developed as a member benefit. ASCO members were going to be able to refer their patients to the website for credible up-to-date information developed by a trusted organization. Three million business cards were printed with the website's URL for members to distribute to their patients. Four years later, the website is a success. It contains quality content, and hundreds of thousands of people visit the site each year. However, it is not used well by ASCO members. Plans are for the site to be promoted more to the public, who seem to be enthusiastic users of it.

The American Cancer Society Call Center in Austin, Texas, is staffed by 400 well-trained counselors who provide a 24-hour, 365-day service. They receive about 2,500 calls a day that are patient related. The counselors link callers to resources according to zip code, but this approach may be limiting insofar as many resources are now virtual. An online service, for example, may be extremely valuable, but it would not necessarily be linked to a caller by zip code. The ACS has very high name recognition with the public and, given the volume of calls and visits to their survivorship-related web content, provides an important dissemination mechanism for information on survivorship.

The ultimate goal in terms of psychosocial services for cancer survivors is for each person at the completion of treatment to have a psychosocial assessment. The distress guidelines developed by NCCN are reasonable. Assessments are, however, appropriate only if resources are available to address the identified needs. Optimally, up-to-date resource materials would be distributed and tailored to the developmental needs of the patient—for example, young adults, older adults, parents. Survivors would then be given guidance on how to use the resources, when to use them, and how to evaluate them. Follow-up with survivors would ensure that appropriate resources were accessed. This is the optimal scenario. At a bare minimum, people should receive at least a resource guide and some basic materials. If every person who is completing treatment could be handed something, that

---

[11]Information on these cancer care programs can be found at: http://www.cancercare.org/get_help/tew_calendar.php.

would put them one step ahead of the game. Further steps could then be taken toward the ideal.

Although admonitions to increase awareness have become a cliché, some awareness campaigns have been very successful, for example, those launched in mid-1980s to raise awareness of breast cancer. An organization like the LAF could probably facilitate this kind of awareness program. Going directly to the survivor is another strategy that has been successful. Women have played a major role in changing the treatment of breast cancer, and they have also changed childbirth practices. Improvements in the management of cancer pain have been made by going directly to the person for whom pain is an issue. Physicians are key to change and also must continue to be targeted through professional organizations to raise awareness of psychosocial resources for their patients. Incentives might considered to aid in implementation efforts.

In conclusion, there are many quality resources, but no systematic method of distributing them and no health care professional identified as being in charge of this particular area of care, especially in community-based practices, in which most people are receiving their care. Lacking also are good evaluations of programs to assess their value.

Discussion

Dr. Lee Newcomer of the UnitedHealth Group started the discussion by asking whether research has shown what steps a new cancer patient takes to find information. Do we know, for example, where patients seek information and their level of reliance on the Internet? Dr. Julia Rowland described some unpublished research on information use that suggests that physicians are key providers, nurses are important, especially during active treatment, and the Internet is actively used by many. Ms. Blum mentioned that the "digital divide" seemed to be decreasing, indicating that Internet services are becoming accessible to more people. When the topic of finding information about cancer was raised in several patient focus groups conducted by Dr. Catherine Harvey, patients often said that they started with a neighbor, a church, a friend, or somebody at work. Information was initially sought through one of these informal networks. In the 10 to 12 communities in which focus groups were held, there was never a mention of a systematic approach to providing cancer-related information. This would seem to be a missed opportunity on the part of both oncology and primary care providers.

Ms. Blum pointed out that many patients do not know how to seek information and do not have the resources even to know where to start. Half of the people who call CancerCare each week have trouble getting transportation to treatment. That is their basic and overwhelming problem.

Dr. Lari Wenzel of the University of California, Irvine questioned whether use of psychosocial resources would increase if good evidence were available on their effectiveness and, more specifically, who benefits and when they benefit. Ms. Blum responded that there is already a robust body of literature showing that a number of psychosocial interventions are effective. Much of the work has been in the context of women with breast cancer and was reviewed in the IOM report on meeting psychosocial needs. Some good evidence exists on the benefits of psychosocial interventions for other diagnostic areas as well.

Dr. Al Marcus of the AMC Cancer Research Center mentioned that a particular challenge from the perspective of a regional cancer center is identifying resources for patients coming to the center from a broad and diverse geographic area. Resources are needed to help patients get local help as they return to their homes. Listing some of the national resources on the care plan should be routine. Another resource, not yet mentioned, is NCI's 1-800-4-CANCER telephone resource, which could also be very important in terms of providing referrals.

Dr. Rowland of the NCI Office of Cancer Survivorship suggested that the cancer-related call centers analyze their data to better understand consumers' and patients' information needs. The NCI cancer information service will do so to determine who is calling and what kind of information is being sought (e.g., prevention, diagnosis, treatment, survivorship, or end-of-life concerns). The LAF and the ACS are also examining the content of their calls. These data can help determine the adequacy of the available information and referral resources.

RECOMMENDATIONS FOR HEALTHY LIFESTYLE BEHAVIORS
Presenter: Dr. Wendy Demark-Wahnefried

Lifestyle factors, such as diet, exercise, and smoking cessation, should be considered in the care plans that are given to cancer patients as they finish their primary treatment. Cancer survivors are at greater risk for cardiovascular disease, osteoporosis, and diabetes, and changes in health behaviors may reduce these treatment-related conditions, cancer-related symptoms, comorbidity, and functional declines. Accumulating evidence also suggests that the pursuit of healthy lifestyles after treatment also may reduce cancer recurrence and improve both cancer-specific and overall death rates.

Only about 20 percent of oncologists provide any sort of guidance to patients on lifestyle issues. When counseling is offered, it is more often for smoking cessation than for diet and exercise. When asked why they do not provide this information, oncologists say that they lack time and are unsure of the science, the appropriate messages, and how to deliver them. Primary care providers have more familiarity and experience in this area. What messages regarding health behaviors have sufficient evidence to support their delivery to cancer patients? What follows is a summary of a background paper prepared for the workshop in the areas of weight management, nutrition and diet, exercise, smoking, alcohol consumption, bone health, protection against skin cancer, and complementary and alternative medicines.[12]

Weight Management: Weight management is a key concern for cancer survivors since there are considerable risks associated with either underweight or overweight status. Anorexia and cachexia are prevalent problems for patients with cancers in advanced stages and certain gastrointestinal, respiratory, and childhood cancers. In these cases, weight gain is recommended to speed recovery, improve well-being, and increase functional status. These patients benefit from information and counseling to improve their nutritional intake. Often this requires additional counseling to increase their physical activity in an effort to stimulate appetite and reduce constipation, and in some cases pharmacologic interventions are required, for example, megestrol acetate.

In contrast, overweight and obesity are risk factors for several cancers, including cancers of the endometrium, esophagus (adenocarcinoma), colon, kidney, and postmenopausal breast cancer. The majority of breast and prostate cancer survivors are overweight or obese, and the high prevalence of overweight among these major subgroups of survivors is a key health concern. Being overweight at diagnosis is a risk factor for subsequent cancers. Weight gain is common during and after cancer treatment and also is linked with progressive disease, second primary cancers, and comorbid conditions (e.g., diabetes, cardiovascular disease) that may play a role in functional decline.

Shown in Figure 4-4 are data on breast cancer survivors enrolled in the Nurses Health Study. Women who increased their body mass index from 0.5 to 2 units were at significantly higher risk for breast cancer recurrence, breast cancer mortality, and overall mortality when compared with women who maintained their weight (represented by the second set of bars from the left). This unit increase in weight is not large and can be anywhere from 3 to 13 lb, depending on a woman's height.

More definitive work needs to be done in the area of energy balance and survivorship because these findings come from longitudinal observational studies. Intervention studies are needed to see if weight reduction and maintenance of healthy weights are effective in reducing cancer recurrence and mortality, as well as comorbidity and functional decline.

---

[12]For more information, see the background paper prepared by Dr. Demark-Wahnefried and Dr. Lee Jones in Appendix D.2.

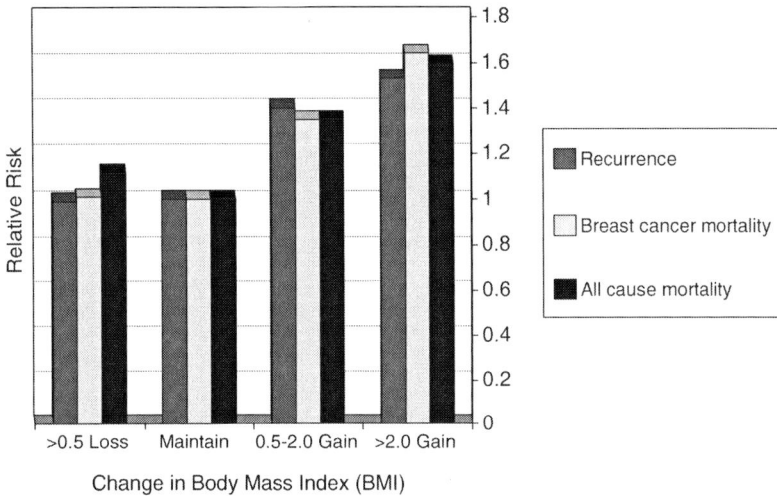

FIGURE 4-4 Outcomes related to weight gain following breast cancer: Results from the Nurses Health Study.
SOURCE: Demark-Wahnefried presentation of information adapted from Kroenke et al., 2005.

Body composition changes that occur during or after treatment also are a concern. Even if cancer survivors are able to maintain their prediagnostic body weight, their body composition often changes, especially during treatment with adjuvant chemotherapy. Figure 4-5 shows changes observed among breast cancer patients who received adjuvant chemotherapy (solid lines) or radiation therapy (dotted lines). The lightly shaded lines show the changes in adipose tissue (in kilograms) from diagnosis to 1 year after diagnosis. The darker lines show changes in lean body mass. Women who received adjuvant chemotherapy had significant increases in fat mass and significant decreases in lean mass, so that even if they were able to maintain weight, they were significantly fatter by the end of the 1-year treatment period. These changes in body composition are equivalent to what would be observed during 10 years of normal aging. This unique form of weight gain, called sarcopenic obesity, has implications for quality of life and metabolically in terms of insulin resistance.

What can the oncologist or primary care provider advise for the patient who come in following treatment with the same prediagnosis body weight, but with complaints that they no longer fit into their clothes and have increased body size? Resistance training is the hallmark treatment for sarcopenic obesity, and recommendation of an exercise program that in-

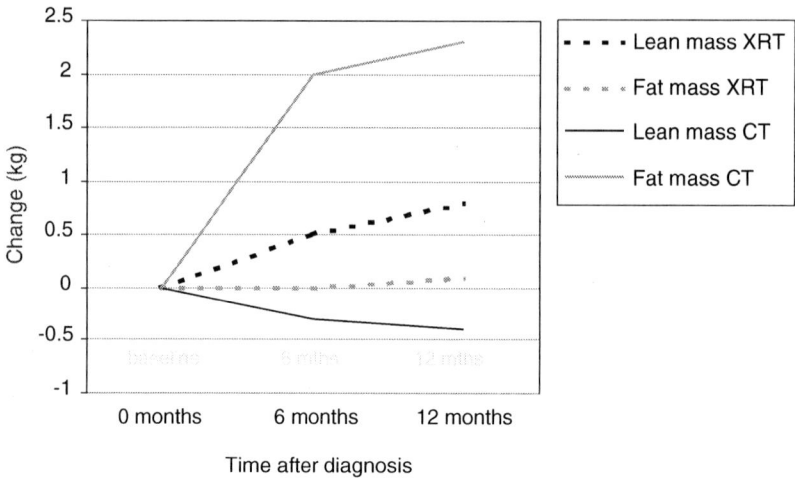

FIGURE 4-5 Body composition changes associated with treatment among women with breast cancer.
NOTE: XRT = x-ray therapy; CT = chemotherapy.
SOURCE: Demark-Wahnefried et al., 2001.

cludes resistance training can be important for regaining lean body mass and resuming previous body habitus.

Figure 4-6 shows the ACS guidelines for weight management. If underweight or at risk for underweight, patients should avoid further weight loss and consider nutritional counseling, physical activity, and the possible use of pharmacologic agents.

Patients of normal weight should try to maintain their weight with exercise and a healthy diet. Overweight or obese patients should be encouraged to lose weight and adhere to guidelines published by the National Heart Lung and Blood Institute (NHLBI). Research is needed to identify weight loss interventions that are effective among cancer survivors.

Nutrition and Diet: ACS guidelines recommend a prudent diet for cancer survivors that includes high proportional intakes of fruits, vegetables, whole grains, and low-fat dairy and lower proportional intakes of meat, refined grains, and high-fat dairy products. This guidance needs to be emphasized, because according to some surveys, fewer than 25 percent of cancer survivors eat at least five servings of fruits and vegetables a day, and fewer than half eat the recommended amounts of saturated fat.

The results of two studies, the Women's Intervention Nutrition Study (WINS) and the Women's Healthy Eating and Living (WHEL) study should

• If underweight or at risk, avoid further weight loss (nutrition counseling, moderate PA & possibly pharmacologic agents)

• If normal weight, strive for weight maintenance (regular aerobic/strength training) & diet focused on nutrient-rich, lower energy density foods & portion control

• If overweight or obese, encourage weight loss – Practical Guide established by NHLBI & NAASO (NIH – Pub 00 -4084)

• More research needed to develop optimal programs of weight loss for cancer survivors

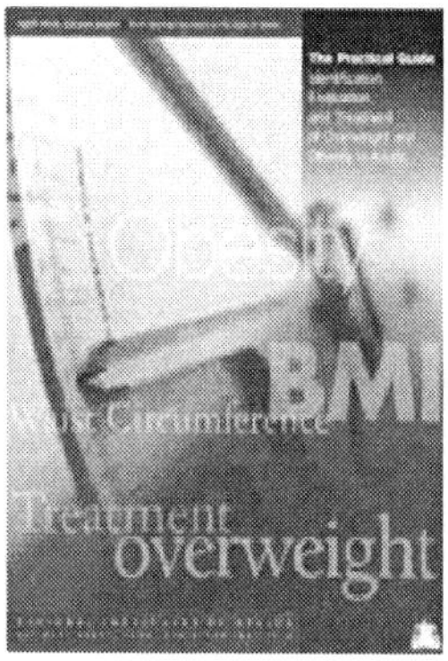

FIGURE 4-6 ACS recommendation for weight management.
NOTE: PA = physical activity; NHLBI = National Heart, Lung, and Blood Institute; NAASO = North American Association for the Study of Obesity.
SOURCE: Demark-Wahnefried, 2006.

provide information to inform future guideline development. WINS is a randomized trial comparing women with postmenopausal breast cancer assigned either to a group asked to adhere to a very low-fat diet (15 percent or less of calories from fat) or a control group that received counseling on a well-balanced diet. Preliminary results of this study suggest a 24-percent risk reduction in recurrence among women in the intervention group compared with the control group, with the greatest reduction among estrogen receptor–negative patients (Figure 4-7).

The WHEL study is currently examining the impact of increased fruit and vegetable consumption and a low-fat diet on breast cancer recurrence and mortality, and results are anticipated in 2008. More research is needed on specific dietary components, for example, soy and flax.

The ACS publication *Nutrition and Physical Activity During and After Cancer Treatment: A Guide for Informed Choices* was first published in 2003, was revised, and was rereleased in fall 2006. In 2004, the AHRQ also published an evidence-based review on physical activity and cancer, *Effectiveness of Behavioral Interventions to Modify Physical Activity Behaviors in General Populations and Cancer Patients and Survivors.*

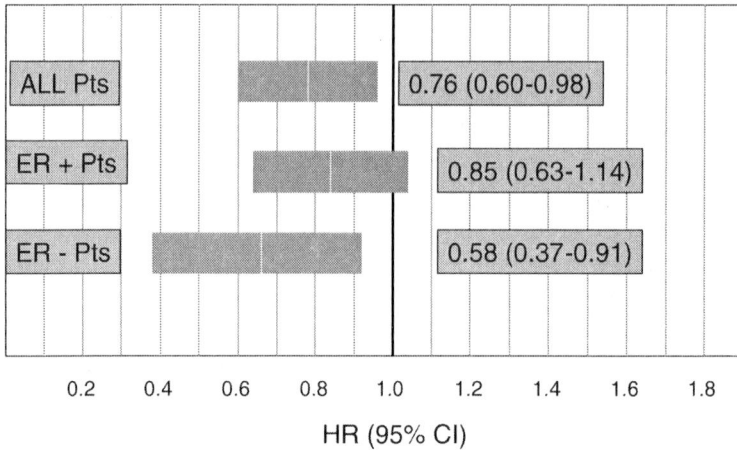

FIGURE 4-7 Preliminary results from the Women's Intervention Nutrition Study on cancer recurrence in postmenopausal women with primary breast cancer (n=2,437).
NOTE: ER = estrogen receptor.
SOURCE: Demark-Wahnefried presentation of information adapted from Chlebowski et al., 2005.

Exercise: Systematic reviews of the literature and consensus reports suggest that exercise is safe for cancer survivors and has consistent positive effects on common symptom management issues, such as vigor, vitality, cardiorespiratory fitness, quality of life, depression, anxiety, and fatigue. A number of groups, including the ACS and the Centers for Disease Control and Prevention (CDC), recommend at least 30 minutes of exercise a day, 5 days a week. There are some patient groups, however, that may need to be evaluated before engaging in this level of exercise. For example, childhood cancer survivors who received anthracycline-based chemotherapy or chest radiation should undergo cardiac screening before starting an exercise regimen.

Data are accumulating to suggest that exercise has a protective effect in terms of cancer recurrence and survival. While data suggest that cancer survivors may exercise somewhat more (9 percent more, according to some surveys) than the general population, most survivors still fail to achieve recommended levels of exercise.

Shown in Figure 4-8 are data on cancer recurrence, breast cancer mortality, and all-cause mortality among a cohort of breast cancer survivors enrolled in the Nurses Health Study according to their levels of physical activity. The sedentary referent group is represented by the far left-hand set of bars. These sedentary women had significantly higher rates of recur-

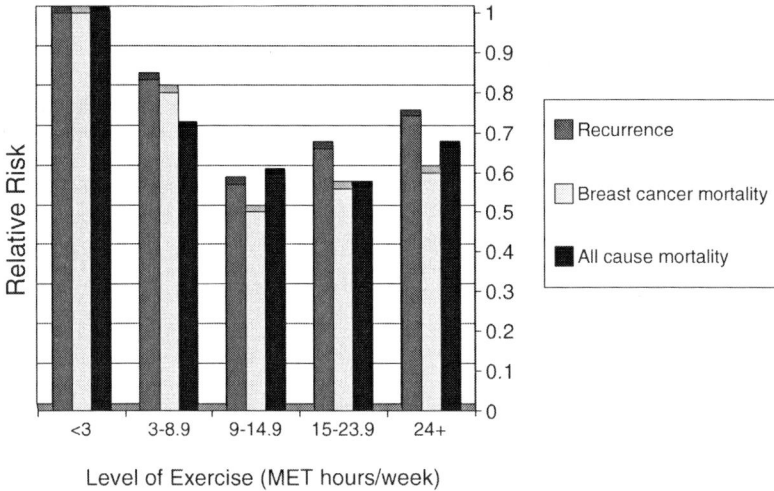

FIGURE 4-8 Exercise and cancer recurrence and mortality: Results from the Nurse's Health Study (n=2,987).
SOURCE: Demark-Wahnefried presentation of information adapted from Holmes et al., 2005.

rence, breast cancer mortality, and all-cause mortality compared with women who had increased physical activity. The cut point of 9 hours per week is similar to the American College of Sports Medicine guidelines, that is, 30 minutes a session, 5 sessions a week. The level of risk reduction observed with exercise in this study is of the same magnitude (or better) than that observed from chemotherapeutic agents. While encouraging, these results must be interpreted with caution, because the data are observational. Randomized intervention studies to evaluate exercise with respect to these outcomes has yet to be conducted.

These promising results are from only one study in breast cancer; however, the *Journal of Clinical Oncology* has recently published two similar studies regarding the association of physical activity and colon cancer outcomes.[13]

---

[13]Meyerhardt JA. et al., 2006. Physical Activity and Survival after Colorectal Cancer Diagnosis. *Journal of Clinical Oncology* 21(22):3527–3534. Meyerhardt JA. et al., 2006. Impact of Physical Activity on Cancer Recurrence and Survival in Patients with Stage III Colon Cancer: Findings from CALGB 89803. *Journal of Clinical Oncology* 24(22):3535–3541.

Smoking: Many cancers are caused by smoking, and persistent tobacco use is associated with complications of treatment, progressive disease, second primary cancers, and increased comorbidity. Smokers diagnosed with smoking-related cancers have relatively high quit rates; however, these smokers often relapse. Clinicians must discuss smoking cessation during the "teachable moments" surrounding diagnosis and treatment and then consistently remind and support patients in sustaining healthy behaviors. The vigilant, long-term follow-up recommended by the U.S. Preventive Services Task Force needs to be applied to cancer survivors. Smokers represent a group in need of attention, because people who smoke often have unhealthy diet and poor exercise habits.

Alcohol Consumption: Alcohol is linked to cancers of the head and neck, kidney and breast. Head and neck cancer survivors who continue to drink have higher treatment-related complications, comorbidity, second primary cancers, and mortality. These patients need to be warned about the risk associated with alcohol consumption and referred to counseling services if necessary.

The prevalence of "risky drinking" (more than 2 drinks a day for men and more than 1 drink a day for women) among most cancer survivors is really no different than that seen in the general population. Higher rates of risky drinking have been noted among survivors of prostate cancer, head and neck cancers, and lung cancer. Moderate alcohol consumption is protective for cardiovascular disease, and the recommendation from the American Cancer Society is that "if you do drink alcohol, do so in moderation."

Bone Health: Bone health is an important survivorship concern because various cancer therapies reduce skeletal integrity (e.g., luteinizing hormone-releasing hormone [LHRH] antagonists, glucocorticoids, select chemotherapeutic agents, radiation therapy). ASCO has published guidelines for breast cancer patients that recommend monitoring bone density and intervening as necessary with pharmacologic agents. For preventive measures, patients should ingest adequate amounts of calcium and vitamin D, undertake weight-bearing exercise, quit smoking, and curb excess consumption of alcohol, protein, caffeine, and sodium. The role of calcium and vitamin D needs further examination because, in the case of prostate cancer, evidence suggests that increased calcium intake may be associated with more aggressive disease.

Protection Against Skin Cancer: Cancer survivors who received X-ray therapy are at higher risk for skin cancer, especially childhood cancer survivors. Thus, skin examinations should be performed routinely. In general, sun protection should be encouraged among cancer survivors. Some controversy has arisen, however, as to the degree of sun protection warranted for survivors of other cancers, given evidence that vitamin D from sun exposure may be protective against some solid tumors and their subsequent progression (e.g., prostate cancer).

Complementary and Alternative Medicine: Complementary and alternative medicine (CAM) includes specific diet and exercise regimens, diet and herbal supplements, acupuncture, massage, and mind-body therapies. No CAM therapies have proven to be beneficial in terms of clinical outcomes; however, some are effective in reducing anxiety (e.g., relaxation therapy). Most cancer survivors use some form of CAM therapy, for example, 60-89 percent of survivors take supplements, and 40-50 percent initiate additional supplements at the time they are diagnosed. Providers need to maintain open communication with their patients regarding CAM, and they should refer patients to reliable sources of information (e.g., the National Center for Complementary and Alternative Medicine). They also should be aware of supplement use with harmful implications (e.g., beta-carotene in smokers and PC-SPES use among men with prostate cancer) so that they can advise their patients accordingly. Additional research is needed to determine the effects of supplements to determine either their potential benefits or adverse events in the survivor population.

In summary, cancer provides a teachable moment for making positive lifestyle changes. Interventions need to be tested to determine how to best capitalize on this opportunity so that healthy behaviors that are initiated are sustained. Oncologists can play a key role in catalyzing behavior change. Primary care providers, nurses, and allied health professionals have key roles to play. Increasingly, Web-based programs, telephone counseling, and mailed interventions may prove to be acceptable and effective in promoting and sustaining lifestyle change. It is very difficult to change lifestyle behaviors, and sustained interventions to ensure long-term adherence are needed.

Cancer survivors are very interested in such lifestyle factors as diet, exercise, and smoking. When asked "How do you like to receive assistance?" survivors report the most interest in interventions that are delivered via the mail, with less interest reported for clinic-based programs, telephone counseling, and computer-based approaches. Recently, however, a telephone-based intervention for smoking cessation in young adults was shown to be highly effective.

A mailed material intervention called Fresh Start has been very successful in changing behaviors of newly diagnosed breast and prostate cancer patients. A new program called RENEW is currently testing a hybrid program of mailed materials (exercise bands, portion-guided tableware and workbooks) and telephone counseling among long-term survivors of breast, prostate and colorectal cancer. Its goal is to facilitate weight loss and diet and exercise behaviors in an effort to improve functional status.

In summary, cancer survivors are at risk for cancer recurrence, comorbidity, functional decline, and decreased survival. Adherence to behavioral health guidelines that have been developed for survivors may help reduce these risks. More research is needed to determine the optimal content, formats, and delivery channels for interventions in these areas. It is clear, however, that sustained lifestyle modification is crucial to achieving optimal health among cancer survivors. Related assessments, education and counseling, and appropriate referrals need to be incorporated into survivorship care planning.

Discussion

Dr. Patricia Ganz questioned whether the education and counseling needed in this area can be accomplished successfully by oncologists. She advised establishing links with primary care physicians, who are providing these interventions for many of their patients. Although it is very important to sensitize the oncology community about these issues, primary care physicians, in following these patients over the long term, will need to be especially vigilant in addressing them. It is critical for the oncologist to say, "This is important," because doctor recommendations are extremely powerful motivators, but at the same time, it is important to somehow establish linkages with other resources.

Dr. Demark-Wahnefried agreed, reinforcing the fact that oncologists play an important role in persuading patients to change their behaviors and in catalyzing appropriate action. If suggestions for behavioral change are made and included in the care plan, primary care physicians will be prompted to raise these issues and to be proactive when it comes to making referrals.

As a primary care provider, Dr. Jean Kutner recommended that oncology providers inform primary care providers of the increased risks facing cancer survivors. Behavioral counseling is very central to what general internists do, especially as preventive health is incorporated into pay for performance initiatives. Primary care providers, however, are unlikely to be familiar with the heightened risks facing cancer survivors.

Dr. Kenneth Schellhase, a family physician from Milwaukee, cautioned that there is no evidence that primary care providers who counsel patients to lose weight are effective. He pointed out that there is actually good evidence that such counseling does not work. Cancer survivors, however, are a motivated group, and so they provide a golden opportunity to test whether, in this context, advice might actually be followed.

PHYSICIAN AND SURVIVOR DECISION SUPPORT USING INFORMATION TECHNOLOGY: THE PASSPORT FOR CARE

Presenters: Dr. David Poplack, Dr. Marc Horowitz, and Dr. Michael Fordis

The Passport for Care is an online national resource for survivors of childhood cancer that is under development by Baylor College of Medicine's Texas Children's Cancer Center and Baylor's Center for Collaborative and Interactive Technologies, in collaboration with the COG through a working group and steering committee.[14]

As discussed throughout this workshop, cancer survivors face the following serious issues:

- Medical late effects;
- Lack of consistent long-term medical follow-up;
- Psychosocial concerns;
- Employment and insurance problems; and
- Discrimination.

Complicating their situation, childhood cancer survivors have frequent changes in health care providers, and they often see primary care physicians who are unfamiliar with survivorship issues. For example, a 28-year-old survivor of Wilm's tumor who received radiation therapy at age 4 and is seeing a primary care provider because he has developed hematuria may not know that this symptom may be associated with his history of cancer treatment. The primary care physician is unlikely to make this connection, especially if the survivor lacks details of his diagnosis and treatment history.

The IOM report identified the need for every survivor to have a Survivorship Care Plan that contains detailed information regarding cancer diagnosis and treatments, recommended follow-up evaluations, preventive practices and health maintenance information, and guidance on available resources related to psychosocial concerns, employment, and health insurance.

The Passport for Care is being developed to provide this care plan information to childhood cancer survivors. It is an Internet-based resource that provides survivors and their physicians or caregivers immediate access to a portable care summary of the survivor's treatment history, individualized guidelines for care, information and links on prevention and healthy lifestyles, alerts to guideline changes and new information on late effects of therapies that the survivor may have received, general news on survivor-

---

[14]For additional information on the Passport For Care, see the background paper prepared by Drs. Poplack, Horowitz, and Fordis in Appendix D.3.

ship, a customized list of national and local resources, provider contact information, and opportunities to participate in research. The passport also provides access to a survivor forum, which allows the survivors to contact others who have had the same disease or who have had similar treatments. There are video stories of individual survivors with the same disease. The Passport for Care is a means of empowering survivors and facilitating their long-term follow-up.

Survivor participation in the Passport for Care will be voluntary and will require consent. One of its most notable features is that the survivor will control the sharing of information, both what is shared and how it is shared. Both the information in the passport and the process of sharing information are secured using encryption technology. The Passport for Care has been designed to be in compliance with requirements of the Health Insurance Portability and Accountability Act (HIPAA).

The Passport for Care will ultimately contain portals for the survivor, the primary care physician, and the pediatric oncology physician following survivors. The portal for pediatric oncology physicians is being developed first in order to meet the needs of providers in the Children's Oncology Group, which treats over 90 percent of the children with cancer in the United States.

The Passport for Care is based on the *Comprehensive Long-term Follow-up Guidelines for Survivors of Childhood, Adolescent, and Young Adult Cancers* that have been developed by COG's nursing discipline and late effects committee. COG members have enthusiastically endorsed broader dissemination and use of the guidelines in helping childhood cancer survivors and other health professionals who provide care to survivors to recognize and manage health risks related to late effects of treatment. However, because of the length of the guidelines and the detail contained in them, clinical utility of the paper-based version of the guidelines on a day-to-day basis in a busy clinical practice is limited. It is precisely for this reason that the Passport for Care, with its ability to generate individualized follow-up recommendations, is anticipated to be attractive to the practicing clinician.

Use of the guidelines is likely to increase when they are accessible through the Passport for Care. It can serve as a clinical guide to the physician in terms of what questions he or she needs to ask the survivor, what the physician should be looking for on the physical examination, what studies need to be done, and how often. Physicians will have access to detailed information embedded with the guidelines, including access to the latest references that relate to any particular recommendation. They will also be able to access links on the COG website that provide detailed information on pediatric cancer and survivorship issues.

It is important to keep in mind that the Passport for Care is not a comprehensive medical record, nor is it intended to be a substitute for an ongoing physician follow-up effort. Workshop participants were shown a brief demonstration of the Passport for Care prototype to illustrate how the passport will be used by survivors and their health care providers.

What is the current status of the Passport for Care? The COG guidelines are now housed in the passport's database and can be easily updated or modified. A consensus has been reached on the elements to be included in the COG care summary, and these elements have been integrated into the passport database. The survivor and primary care portals are being completed, and pilot testing is scheduled for selected COG clinics in early 2007. An evaluation will be conducted to validate the feasibility, utility, and impact of the Passport for Care on the follow-up of long-term survivors.

The passport as envisioned will play an important role in research. It will serve as a way to recruit survivors into studies and will also provide opportunities for educational and outcomes research. In terms of training, continuing medical education credits could be given to those physicians who use it.

What are some of the challenges faced in developing the Passport for Care that are relevant when considering such a tool for survivors of adult cancer? The first and most important prerequisite for such a tool is having evidence-based guidelines and adapting them to online use. A care summary is then needed. A major problem in the development of the Passport for Care has been securing financial support. Most representatives of federal funding agencies, although excited about the passport, do not have funding mechanisms to support the development of these sorts of applied tools. More readily available is funding for research to demonstrate the value of the passport. For its development, support has come from a variety of organizations, including the LAF, Ronald McDonald House Charities, and the Hearst Foundations. What is needed for the long term is a source of support to maintain this type of resource. Possibilities being considered include the development of a survivorship foundation or an endowment that would allow us to maintain and improve this technology over the long term. The Passport for Care represents a paradigm and a model that could potentially be applied to survivors of adult cancer. Adult oncology care differs markedly from pediatric oncology care. Nevertheless, it is likely that the Passport for Care could eventually be adapted for survivors of adult cancers.

Discussion

Dr. Peter Raich of Denver Health Medical Center applauded how the Passport for Care has been designed to meet the needs of survivors while at the same time facilitating entry into clinical trials. Such a system for adults, even using some of the templates under discussion at the workshop, could potentially increase clinical trial enrollment among adults, which now stands at 3 to 5 percent. Dr. Poplack is optimistic that the passport can be adapted for survivors of adult cancer, but he cautioned that "the devil is in the details." In the context of adult cancer, he advised starting with a discrete population of patients, for example, breast cancer survivors. For this group, evidence-based guidelines can be developed and integrated into a passport-like tool that can be tested as a "proof of principle."

Dr. Shapiro congratulated the passport developers for their outstanding work and pointed out that the Passport for Care comprehensively applied principles embodied in the IOM report. He asked how the passport works in practice, for example, "Who inputs data into the system?" Dr. Poplack responded that, in the COG, the care summary information can be entered by oncology physicians, nurse practitioners, or certified research administrators. The physician checks and verifies the information. This aspect of the passport is key, because the underlying algorithms use this information to generate the individualized guidelines. Once the treatment summary information is entered, the rest is automatically generated.

Dr. Poplack reiterated the monumental nature of the guideline development process. While difficult, the process of adapting the guidelines into the standard format required by the passport system has improved the guidelines.

Dr. Ganz asked about interoperability and wondered if oncology providers could download guideline recommendations from the passport system into the physician's own electronic record. Dr. Poplack described how physicians can read or can access and retrieve information electronically and then can use it in their own systems. The passport will be interoperable, and one of the goals will be to have automatic population of the passport with information that is entered into the treatment summary record. The COG has developed a very comprehensive care summary that, once completed, will be linked with the Passport for Care.

REACTION

Dr. Lawrence N. Shulman

As an invited reactant to the presentation given by Dr. Poplack and his colleagues on the Passport for Care, Dr. Shulman credited the pediatric community with leadership in all aspects of survivorship. Examples include not only the Passport for Care effort, but also early adoption of survivorship clinics and an organized system to develop comprehensive guidelines. In his view, incorporating information technology into adult care systems presents some unique challenges. Dr. Shulman shared some of the lessons he has learned over the 15 years he has applied information technology solutions to improving adherence to guidelines and ensuring patient safety.

- Tools to create a Survivorship Care Plan must have a high usability rating by the physicians, nurses, and certified research administrators who are going to be completing it. Without their acceptance, the system will not be adopted.
- Tools must be easily changeable as new information becomes available. Programmers or analysts must be able to enter new information into the system overnight to reflect the latest scientific evidence.
- Decision support should be a component to improve the output and benefit of the tool.
  - In relation to completion of forms: knowing the last bit of data should lead to entry of the next, for example, choosing breast cancer should lead to breast cancer chemotherapy and hormonal regimens and breast radiation options.
  - In relation to delineation of risks and recommendations: selecting certain treatments should preselect risks and follow-up recommendations.
- Development of tools should be iterative: if you try to develop and deploy the perfect system, you will never implement any system. Start simple and develop a system that can grow and improve with experience.
- Tools must be widely available for practicing clinicians in both academic and community settings, for those using and not using electronic medical records. The vast majority of adult patients get their care in community-based programs.
- Tools should have customized output that may be different for patients, referring physicians, and oncology records.
- Tools should be able to use disease- and treatment-specific information as decision supports to develop individualized risk assessments and follow-up care recommendations.
- Tools might incorporate information for which there are different levels of evidence. The level of evidence may be specified.
- Clinicians completing the form should be able to edit statements regarding risks and recommendations on assessments.
- As risk factor and patient-specific information changes, the tool needs to be able to incorporate new data, revising risk assessments and recommendations.
- Tools should supply risk assessments and recommendations around:
  - medical issues specific to individual cancer and treatment history;
  - psychological issues and support; and
  - routine health care, as indicated.

Dr. Shulman presented slides showing a pilot tool being developed at the Dana-Farber Cancer Institute. It represents a simple approach and a place to start in adult survivorship care. The first slide shows the entry of the diagnosis of Hodgkin's lymphoma (Figure 4-9).

Once the diagnosis is entered, the chemotherapy page pulls up the specific chemotherapies that are used for that cancer (Figure 4-10). The provider can check the agents and then enter the total doses.

The radiation page profiles what the Hodgkin's lymphoma patient is likely to have gotten, and the provider specifies the doses and the dates (Figure 4-11).

The information provided on chemotherapy and radiation therapy is summarized on a treatment summary page (Figure 4-12).

An assessment/problem list is then generated based on the patient's age, sex, and treatments (Figure 4-13). The provider can then go down the list and check risks—for example, in this case, azoospermia, cardiomyopathy, coronary artery disease, depression and anxiety, and risk of second cancers. The provider can indicate that the patient's risk has been ruled out or that the patient has the listed problem.

Once the provider has identified the pertinent risk factors, information and recommendations can be generated in a bulleted format (the information shown in the figure is in draft form and is shown only to illustrate how the system might work) (Figure 4-14).

A patient summary can be generated and printed. This draft example is written in patient-friendly language and is called an oncology long-term follow-up summary (Figure 4-15). It instructs the survivor to share the summary the doctors and to keep it in their personal files.

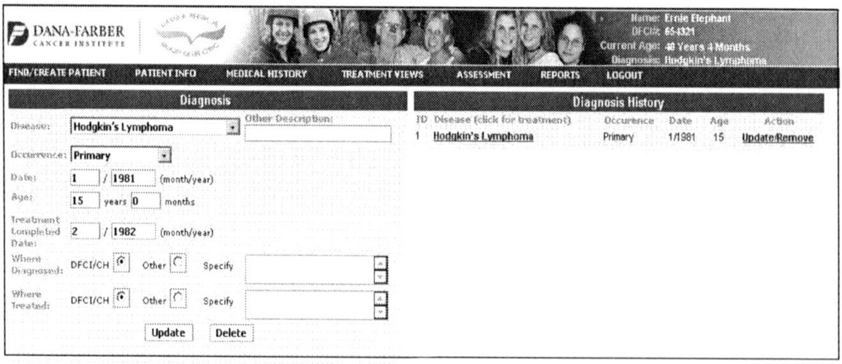

FIGURE 4-9 Diagnosis entry.
SOURCE: Shulman, 2006.

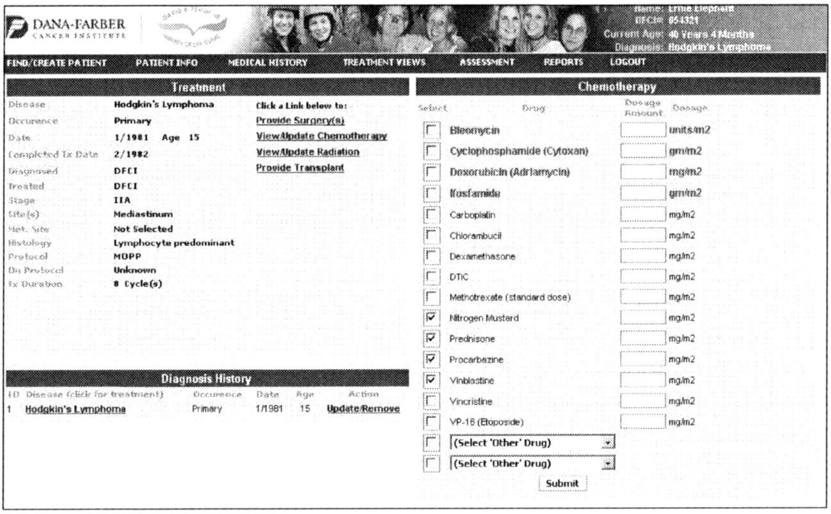

FIGURE 4-10 Chemotherapy entry.
SOURCE: Shulman, 2006.

A summary suitable for distribution to the primary care provider can also be generated (Figure 4-16).

Dr. Shulman raised several questions for the workshop participants to consider regarding implementation:

• Will physicians and nurses want to use such a tool? Will its potential value make them feel that its use is worthwhile? Will peer pressure motivate its use?

• Could the treatment summary become the equivalent of a clinic note or admission note and be considered a part of normal practice?

• Could the treatment summary be required by regulatory agencies such as the Joint Commission on the Accreditation of Healthcare Organizations?

• Could the use of this tool be tied to pay for performance and reimbursement to improve the quality and rationality of follow-up care? Payers and insurers want well-codified care plans.

• Could patients help push this as an expectation of their care?

Dr. Shulman described mechanisms to encourage the development of information technology that will facilitate survivorship care. A centralized,

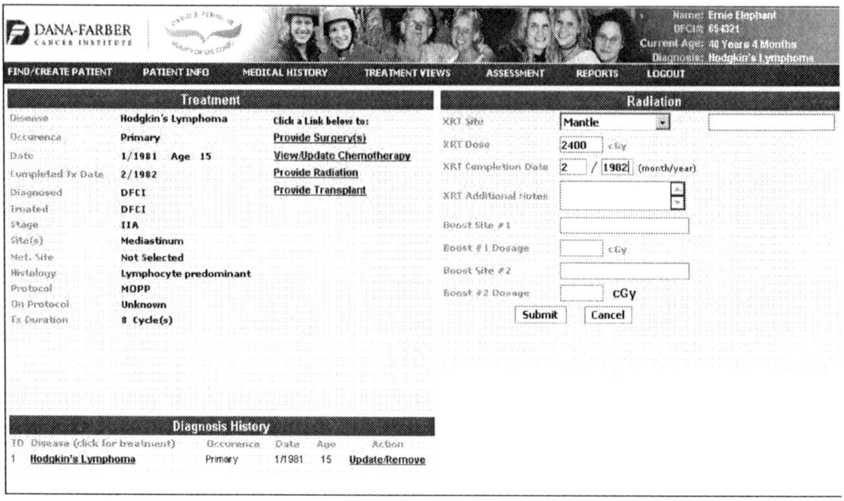

FIGURE 4-11 Radiation entry.
SOURCE: Shulman, 2006.

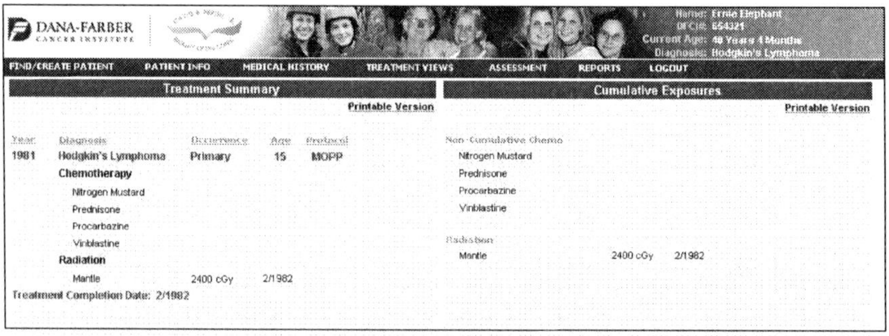

FIGURE 4-12 Treatment summary.
SOURCE: Shulman, 2006.

national effort, similar to the COG guideline development project, is needed in adult oncology. Teams will need to be assembled by cancer type to achieve consensus on the content of the care plan—for example, the chemotherapy and radiation therapy regimens that need to be included, the risks for late effects, and recommended follow-up. This collaborative effort might be similar to the NCCN's efforts to develop guidelines. There is a need to start simply but on a platform that will facilitate enhancements with time.

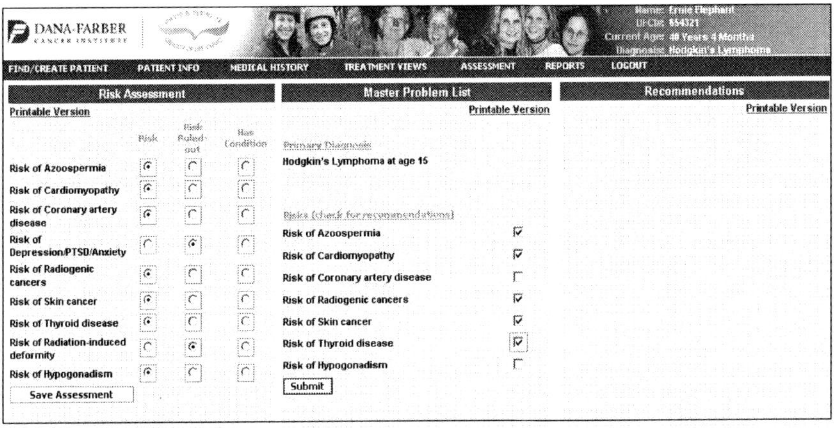

FIGURE 4-13 Assessment/problem list.
SOURCE: Shulman, 2006.

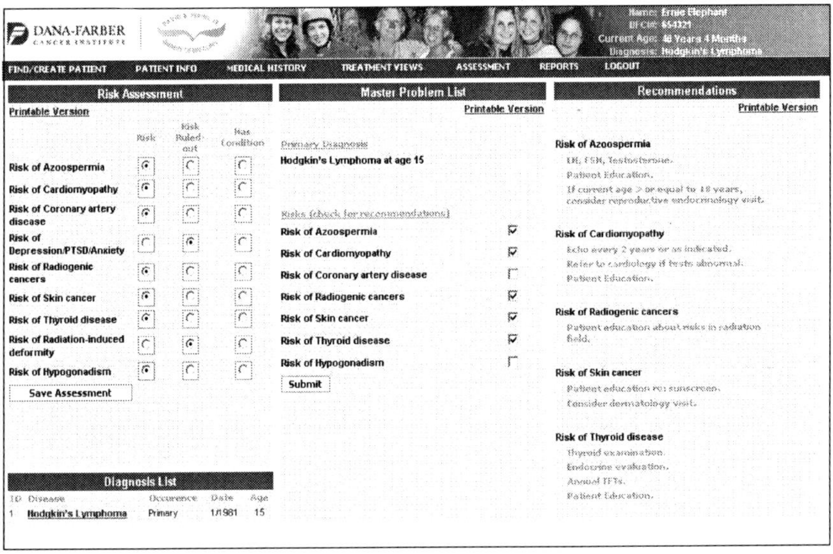

FIGURE 4-14 Recommendations.
SOURCE: Shulman, 2006.

DANA-FARBER CANCER INSTITUTE

Summary: Disease Treatment and Follow-Up
Medical Record Number: DFCI 654321

Ernie Elephant

This is your pediatric oncology long-term follow-up summary which should be shared your doctor(s) and kept in your personal files.

Diagnosis: Hodgkin's Disease
Date of Diagnosis: 1/1981 **Age at Diagnosis:** 15

Treatment Summary:

1. **Surgery:** None
2. **Radiation Therapy:** Mantle (2400 gCy)
3. **Chemotherapy:** Nitrogen Mustard; Prednisone; Procarbazine; Vinblastine
4. **Transplant:** None

There are specific risks and recommendations for your medical follow-up based on your disease and the treatments that you received.

Risk of thyroid problems: The therapy you received increases your risk of developing thyroid problems. It is recommended that you annually have blood tests called Thyroid Function Tests (TFTs) and you have a physical examination of your thyroid gland.

Risk of skin cancer: The radiation you received to treat your Hodgkin's Disease increases your risk of developing secondary skin cancer in the treatment field. Our recommendation would include a regular yearly dermatology screening. It is also important to limit the amount of unprotected sun exposure you receive. Using sunscreen with an SPF of 15 or greater on any exposed skin anytime you are outdoors would also be recommended.

Risk of cardiac complications: The radiation and chemotherapy that you received can cause complications with your heart vessels and valves. We recommend that you get a baseline echocardiogram and a "stress echo" at age 35. We recommend being followed by a cardiologist if there are any abnormalities in your cardiac tests.

Risk of low sperm count: Chemotherapy can cause damage to sperm producing cells. You can have testing of sperm count (a semen analysis), if there are abnormalities, you can meet with a reproduction specialist to learn about your options for reproduction. If your sperm count is found to be normal, you are at very low risk of this becoming a problem later.

FIGURE 4-15 Patient treatment summary.
SOURCE: Shulman presentation, 2006.

A central organization needs to be established to assume this task. It will need an administrative arm, clinical teams, and an information technology group that manages the development of the tool. Funding will have to support this effort—including the development, implementation, maintenance, and evaluation costs.

REGIONAL APPROACHES TO CANCER SURVIVORSHIP PLANNING

Presenter: Dr. Tim Byers

As clinicians become engaged in survivorship care planning and as tools are developed to aid them, it is important to be thinking about the role of organizations and institutional systems at the state, regional, and local

DANA-FARBER CANCER INSTITUTE

Summary: Disease Treatment and Follow-Up
Medical Record Number: DFCI 654321

Primary care provider summary and recommendations

Name: Ernie Elephant **DOB**: 1/1/1966 **Current Age**: 40

Diagnosis: Hodgkin's Disease
Date of Diagnosis: 1/1981 **Age at Diagnosis:** 15

Treatment Summary:
1. **Surgery:** None
2. **Radiation Therapy:** Mantle (2400 gCy)
3. **Chemotherapy:** Nitrogen Mustard; Prednisone; Procarbazine; Vinblastine
4. **Transplant:** None

Risks and recommendations based upon exposures:

Potential Radiation-Associated Thyroid Problems: Thyroid examination, endocrine evaluation and annual Thyroid Function Tests (TFTs) to rule out nodules, hypo and hyperthyroidism which have been observed in survivors of mantle radiation.

Risk of Skin Cancer after Radiation: Dermatology evaluation. Patient education about sun exposure and sunscreen use.

Risk of Radiation-induced cardiac disease: Echo at baseline with referral to cardiologist if any abnormalities are noted. Stress echo at age 30. Aggressive management of other cardiac risk factors given the observed increased risk of coronary artery disease seen in survivors of mantle radiation.

Risk of azoospermia: Suggest semen analysis. LH/FSH elevations or abnormal testicular exam may suggest oligo or azoospermia without semen analysis results available. Sex hormone production likely to be preserved, but testosterone levels may be helpful.

FIGURE 4-16 Primary care provider (PCP) summary.
SOURCE: Shulman, 2006.

levels.[15] These could be involved in both responding to and perhaps motivating national opportunities. A recent example of this interplay between local and national opportunities is the decision by the companies making Coca-Cola and Pepsi-Cola to remove high-calorie carbonated beverages from U.S. schools. This national solution was reached because of activities at the local level. It became clear to drink manufacturers that they were going to lose their access to schools city by city, and so a number of bottom-up efforts created a top-down solution. Both kinds of solutions will be necessary to improve U.S. cancer survivorship care. There are going to be national efforts, but also some state, regional, and local ideas and demonstration projects that will emerge.

---

[15]For additional information on regional approaches to cancer survivorship planning, see the background paper prepared by Dr. Byers in Appendix D.4.

State-level cancer control efforts are beginning to focus on cancer survivorship. Across the country there are 44 states with comprehensive cancer control plans. The CDC has a strategy to capitalize on their state-based investments in epidemiologic surveillance, tobacco control, and breast and cervical cancer screening. They are providing support to states to help them coordinate these varied efforts into cohesive and comprehensive cancer control programs.

States have received assistance for planning, but they now face the challenge of implementing their plans with limited support. Most have specified that they want to cut cancer death rates, decrease smoking, address the problems of obesity and physical inactivity, and increase screening for cervical and breast cancer. Without the necessary federal support, the 44 states that are implementing their plans are trying to identify new sources of support and partners. In response to a question that Dr. Byers posed to the audience about involvement with state plans, about 10 percent of the workshop participants indicated that they were well engaged with their state's cancer control program, two-thirds indicated that they were unfamiliar with their state's plan, and the balance fell somewhere in between.

Dr. Byers introduced Dr. Loria Pollack, a medical officer at CDC, and asked her about its vision for state cancer programs over the next 5 years. Dr. Pollack indicated that CDC sees itself as providing an impetus, guidance, and expertise to states as they design their own plans. CDC does not want to dictate how states create their plans or what goes into them. CDC has provided guidance to address the entire continuum along the cancer trajectory, from prevention and early detection to palliative and end-of-life care. The budget for comprehensive cancer control planning has gone up, but more and more states, tribes, and territories are getting this support.

CDC encourages states to create coalitions of clinicians, public health departments, businesses, and advocacy organizations. The comprehensive cancer control plan is an impetus to bring these divergent groups together. CDC expects the partners to also provide some funding. In Georgia, tobacco settlement money has gone into the planning efforts. In Connecticut, $6 million has been directed to cancer planning from the state budget, the hospital fund, and other sources. CDC takes a background role as these coalitions take ownership of the cancer control plan to serve their own communities.

Dr. Byers noted the existence of a wide gap between public health and clinical care in the United States, resulting in some state coalitions lacking the necessary clinical partners. Most of the systems involved in care for cancer patients are not represented in the cancer coalitions. Creative ways to engage clinicians are needed. The cancer plans, in order to be considered comprehensive, need to diversify to include clinical perspectives. A content analysis of the 44 state plans shows that tobacco control, epidemiologic surveillance, and cancer screening goals are all well represented. There is very little coverage of clinical issues.

There is an enormous opportunity to use the state cancer planning groups and the state cancer coalitions to move survivorship care planning forward into demonstration projects. Every one of the 44 state cancer plans mentions cancer survivorship as an important issue. Most of these plans mention survivorship only briefly. There are at least two states, Oregon and Minnesota, that have some focus on cancer survivorship planning. All of the states recognize that they need to do more to address the needs of cancer survivors, and they are looking for something specific to do. Including survivorship care issues in the state plans may engage some of the clinical partners who have not yet come to the table, especially if they can participate in a specific demonstration project. Survivorship as a public health issue is something that both NCI and CDC have been talking about, and the LAF is now joining with both of those organizations to try to move this forward.

There are opportunities in the short term to have demonstration projects in partnership with public health agencies and some of the NCI-supported cancer centers. There are 39 comprehensive cancer centers around the United States whose primary mission is cancer research. Each one of them has an unfunded mandate to earn that adjective "comprehensive" in its name and provide community service through education and outreach.

In the short term, NCI-designated comprehensive cancer centers, CCOPs, and other cancer care systems could take a look at their clinical trials and examine the opportunities to answer questions related to cancer survivorship. Dr. Raich, asked to comment on this suggestion, pointed out that few adult cancer patients participate in clinical trials and that relatively few trials have been designed with survivorship issues in mind. Nevertheless, these programs could provide excellent settings for doing pilot studies in cancer survivorship care planning. The big obstacle is funding such demonstration projects. CCOPs can receive "cancer control credits" for conducting this kind of research, and this may represent a small motivator for them to get involved.

Dr. Byers mentioned that many patients leaving clinical trials are not given a Survivorship Care Plan at the conclusion of their treatment, and they probably should have such a plan. This could be a good place to pilot test paper- or Web-based versions that have been discussed. Cancer centers are supposed to be innovative and cutting edge, and the treatment provided as part of any trial is very well defined. This and the fact that quality-of-life outcomes are often measured as part of trials would seem to make this an ideal place to start.

Other opportunities for demonstration programs at the state or regional level may be through the Centers for Medicare and Medicaid Services' (CMS) quality improvement organizations (QIOs). QIOs may examine claims data to identify problems and work in concert with providers to improve care. Some cancer quality programs have been undertaken, but most of the successful efforts have been in the area of cardiovascular disease and diabetes management. A QIO-run demonstration project would be very natural because they already work closely with providers to monitor and evaluate care. A joint project could be undertaken by two or three of them around the country. If the demonstration project were successful, both operationally and in terms of improved outcomes, then it would be expected to become a standard of care. Once a program was established in Medicare, other payers would be likely to come on board.

Sometimes local health care systems can have an enormous impact. For example, if the Mayo Clinic adopts a new policy, then southern Minnesota is affected as a region. When the Marshfield Clinic moves ahead with a new program, then central Wisconsin is affected as a region. This is also the case with large managed care programs such as Kaiser Permanente.

In summary, in terms of the various organizations that can affect state and regional approaches to survivorship care planning, state public health departments have a key role to play. They are the conveners of the state-level cancer control programs. The state public health agencies will have to learn how to accommodate multisectorial involvement, especially private-sector involvement and leadership in improving the cancer situation in states. State health agencies must be active partners in the process, but they will need to step aside to let others move the process forward. Comprehensive cancer centers have an important role to play, but they will need to avoid ivory tower approaches and design demonstrations projects that have a business model for the private sector so that they can be sustainable. QIOs have statewide reach. They are generally not active partners in state cancer programs, but there is an immediate opportunity for CMS to conduct demonstration projects and affect state-level practice along these lines. Health professional societies tend to be more national than local, but in some areas there are some active local health professional societies that might come to bear on this.

To move the agenda forward, cancer survivorship planning should be a key element in every state comprehensive cancer control plan. Inclusion in the plan does not ensure its implementation. However, if there are actionable items in the plans, and if there is interest in the community, then putting some specific goals and objectives into plans for cancer survivorship care planning could be very helpful.

Should the plan say that, statewide, by the year 2010 everybody is going to have a care plan? That might be a long-term vision, but the most useful action item for the next 2 to 3 years would be to conduct some demonstration projects, evaluate them, publicize the results, and then move toward standardizing the practice. It may be the case that the imperative for care planning will be established nationally in the next two to three years, but it is also likely that local initiatives will be needed to motivate change at the national level. As demonstrations are proceeding, business models must be developed to sustain survivorship care planning.

Dr. Demark-Wahnefried suggested that for states to take an active role, CDC will have to encourage demonstration projects on survivorship. Dr. Pollack said that while CDC is very interested in this area, they have no dedicated funds for survivorship projects.

Dr. Byers pointed out that CDC does not have the resources for 98 percent of the items that are in cancer plans. This is why diversification is necessary. Dedicated tobacco tax revenues, the private sector, and nongovernmental organizations can be mobilized to support the implementation of these plans.

Dr. William Kraybill identified another potential partner in state or regional cancer control, the American College of Surgeons' Commission on Cancer (ACS-COC). Most large and small cancer programs around the country are organized in a multidisciplinary fashion and abide by a set of standards promulgated by the ACS-COC. They are partially funded by the American Cancer Society and are likely to be enthusiastic about moving survivorship forward. Dr. Byers agreed and suggested that the combination of the American Cancer Society, the ACS-COC, and the state tumor registries represent a potentially powerful triad that has not been fully taken advantage of.

Dr. James Talcott characterized survivorship as crosscutting and mentioned organizational barriers that make it difficult to cut across disease entities. Academic medicine is often organized by disease, and often, one must duplicate effort for breast cancer, prostate cancer, lymphoma, and every other oncology subspecialty. It is sometimes hard to engage in activities that cut across diagnoses. There are almost no opportunities for researchers to work with other investigators who are doing the same thing "one disease over."

Finally, Dr. Byers discussed how the traditional public health role of surveillance could be enhanced to further survivorship care planning. Perhaps methods could be devised to routinely monitor outcomes of confusion, anxiety, fatigue, dissatisfaction with care, and poor quality care. Survivorship-related quality-of-care measures could include those related to poor transitions in care or underuse of tamoxifen among women with breast cancer who were prescribed the medication. Cancer registries could be monitoring outcomes after cancer apart from death and (in some) recurrence. Demonstration projects on enhanced cancer registration to capture some of these data elements could be considered. Extending cancer registration into these areas on a fairly routine basis would help to shine a light on the problem.

In summary, Dr. Byers reiterated the value of working with state cancer programs to build survivorship issues into the comprehensive cancer control plans. This planning effort should be moved out of public health agencies, so that public health is a partner but not a convener of these plans. Extending the public health function of surveillance to include cancer outcomes that are common and important to cancer survivors should be considered and tested. Demonstration projects could be initiated soon to begin to test these ideas and processes and to move them forward.

5

Pilot Tests and Assessment
of Their Impact

INTRODUCTION

Moderator: Dr. Julia Rowland

This session of the workshop addresses pilot tests of survivorship care planning and efforts under way to assess their impact. Craig Earle describes the LIVESTRONG™ Survivorship Center of Excellence Network, which is supported by the Lance Armstrong Foundation. The role that the American Society of Clinical Oncology's Quality Oncology Practice Initiative (QOPI) could potentially play to improve survivorship care is then discussed by Patricia Ganz. Martin Brown illustrates the potential for research networks to promote applied survivorship research with the success of the National Cancer Institute's HMO Cancer Research Network in carrying out cancer-related health services research. Peter Bach then describes the Centers for Medicare and Medicaid Services' (CMS) 2006 Oncology Demonstration Program as an effort to learn more about the status and quality of contemporary cancer care. Lastly, Craig Earle returns to present a comprehensive evaluation and research agenda for survivorship research.

LIVESTRONG™ SURVIVORSHIP
CENTER OF EXCELLENCE NETWORK

Presenter: Dr. Craig Earle

The Lance Armstrong Foundation (LAF) plans to accelerate progress in addressing the complex needs of the rapidly growing number of cancer survivors through a collaborative network established to meet the following goals:

- Transform how survivors are perceived, treated, and served;
- Help create a body of knowledge, understanding, and evidence;
- Develop and deliver evidence-based treatment and care interventions;
- Increase the quality and integration of survivorship services;
- Strengthen linkages between survivorship services and primary cancer treatment and care;
- Increase accessibility to services among ethnically diverse and underserved survivors;
- Create insurance and reimbursement mechanisms to cover survivors' care and services; and
- Help find sources of support to sustain survivorship centers over the long term.

In establishing these goals, the LAF recognized the complexity of survivorship care, the relative lack of experience with long-term survivorship care, and the lack of training available for providers of survivorship care.

Centers of excellence have been established in five locations: (1) Memorial Sloan-Kettering Cancer Center in New York City; (2) Dana-Farber Cancer Institute in Boston; (3) Fred Hutchinson Cancer Research Center in Seattle; (4) the University of Colorado in Denver; and (5) the Jonsson Comprehensive Cancer Center at the University of California, Los Angeles. These centers will be involved in the following activities:

- Collaborative clinical, biomedical, psychosocial, and health services research;
- Accessible, relevant, and integrated quality care and services;
- Development and testing of new medical, psychosocial, and behavioral interventions;
- Dissemination and delivery of new information, interventions, and best practices to those in need; and
- Training the next generation of health care professionals, social service providers, and researchers.

Each center of excellence will develop its own network of community-based centers, which will provide direct services locally to survivors in traditionally underserved areas. Figure 5-1 shows the interactions among the LAF, the centers of excellence, and their affiliated network of community-based centers.

The LAF invited selected cancer centers to respond to a "closed" request for proposals (RFP). The following additional four cancer programs

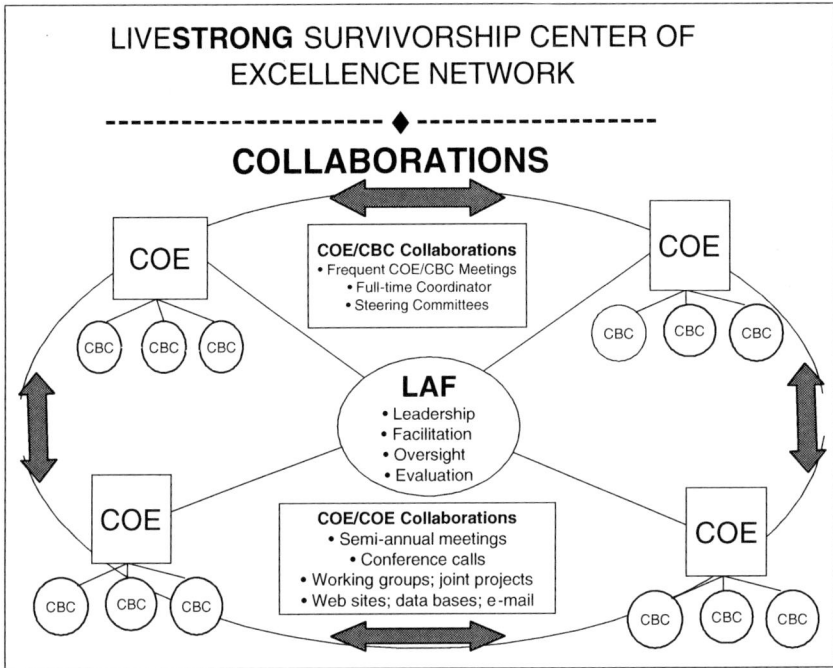

FIGURE 5-1 Interactions among participants in the Lance Armstrong Foundation Center of Excellence Network.
SOURCE: Earle, 2006.

are not officially part of the network but have received support to develop their survivorship programs:

- Cook Children's Medical Center in Fort Worth, Texas;
- University of Pennsylvania in Philadelphia;
- Nevada Cancer Institute in Las Vegas; and
- Rainbow Babies and Children's Hospital in Cleveland, Ohio.

The plan is to harness the expertise, experience, creativity, and productivity of the leading centers and have them share their knowledge and resources to improve the delivery of services to survivors. This collaboration is expected to accelerate the progress in cancer survivorship. The development of a standardized Survivorship Care Plan is one of the priorities of the network. The centers have a coordinated development plan under way to pilot test templates at the centers of excellence and their community-based partners. This program will serve as a large laboratory to promote quality cancer survivorship care.

Discussion

Dr. David Poplack of Texas Children's Cancer Center asked Dr. Earle about planned initiatives in the area of education and training, pointing out that awareness of survivorship issues and care is absent from most contemporary programs. In fact, it is possible for a pediatrician to go through training and never rotate through a hematology or oncology unit. Dr. Shulman of the Dana-Farber Cancer Institute confirmed that at his institution the house staff are spending less and less time in cancer medicine and are spending almost no time in the ambulatory setting, which is where survivors are seen. There is a training system in place that will graduate a group of primary care doctors who have essentially no experience in this area.

Dr. Earle acknowledged the importance of training, adding that physicians need not become experts in oncology, but they need at least to recognize what the potential issues are when dealing with a cancer survivor and have some idea of what to do and whom to refer to. The Dana-Farber Center of Excellence is affiliated with a rural oncology practice in New Hampshire and is collaborating with an urban community health center and centers in New England that deliver pediatric cancer care. Specialists in the center will be working with community-based primary care physicians, pediatricians, and pediatric oncologists to raise awareness of survivorship issues and how to address them.

Dr. Lee Newcomer of the UnitedHealth Group asked Dr. Earle to describe how the Centers of Excellence would know if they were successful in 3 years and how they planned to measure the achievement of success. The centers have been measuring patient satisfaction and acceptance as well as knowledge gained following interactions with the clinic. Dr. Earle recognized the importance of looking at some other outcomes, such as anxiety, and those relating to the coordination of the transition out of cancer therapy. Dr. Lawrence Shulman suggested that the measure of the network's success will be the pace of accomplishment and the creation of collaborative efforts. Ms. Mary McCabe added that, in terms of outcomes or metrics for success, the collaborators from Memorial Sloan-Kettering decided to start with two very simple but realistic aspects of the program, feasibility and acceptability. The program changes the paradigm of care and extends it to include the survivorship period. Important questions are, "Can this be done in a cancer center?" and "Is it acceptable to the patients, the physicians, the nurses, and the referring primary care providers?" A survey will be conducted of these stakeholders to assess reactions to the program. Another metric to be used is adequacy of screening among cancer survivors followed in the institution.

In response to a question about future solicitations and participation in the LAF effort, Ms. Caroline Huffman said that a steering committee is providing guidance and that, at this point, LAF plans to keep the closed RFP model. The Centers of Excellence Network is viewed as bold and filled with tremendous possibilities, but the immediate plans are to concentrate on getting the network launched and initiating the ambitious collaborative projects.

When questioned about educational materials used in the centers of excellence clinics, Dr. Earle reported that, although they were not using the Lance Armstrong LIVE**STRONG**™ notebook, they are incorporating all of its elements in structured letters to patients that include the treatment plan, the treatment summary, and the survivorship care plan. Structured consultation notes are sent to the primary care providers and the oncologists involved. Mr. Richard Boyajian added that the team at the Dana-Farber Cancer Institute is involved with BlueCross and BlueShield in the development and evaluation of a transition notebook for use among breast cancer survivors.

Clinics in this network will be working toward developing and testing a single template, rather than having each of the centers developing its own. An attempt is being made to satisfy both the academic and community-based providers.

Ms. Kathy Smolinski, representing the Association of Oncology Social Work, asked whether there are staffing standards for the centers of excellence. Dr. Earle responded that there were no standards, and that each center has developed staffing levels for its own setting. The program started with limited evidence and experience at hand. A tremendous amount has been learned in the past year and a half, as the clinic has taken on this relatively new area of survivorship care. Ms. McCabe, from the Memorial Sloan-Kettering Center of Excellence, added that while each of the centers has taken an institutional approach to what might work, the barriers and the goals for each of the centers are the same. This common purpose is behind the collaboration on specific tasks, such as the care plan and adherence to screening. There are some important areas in which there is agreement, but at the same time there is a realization that one size does not fit all. Dr. Earle mentioned that the issue of acceptability of survivorship clinics among oncology physicians is a critical one. Some physicians are very threatened by the idea of a specialized survivorship clinic, worrying that they will lose their patients if such a program is available.

Dr. Patricia Ganz of the University of California, Los Angeles described the diversity represented in the five centers of excellence. Three are free-standing cancer centers, and two are state-funded university programs. All are comprehensive cancer centers, but they vary in their level of resources. The kinds of models that each center develops will reflect this diversity and that which exists in the various community-based partners. Oncology care delivered in America varies greatly by geography and setting, and different models of excellence are likely to emerge to suit specific environments.

QUALITY ONCOLOGY PRACTICE INITIATIVE

Presenter: Dr. Patricia Ganz

Several years ago, as the American Society of Clinical Oncology (ASCO) embarked on the National Initiative on Cancer Care Quality (NICCQ), it became very apparent to the highly skilled health services researchers who were running that project how arduous it was to collect oncology data from medical chart reviews. The study involved reviews of 1,600 patients in multiple cities. Unlike other data collection efforts related to diabetes, arthritis, and heart disease, the review of oncology care was complicated by records being in multiple places, completed by different kinds of providers, and organized in a nonstandard fashion. The record abstractors felt lucky if the record included an initial consultation note that might have spelled out the planned treatment or a flow sheet that captured the course of treatment received. Often, however, a nurse abstractor had the arduous task of going through every page of the record to find out what drug doses were delivered and if a doctor followed the recommended prescription for the adjuvant therapy.

It became clear to ASCO that if the professional society was going to advance quality-of-care assessment, there needed to be a better way of getting this kind of data in a systematic way. With the publication of the Institute of Medicine (IOM) report on cancer survivorship, it became clear that survivorship care planning depends on having accurate and accessible diagnostic and treatment information.

Dr. Deborah Schrag discussed in her presentation the steps that have been taken to establish the content for the treatment summary (see Chapter 2). To test the draft template, five oncologists involved in ASCO's QOPI volunteered to try it in their group practices. Two versions were tested in practices, most of which did not have an electronic medical record; a paper-and-pencil and a dictatable form. Both formats seemed relatively easy to use. The dictated form obtained more information because physicians may have felt obligated to go back through the chart and dictate it as they would a discharge summary. The paper version was completed more quickly than the dictated form.

Disease-specific formats are undergoing development to be tested further within the QOPI network because there are common regimens for treatment that can be prefilled, making completion of the form easier. For hematologic cancers, it may be difficult to decide when a patient needs an end-of-treatment summary, since for many of those individuals the disease may be chronic in nature.

Based on this pilot work, it is clear that more work is needed on the treatment summary. Physicians pilot testing the form felt strongly that it needs to be brief. The form needs to synthesize succinctly what went on without summarizing the entire chart. That said, some medical oncologists have indicated that they want the information to be comprehensive and complete so that the form could meet other recordkeeping requirements. It will be critical to communicate the purpose and intent of the treatment summary so that the appropriate elements are included on the standardized template.

In terms of next steps, plans are to revise the forms and then broaden the participation into more QOPI practices. The development process will be iterative and will involve getting buy-in from all users. Physician and nurse buy-in is a prerequisite to success. Ultimately, the design of the template has to be adapted for electronic medical records. ASCO is actively pursuing development of an oncology electronic record because those that are available for primary care physicians are not well suited for oncology.

Dr. Rowland commented on the strictly medical content of the draft templates and wondered what would happen if one added a psychosocial component. Dr. Ganz responded by pointing out that the template is meant to be a conversation piece. Like the informed consent form, it is not just signing the document that is important. Transfer of information depends on the verbal communication, the other supplementary materials given to the patient, and then the reiteration of the information at every visit. Even though the form is short, the piece of paper should be associated with a very lengthy conversation, and it is something that the patient takes away. These tools can serve as a catalyst for these in-depth conversations. The written records are especially important, because patients do not always have access to their medical records and may need them in the case of natural disasters or doctors closing their practices. Having a concise synoptic statement of what went on can go a long way to facilitate the conduct of conversations.

Some doctors are better at engaging in these conversations than others. Perhaps survivors can be encouraged and activated to ask at the end of treatment "Well, how am I going to be followed now? How are you going to know if my cancer is coming back?" When these questions arise, physicians will at least have a document with the medical aspects of care spelled out. We hope it is going to be backed up in many practices with the resource information that Ms. Diane Blum described in her presentation (see Chapter 4). Physicians, as part of their posttreatment conversation should be ready to say, "By the way, I know this is a very stressful period; would you want to talk to the social worker who works with me or the support group that I think would be helpful to you?" Setting time aside to have a conversation is what the Survivorship Care Plan template will facilitate. It is a starting point, and there is agreement that we have to get started.

Dr. Michael Fordis of Baylor College of Medicine mentioned the possibility of granting credit for continuing medical education (CME) as an incentive for using the Survivorship Care Plan template. Some CME credits are being granted to individuals who are participating in quality improvement initiatives. Maintenance of certification was mentioned as another potential incentive, but the experience nationally is that relatively few providers participate in quality programs in response to this incentive. Dr. Ganz pointed out that there is a large group of physicians who completed their training more than 10 years ago and who are now required to do something for their American Board of Internal Medicine recertification. This may provide an impetus for some to participate in the QOPI project. The initial cohort of QOPI participants was motivated by competition and an interest in peer evaluation. Once there is agreement on the treatment summary, its completion could be considered for inclusion in the QOPI quality measure set. This may occur in the next 2 to 3 years. ASCO is discussing with the National Committee for Quality Assurance (NCQA) the potential for a physician certification program in oncology, which could be based on the QOPI initiative.

Dr. Al Marcus of the AMC Cancer Research Center agreed with the need for treatment summaries and care plans as recommended in the IOM report and elsewhere. He pointed out that pilot tests are under way to assess usability and feasibility, but in the long term he thought that these care plans must be evaluated for their effects on important survivorship outcomes. Such evidence will be needed to persuade payers and others that survivorship care planning is an essential component of care.

THE HMO CANCER RESEARCH NETWORK

Presenter: Dr. Martin Brown

The Cancer Research Network (CRN) is a cooperative agreement supported by the National Cancer Institute. It consists of research organizations affiliated with 12 large nonprofit health maintenance organizations in the United States, including:

- Six Kaiser Permanente affiliates (Southern California, Northern California, Oregon, Hawaii, Georgia, and Colorado);
- Group Health Cooperative, Seattle, Washington;
- Lovelace Sandia Health Clinic, Albuquerque, New Mexico;
- Henry Ford Health System, Detroit, Michigan;

- Health Partners, Minneapolis, Minnesota;
- Harvard Pilgrim Health Care, Boston, Massachusetts;
- Meyers Primary Care Institute, Worcester, Massachusetts.

The CRN is a resource for which there are potential partnerships for survivorship research. The network, originally funded in 1999, has been approved for renewal. Support will depend on peer review and the budget of the National Cancer Institute (NCI) in 2007. If all goes well, this network will be an available resource for at least 5 more years. The network is ideally suited for pilot testing a treatment summary and care plan, because the researchers in this network have access to health care systems that will provide care to 15 million individuals by 2007. There were 37,503 incident cancers in the network in 2003. CRN is especially well suited for studies of survivorship and long-term outcomes because the majority of health maintenance organization (HMO) members diagnosed with cancer remain enrolled. Five-year retentions rates were 84 percent.

Most of the health systems involved in the CRN have integrated delivery systems and are on the cutting edge of having comprehensive and integrated health information technology systems. These networks already have automated data on enrollment, utilization, laboratory, pharmacy, and hospitalizations. They are all in the third or fourth year of installing electronic medical records, and most of them are using the same vendor for the electronic medical record. An oncology module is under development and will be used across the network. All the networks are in the process of building extensive Web applications to connect the management, the providers, and the patients of these networks. All of these resources are potentially available for researchers who want to conduct intervention studies or surveillance studies. Many of the sites have established linkages to local Surveillance Epidemiology and End Results (SEER) tumor registries or maintain a local tumor registry.

There are several components of existing studies that relate to survivorship. For example, one study assessed the efficacy of prophylactic mastectomy for women at high risk for breast cancer. From that study a follow-up cohort was constructed, and those women are being questioned about their survivorship experience. Other studies are assessing psychosocial issues, late effects of treatment, and palliative and end-of-life care. The network has established a survivorship interest group, so there is interest and experience in this area. External members are welcome to join the survivorship special interest group.

The network is open to the general research community. External investigators can propose studies to the network. The network has an informatics resource that can do quick turnaround feasibility analyses to determine how many patients are available, what kind of information is available on these patients through electronic medical records, what type of patient is not available, and types of information that would require chart review or a special survey.

A study can proceed if it is feasible, there is an interested scientific partner in the network, and funding is available. Numerous studies have been undertaken in collaboration with outside investigators. To make the CRN more accessible to outside investigators, NCI is mandating in the renewal requests for applications that additional resources go into a collaboration core, which will have dedicated resources to facilitate even quicker and better kinds of studies. NCI is considering the possibility of a funded competitive supplemental program dedicated to researchers who want to do collaborative studies. This would be something of a fast-track mechanism for getting these collaborative studies up and going.

A recent issue of the *Journal of the NCI Monograph* (No. 35, 2005) is exclusively devoted to the CRN. It includes a very detailed description of its structure, function, and governance and about 18 research articles, some of them related to survivorship research.

Discussion

Dr. Rowland highlighted an attractive feature of the CRN, that investigators may access family data because families are usually enrolled in the systems of care. A study can therefore include outcomes not only of the survivor, but also of the secondary survivors' health care utilization. The CRN also allows assessments of the costs associated with interventions and with utilization. This is a unique platform to ask some of the very questions that have been raised during the workshop about the role of care plans and their potential benefits for patients and their families, payers, and society.

Dr. Tim Byers, of the University of Colorado Cancer Center, asked Dr. Brown to comment on the availability of funding to support external investigators who wish to collaborate with the CRN. Dr. Brown expects that when the new grant starts up again in March 2007, there will be substantial pilot funds in the grant. However, if an investigator wants to do a major study in collaboration with the CRN, they will have to apply for RO1 funding through the usual processes. The competitive supplemental funding mechanisms mentioned may be available in a year or two. Some other funding mechanisms might be relevant. One is a program announcement for economic studies. It does not have any funds associated with it, but these program announcements have been very useful in channeling grants to the right program directors and study sections. The applicants are advised to some degree, and they have been quite successful. Cathy Bradley has done some very interesting work on the employment experience of cancer survivors. She has had several grants funded through this program announcement.

There is also a program announcement on the use of health claims data for health services research. This has been used primarily to fund research using the SEER-Medicare database, which is maintained by NCI, but it could also be used for analyses of other types of health claims

THE CENTERS FOR MEDICARE AND MEDICAID SERVICE'S 2006 ONCOLOGY DEMONSTRATION PROGRAM

Presenter: Dr. Peter Bach

CMS conducts demonstration projects to identify and evaluate new approaches to health services delivery and/or reimbursement. There are many examples of demonstration projects turning into programmatic initiatives. One example is Medicare Advantage, which is a system in which private plans receive a capitated payment amount for each Medicare beneficiary who chooses to receive all their care from the plan. The Medicare Part D program, which pays for prescription drugs, also began as a demonstration program. CMS is actively experimenting with different strategies, for example, paying for quality metrics or paying for efficiency, in an effort to move toward a delivery system that enhances quality and is patient centered.

An oncology demonstration program began in 2005 to evaluate the use of billing codes to gather data on cancer patient symptoms. Oncologists submitted symptom G codes in association with codes used for infusion chemotherapy administration. Under Medicare's fee-for-service system, a doctor submits a bill on a form (called the 1500 form) and codes are filled in at the bottom of that bill signifying the patient's diagnosis and the services delivered. For this demonstration, CMS created additional codes to capture physician assessments of pain control, nausea and vomiting, and fatigue. Physicians were paid $130 for reporting on these three symptoms in association with a chemotherapy treatment visit. By the end of the year, more than 80 percent of oncologists were submitting data on chemotherapy patients' symptoms using these billing codes. This demonstration provided the proof of principle that the billing system could work to capture data on important patient outcomes. Mathematica has a contract to evaluate these data and summarize lessons learned from this demonstration.

The 2005 demonstration was limited to patients undergoing intravenous chemotherapy, and there was interest in broadening the scope of measurement to extend to all cancer patients along the continuum of care. In addition, there was an interest in developing longitudinal measures of efficiency, that is, getting similar or better outcomes and well-coordinated

---

BOX 5-1
Cancer Types Covered in the CMS
2006 Oncology Demonstration Project

1. Lung
2. Breast
3. Prostate
4. Colon
5. Rectum
6. Gastric
7. Pancreatic

8. Esophageal
9. Ovarian
10. Head and neck
11. Chronic myelogenous leukemia (CML)
12. Non–Hodgkin's lymphoma (NHL)
13. Multiple myeloma

SOURCE: Bach, 2006.

---

care for less cost. Longitudinal data are also need to assess alternative payment mechanisms, such as prospective or capitated payment.

Several steps have been taken in 2006 to augment the oncology demonstration program. In 2006, the demonstration will apply to nearly all oncology patient visits, insofar as it will rely on evaluation and management codes (called E&M codes) instead of G codes. Physicians use E&M codes for doctor-patient interactions when the focus is on problems and care planning. This shift in emphasis also removed the incentive for intravenous treatments in place of alternative therapeutic choices, such as oral chemotherapy.

Under the 2006 demonstration, physicians submit claims for every E&M visit, a process that creates a longitudinal record of claims. CMS is paying $23 for each of these reports. This reimbursement level is lower per claim ($130 in 2005), but physicians can apply the E&M code to more of their patients. New measures have been incorporated into the 2006 demonstration, including disease status, visit focus, and guideline adherence for each patient, on each visit. CMS created codes for 13 cancers, representing about 85 percent of Medicare payments to hematologist oncologists and medical oncologists (Box 5-1).

CMS created a set of stratification disease status codes for each of these 13 cancer types. There is a total of 60 disease status codes with three to seven codes per cancer type.

Having measures of disease status was felt to be more valuable than having information on stage alone. A patient's disease status can change over time. The six disease status codes for colon cancer shown in Figure 5-2 incorporate information on stage.

The colon cancer codes include five categories representing a hybrid of stage of presentation and current disease status, for example, presence of

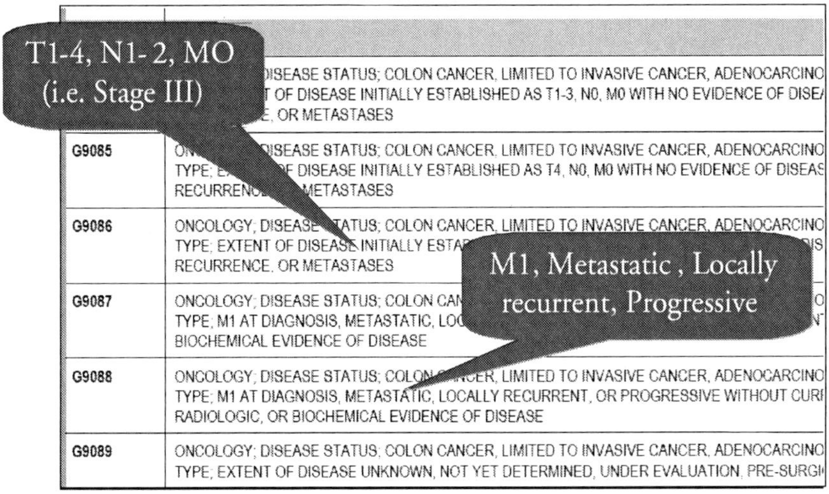

FIGURE 5-2 Colon cancer disease status codes.
SOURCE: Bach, 2006.

recurrence or metastases. In creating these categories, there was some lumping and some splitting. Code G9086, for example, is stage III colon cancer after surgery, representing an important subgroup of patients who benefit from adjuvant chemotherapy. In contrast, code G9088 represents a mix of patients, ones presenting with metastatic disease as well as ones developing local recurrences and metastatic disease after diagnosis. The sixth category, code G9089, represents the situation when extent of disease is unknown, is not yet determined, or under evaluation.

Oncology visits typically address multiple issues, and, under the demonstration, clinicians are asked to code one of the following six activities as the predominant focus of the visit:

1. Work-up, evaluation, or staging;
2. Decision making, supervising therapy, or managing toxicity;
3. Disease surveillance;
4. Expectant management;
5. Palliative therapy or end-of-life care (life prolongation not anticipated); or
6. Other.

The 2006 demonstration also asks clinicians to report on their adherence to clinical practice guidelines issued by the National Comprehensive

Cancer Network (NCCN) and the American Society of Clinical Oncology. Much of cancer care for the 13 cancer types included in the demonstration is addressed by the guidelines of these two organizations. Clinicians, in reporting whether or not they have adhered to guidelines, can use one of the following response categories:

- Yes, treatment adherent to guidelines;
- No, patient on institutional review board (IRB)–approved clinical trial;
- No, treating physician disagrees with guideline recommendations;
- No, patient prefers alternative or no treatment;
- No, patient comorbidity or performance status precludes guideline treatment;
- There are no guidelines relevant to patient's condition;
- No, another reason.

The focus of CMS on guideline adherence is based on the belief that guidelines capture the current standards for most of cancer care. Most of the guidelines are evidence based, and the extent of the evidence supporting them is well annotated. When the guidelines are not evidence based, they are at least based on a consensus of current opinion. In addition, using guidelines is advantageous because they are generally kept up-to-date. Trying to use CMS codes to keep up with changing standards of oncology care would be difficult. An alternative to asking about guideline adherence would be to measure directly the application of particular elements of care for selected patient subgroups. Sometimes, such direct measures are embedded in the guidelines. Included in the NCCN guidelines, for example, is that stage III colon cancer patients after surgery should be offered adjuvant chemotherapy.

This demonstration will help CMS learn whether asking about guideline adherence is an effective way to measure quality of care. The demonstration will allow CMS to determine when physicians disagree with guidelines, what clinical situations are not well addressed, and when patients elect alternative treatments. Answers to these questions could inform medical educators, guideline developers, cancer advocacy and education, and research policy.

More needs to be learned about how patient preferences affect treatment decisions. If the 2006 demonstration data show that patients are making choices that run counter to current guidelines, for example, refusing radiotherapy when it is recommended, there will have to be further analyses to understand what factors underlie these decisions. Does this reflect patient preference, or does it represent the fact that there are no accessible radiotherapy facilities?

Dr. Bach provided an example of how the 2006 demonstration project measures adherence to the standard of offering stage III colon cancer patients adjuvant chemotherapy after surgery. To determine the proportion of patients for whom appropriate care is provided, a rate is assembled with a numerator and a denominator. The denominator includes patients with an ICD-9 code for colon cancer as well as the disease status code indicating stage III cancer. The focus of the visit would be coded "supervising treatment." In this case, the physician would need to report whether their treatment conformed to the relevant guideline for treatment. They could indicate that the patient's treatment adhered to guidelines or that the patient preferred alternative or no treatment. The physician reports can be validated using claims data. CMS pays for individual chemotherapies using J codes, so in this example, these claims can be used to assess whether adjuvant chemotherapy is actually provided. A preliminary look at data from January and February 2006 indicates that adjuvant therapy is provided in about 82 percent of cases of stage III colon cancer, according to physician reports. About 6 percent of patients are refusing this therapy.

The CMS 2006 oncology demonstration will provide some needed basic information on disease status and treatment patterns. This is information that even the cancer registries cannot provide. There may be opportunities to learn more about the frequency and timing of recurrence and cancer progression. The data may also provide valuable information on the proportion of care directed at palliation. Very preliminary data from the demonstration suggest that between 1 and 2 percent of cancer visits have palliation as a primary focus.

The CMS 2006 demonstration also permits some examination of the quality of cancer care. We will be able to document the extent to which oncologists are at least self-reporting that they are following practice guidelines. It may be possible to generate feedback reports to physicians to inform them how their practices compare with peers. Ultimately, the demonstration may form the basis for publicly reported information on oncology practices. A report card format could be used to present comparative information on local oncology practices. These hypothetical applications will require much more experience and evaluations of preliminary efforts. This demonstration may also help to build the groundwork for estimating prospective costs for disease management and for providing benchmarks for measures of efficiency.

Dr. Bach asked the workshop audience to consider whether the 2006 CMS oncology demonstration represents the right approach to measurement. A strength of the demonstration, in his view, is the reliance on guideline-based standards from the oncology community. The demonstration represents a departure from other CMS efforts, for example, the physician voluntary reporting program, in which internal standards have been developed.

There are many challenges ahead. Coordinating the codes and the guidelines represents a technical challenge. Importantly, the guidelines that are used in the program must be free of conflicts of interest. Agreement among stakeholders will need to be reached to determine how assurances for conflict-free guidelines can be made.

Discussion

Dr. James Talcott began the discussion by raising a concern about basing the oncology demonstration on guidelines that are both evidence based and based on expert opinion. There is sometimes a blurring of the distinction between these two types of guidelines. When experts are convened to develop guidelines, the recommendations for care often end up reflecting how these experts happen to practice. The consensus guidelines may not be consistent with evidence. Dr. Talcott also wanted clarification on potential conflicts of interest. Are the concerns related primarily to financial conflicts of interest? There is also an embedded self-interest of experts on the guideline committees that needs to be considered. Dr. Talcott asked if CMS has thought about the dependence on consensus guidelines as part of the CMS 2006 demonstration.

Dr. Bach responded that more rigor is needed in terms of the content of the guidelines, how CMS characterizes the guidelines, and how the doctors evaluate whether or not they are following them. How to balance the use of consensus-based standards versus evidence-based ones is very important. Presumably, the guidelines will improve as they receive more scrutiny. In many areas of oncology practice, there are limited data with which to determine best practices. This reflects a shortcoming of the current knowledge base, and the CMS demonstration is likely to help drive the development of further knowledge.

Dr. Sheldon Greenfield pointed out that physicians' adherence to guidelines is usually not based on reports from the physicians who are being evaluated. Is it possible that the CMS 2006 demonstration is bringing about changes in practice by raising physicians' awareness of available clinical practice guidelines? Dr. Bach agreed that there may be such an effect, whereby practices are influenced by the very act of measuring their performance. This "Hawthorne" effect is likely to diminish over time. There were many hits on the NCCN guideline website following the announcement of the 2006 demonstration. CMS expects clinicians to be familiar with the guidelines. Hospitals self-report their adherence to quality measures, and audits of the validity of these reports have been largely positive but mixed.

CMS will have to conduct validation studies through analyses of administrative records and some fieldwork.

Dr. Ganz asked whether participation in the 2006 demonstration is as high as that observed in the 2005 demonstration. What is required of physicians in 2006 is much more challenging. The reporting categorization and coding scheme is more complex and time-consuming in 2006. Dr. Bach replied that while data are preliminary and from only the first few months of the demonstration, participation appears to be high, with greater than 80 percent of physicians reporting data.

In the context of developing treatment summaries and care plans, Dr. Ganz asked if in 2 to 3 years agreement is reached on content and format, whether the use of these documents could be ascertained in the CMS demonstration system. Dr. Bach indicated that it would likely be relatively easy to integrate use of care plans into the demonstration, especially if a recommendation for the use of treatment and care plans were incorporated into recognized practice guidelines. Dr. Bach pointed out that the focus of the visit coding used in the 2006 demonstration has not broken out survivorship care planning. Ideally, one would like to be able to identify this aspect of care, but the rules of E&M coding are complex, and changing them can be quite involved. It is easier to nest this sort of information into the existing codes for focus of the visit.

Dr. Byers asked whether CMS's quality improvement organizations (QIOs) could play a role in developing and demonstrating the effectiveness of treatment and care plans. Dr. Bach agreed that the QIOs could be a vehicle for independent demonstration projects. There are many examples of pilot projects carried out in a single state QIO. For example, studies have been conducted to see if mailing people fecal occult blood testing cards improves screening rates. QIOs have a quality measurement infrastructure that allows them to conduct such studies. QIOs are guided in their activities by a nationally established scope of work. Over time, it may be possible to incorporate aspects of survivorship care into those overarching goals set for the program. Before CMS would act to incorporate treatment and planning into programmatic initiatives, there would need to be evidence on effectiveness and related costs.

Dr. Byers asked if there were ways to identify the potential misuse of certain therapies. He pointed out that CMS sometimes pays for treatment that is contraindicated according to guidelines. Trastuzumab (Herceptin), for example, is sometimes prescribed for uses for which there is no evidence that it is effective. Dr. Bach responded by stating that CMS does not have a national coverage determination on Herceptin. This means that CMS does not regulate its use at the national level. The use of Herceptin is managed by CMS contractors, the local carriers. It is within their contractual discretion to monitor the appropriateness of drugs and tests. CMS will pay for

Herceptin for its listed off-label use in compendia. If CMS makes a national coverage determination on an intervention, then payment policies can be enforced. For example, CMS will not pay for an implantable cardiac defibrillator for anyone with an ejection fraction over 35 percent.

AN EVALUATION AND RESEARCH AGENDA

Presenter: Dr. Craig Earle

The IOM asserted in its recent report that survivorship care plans have strong face validity and can reasonably be assumed to improve care unless and until evidence accumulates to the contrary. The report recommended moving forward with implementation and at the same time engaging in applied research to define optimal models of delivery and quantify effects on survivors' health and well-being. In the IOM report there is a strong recommendation for action and also a charge going out to the research community to accumulate the evidence surrounding use of survivorship care planning. Creating survivorship care plans is time-consuming and requires work from busy clinicians. Understanding the benefit to patients as well as the costs to health systems and providers will be important factors in disseminating survivorship care planning.

Research is needed to determine how the entire Survivorship Care Plan, in addition to the following elements of it, affect outcomes:[1]

- Treatment summary;
- Description of possible clinical course (e.g., expected recovery from acute toxicities);
  - Surveillance plan for recurrence and late effects;
  - Psychosocial issues and available resources; and
  - Lifestyle recommendations.

There are research questions associated with each of these elements. Are all of these elements needed for all cancer survivors? Are psychosocial interventions as important for a stage II colon cancer as they are for a woman with advanced breast cancer? Is the transition to survivorship really a teachable moment, or is it the case that lifestyle issues would be better addressed by a primary care provider 6 months later? These are empirical questions that need to be answered.

Research outcomes that could be considered occur at both the patient level and the systems level (Table 5-1).

---

[1]This presentation is supplemented by a commissioned background paper prepared by Dr. Earle (see Appendix D.5).

TABLE 5-1 Research Outcomes to Be Evaluated in Survivorship Research

Patient-Level Outcomes	System-Level Outcomes

• Knowledge
• Satisfaction
• Symptoms
  – Anxiety, depression
  – Physical
• Quality of life
  – Physical, psychosocial, and/or spiritual wellbeing, perceived health and functional status
• Survival
	• Communication/coordination
	• Practice patterns
	• Processes/quality of care
	• Efficiency
	  – Resource utilization, time, cost

SOURCE: Earle, 2006.

The IOM survivorship focus groups indicated that satisfaction with care would improve with survivorship care planning. Some patients have the feeling that they have been abandoned by their oncologists. While there is a perception that doctors are not doing much for them in the posttreatment period, in reality, many things are being done. Perhaps providers need to discuss with patients what follow-up steps are being taken on their behalf. Explicitly sitting down and saying, "Here is what I have been doing for you; here is what I have been checking in your blood work in advance of your visit" might improve the patient's communication, knowledge, and satisfaction.

Evaluating how survivorship care planning affects anxiety or depression is critically important, because while such planning is likely to address these issues for most patients, it may increase anxiety or depression for others. Implementing parts of the Survivorship Care Plan may assist in identifying late effects of cancer treatment, and if interventions are available there is the possibility of relieving symptoms and improving quality of life, functional status, and survival. Implementing surveillance strategies might identify second malignancies earlier or recurrences of cancer at a time when interventions could be beneficial. Survival could be considered as an outcome of studies evaluating survivorship care plans. However, surveillance studies require very large sample sizes to detect what are likely to be very small differences, and so survival may not necessarily be the main outcome by which to judge the success or failure of survivorship care planning.

There are also systems-level outcomes that can be considered in evaluations of survivorship care planning. These include communication and coordination of care studies that could focus on potential improvements in linkages between specialty and primary care, as well as increased involvement of primary care physicians in posttreatment care.

Practice patterns and processes and quality of care—for example, whether appropriate mammography surveillance occurs following breast cancer treatment—could be affected by survivorship care planning and should be evaluated. Efficiency is a very important measure. Better coordinated, well-planned care is probably less costly. Care planning may help to avoid duplication of follow-up tests or unnecessary tests. If patients are well informed of their potential risks for late effects or recurrence, they may not receive MRIs for headaches or other tests that are not likely to be informative. Survivorship care planning could, however, result in care that is more expensive given the time and resources that will be needed to create and then implement the plan. Care planning would also result in people receiving tests who, without care planning, would not have received recommended surveillance. That is going to add to cost, one hopes with benefit, but it will add to cost. How survivorship care planning affects resource use and costs is an important area of research.

In testing survivorship care plans, attention will have to be paid to the needs of subpopulations. Individuals with different cancers may have distinct issues to be addressed. Age, race/ethnicity, socioeconomic status, and geography could all affect the optimal format and content of a care plan. For example, the format that might work best for an adolescent or young adult cancer survivor is probably different from a format suited to an elderly person with prostate cancer or colon cancer. The health of patients affects the health of their family members and other caregivers and so it is reasonable to also look at the effects of survivorship care planning on caregivers.

There are many researchable questions around the setting and personnel required for survivorship care planning. Demonstrations are needed to evaluate whether the responsibility for care planning should rest primarily with the oncology specialist, perhaps in conjunction with a nurse practitioner, a team in a dedicated survivorship clinic, or through a shared care model between the oncology and primary care provider. The optimal care delivery model will be likely to vary according to patient preference and circumstance. Demonstrations may also be tested to evaluate methods to financially support the delivery of services.

Various formats for care plans can also be tested, for example, structured oral consultations, written paper copy, or electronic formats. How structured or flexible the format needs to be to accommodate different clinical practices also needs to be assessed. Critical is determining the minimum essential elements of the care plan. Feasibility studies will be needed to see if some parts of the care plan can be automatically generated, for example, from electronic pharmacy record systems. It may be feasible to develop and test Web-based systems that are accessible by both patients and their care providers.

Several types of research study designs may be applied to these various questions. Qualitative research, such as focus groups and interviews, can identify potential barriers to implementation and strategies to overcome them. Observational studies, such as cross-sectional surveys of patients, may be instructive to assess knowledge, needs, and gaps in care delivery. Answers to some questions pertaining to surveillance patterns may be ascertained through medical record review or analyses of administrative data. Prospective cohort studies may also be informative. For example, a cohort study that included a baseline measurement of knowledge, anxiety, or other outcome of interest and then provided patients with all or part of the Survivorship Care Plan could help determine how that variation in plan content affects outcome.

Quasi-experimental studies, in which the experience before and after administering care planning is assessed, could be informative. There may also be some natural experiments in which comparisons could be made between clinics that, for example, implemented just the treatment summary and those that implemented both the treatment summary and the care plan.

Finally, randomized controlled trials could be conducted on aspects of patient follow-up. Such trials are expensive and logistically difficult, but they are very informative. Eva Grunfeld is an investigator who has completed several trials on alternative follow-up strategies for women with breast cancer.[2] Clinical trials would provide the best evidence on how outcomes are affected by survivorship care planning. For the questions pertaining to economic resource utilization, trials may be the only mechanism to obtain good estimates. One of the challenges to conducting randomized trials will be contamination. If randomization occurs at the level of a patient, a physician who is providing care planning to some patients and not to others is probably going to improve the survivorship care planning that they do with all patients. Because the IOM and other groups have recommended survivorship care planning, there may also be ethical issues if some patients are randomized to a group that does not receive care plans.

---

[2]Grunfeld E. et al., 2006. Randomized trial of long-term follow-up for early-stage breast cancer: a comparison of family physician versus specialist care. *Journal of Clinical Oncology* 24(6):848-55. Grunfeld E. et al., 1999. Comparison of breast cancer patient satisfaction with follow-up in primary care versus specialist care: Results from a randomized controlled trial. *British Journal of General Practice* 49(446):705-710. Grunfeld E. et al., 1999. Follow-up of breast cancer in primary care vs specialist care: Results of an ecomonic evaluation. *British Journal of General Practice* 79(7-8):1227-1233. Grunfeld E. et al., 1995. Evaluating primary care follow-up of breast cancer: Methods and preliminary results of three studies. *Annals of Oncology* 6(Suppl 2):47-52.

Any trial will probably have to test different levels or intensities of care planning. In this case, large sample sizes will be necessary to detect differences between groups.

In conclusion, rigorous systematic studies are necessary in order to determine what works and what does not work in survivorship care planning. The IOM report called for increased support for research and demonstration projects. The goal is to have good evidence on which to base guidelines and standards of care and thereby improve care delivery and optimize the health of survivors.

Discussion

Dr. Raich of Denver Health Medical Center suggested that multiinstitutional, interdisciplinary collaborations will be needed to strengthen the capacity to address the many research questions raised by Dr. Earle. Dr. Earle agreed that a large collaborative venture was probably needed to address the many challenges posed by this research. He noted, however, that such collaborative networks were difficult to organize and fund. Dr. Smita Bhatia of City of Hope Comprehensive Cancer Center emphasized the need to learn from the experience of the pediatric oncology community, which has organized a team effort to create care summaries and guidelines.

6

Wrap-up Session

Ms. Ellen Stovall thanked the workshop speakers and participants for a very informative meeting. On behalf of the sponsoring organization, the National Coalition of Cancer Survivors, she thanked the workshop's partnering organizations, the Lance Armstrong Foundation and the National Cancer Institute.

Dr. Sheldon Greenfield summarized the main themes that emerged from the workshop. According to the discussions, he concluded that the Survivorship Care Plan should: (1) recognize the interests of stakeholders, including patients, primary care physicians, nurses, and insurers in its development; (2) be portable and provided in both paper and digital formats; (3) be designed in collaboration with the potential users, for example, patients, physicians, and nurses; (4) include a set of elements that represent a minimum standard, allowing individual providers the opportunity to tailor the care plan to their circumstances; (5) optimally be shared with patients, starting with the treatment plan at the time of diagnosis and continuing with a follow-up care plan at the conclusion of primary treatment, amended as needed over time; (6) be used as a communication tool to enhance the patient-physician relationship and assist in addressing survivors' psychosocial concerns, with appropriate referrals to supportive services; and (7) be designed as a dynamic tool that will evolve as evidence from research and demonstration projects emerges.

Ms. Stovall noted the great interest expressed by cancer survivors to have survivorship care plans and improved communication with their providers. She also acknowledged the many challenges ahead that were raised by workshop participants, for example, how to develop survivorship care planning as a standard of care, how to support the generation of empirical evidence to discover how best to implement survivorship care planning, and how to pay for this service to ensure its availability. While some of these challenges seem daunting, she was encouraged by the success of the pediatric oncology community in collaboratively developing survivorship guidelines and innovative tools to implement survivorship care planning.

She concluded that the workshop had galvanized support for survivorship care planning and was reassured that the many adult cancer survivors in need of this service will have it available to them. Ms. Stovall stated that the patient advocacy community will be taking the important themes emerging from the workshop and entering into productive collaborations with physicians, nurses, social workers, insurers, and other stakeholders to ensure progress in implementation efforts.

APPENDIXES

Appendix A

Workshop Agenda

Implementing Cancer Survivorship Care Planning
An Institute of Medicine, National Cancer Policy Forum Workshop
Sponsored by the National Coalition for Cancer Survivorship in
Partnership with the Lance Armstrong Foundation and
the National Cancer Institute

Date: May 15 and 16, 2006
Location: The Marriott Georgetown University Conference Hotel
3800 Reservoir Road NW, Washington DC

Workshop purpose: Review next steps to implementing survivorship care planning focusing on: templates for treatment summaries and care plans; overcoming barriers facing providers and health care systems; and pilot tests.

Monday, May 15, 2006

8:30-9:00	Breakfast
9:00-9:15	Welcome and Introductions
	Sheldon Greenfield and Ellen Stovall

Session I: **Survivorship care planning: overview**
9:15-9:45 *Patricia Ganz*-Implementing the survivorship care plan
9:45-10:30 *Deborah Schrag*-The status of treatment summaries for oncology care

10:30-10:45 Break

Session II: Perspectives on survivorship care planning
10:45-12:30   *Presentation of IOM-commissioned qualitative research*
                 • Survivors-*Rebecca Day and Reynolds Kinzey*
                 • Nurses-*Catherine Harvey*
                 • Physicians-*Annette Bamundo*

12:30-1:30   Lunch

1:30-5:00   *Discussion*
                 • What are the essential elements of the care plan? Will
                   a single template work?
                 • Who is responsible for creating the plan and discuss-
                   ing the plan with patients?
                 • What are the respective roles of oncology/primary care
                   and physicians/nurses?
                 • What economic strategies could encourage implemen-
                   tation of care planning?
                 • What barriers exist to creating the care plan? How can
                   they be overcome?

                 Moderator: Sheldon Greenfield

Tuesday, May 16, 2006

8:00-8:30   Breakfast

Session III: **Implementation issues**
8:30-10:30   Resources for completing the care plan
                 • *Kevin Oeffinger and Charles Shapiro*-Survivorship
                   guidelines
                 • *Diane Blum*-Psychosocial support resources
                 • *Wendy Demark-Wahnefried*-Recommendations for
                   healthy lifestyle behaviors

10:30-10:45   Break

10:45-11:30   Information technology
                 • *David Poplack, Marc Horowitz, and Michael Fordis*-
                   Passport for Care, an online resource for survivors
                   of childhood cancer
                 • Reactant: *Lawrence Shulman*

11:30-12:30   Public health approaches
- *Tim Byers*-Regional approaches to cancer survivorship planning

12:30-1:30   Lunch

Session IV: **Pilot tests and assessment of their impact**
1:30-3:15   Implementation through practice networks
- *Craig Earle*-LIVESTRONG Survivorship Center of Excellence Network
- *Patricia Ganz*-ASCO's Quality Oncology Practice Initiative (QOPI)
- *Martin Brown*-The HMO Cancer Research Network (CRN)
- *Peter Bach*-CMS's 2006 oncology demonstration program

3:15-4:00   *Craig Earle*-An evaluation and research agenda

Session V: **Wrap-up**
4:00-5:00   *Moderators: Patricia Ganz, Caroline Huffman, Julia Rowland, and Ellen Stovall*

Appendix B

Participant Names and Affiliations

Noreen M. Aziz, MD, PHD, MPH, National Cancer Institute
Peter Bach, MD, Centers for Medicare & Medicaid Services
Annette Bamundo, Bamundo Qualitative Research
Michael Bergin, National Coalition for Cancer Survivorship
Smitia Bhatia, MD, City of Hope Comprehensive Cancer Center
Judith Blanchard, MS, National Coalition for Cancer Survivorship
Diane Blum, MSW, CancerCare Inc.
Richard N. Boyajian, RN, MS, Dana Farber Cancer Institute
Martin Brown, PhD, National Cancer Institute
Patricia Buchsel, RN, MSN, FAAN, University of Washington School of
    Nursing
Tim Byers, MD, MPH, University of Colorado Cancer Center
Jackie Casillas, MD, MSHS, David Geffen School of Medicine at UCLA
Charles Catcher, MD, New Hampshire Oncology-Hematology
Carol P. Curtiss, MSN, RNC, Massachusetts Pain Initiative
Sarah Davis, JD, MPA, University of Wisconsin Law School
Rebecca Day, Kinzey & Day Market Research
Wendy Demark-Wahnefried, PhD, RD, LDN, Duke University Medical
    Center
Molla Donaldson, DrPH, MS, American Society of Clinical Oncology
Craig Earle, MD, MSc, Dana-Farber Cancer Institute
Betty R. Ferrell, PHD, RN, FAAN, City of Hope National Medical
    Center
Michael Fordis, MD, Baylor College of Medicine

Debra L. Friedman, MD, Fred Hutchinson Cancer Research Center
Martha E. Gaines, JD, LLM, University of Wisconsin Law School
Patricia A. Ganz, MD, UCLA Jonsson Comprehensive Cancer Center
Mark Gorman, National Coalition for Cancer Survivorship
Elizabeth Goss, Ropes & Gray
Sheldon Greenfield, MD, University of California at Irvine
Stacia Grosso, MA, National Coalition for Cancer Survivorship
Wendy S. Harpham, MD, FACP, Author/Speaker/Patient Advocate
Catherine Harvey, RN, DrPH, The Oncology Group
Pamela J. (PJ) Haylock, RN, MA, Oncology Consultant and Doctoral
    Student, School of Nursing, University of Texas Medical Branch,
    Galveston
Marc Horowitz, MD, Texas Children's Cancer Center
Caroline Huffman, LCSW, MEd, Lance Armstrong Foundation
Linda Jacobs, PhD, CRNP, Abramson Cancer Center of the University of
    Pennsylvania
Sherry Kaplan, PhD, University of California at Irvine
Suzanne Kho, Lance Armstrong Foundation
William G. Kraybill, MD, Roswell Park Cancer Institute
Jean Kutner, MD, University of Colorado Health Sciences Center
Wendy Landier, RN, MSN, CPNP, CPON, City of Hope National
    Medical Center
Susan Leigh, BSN, RN, Cancer Survivorship Consultant
Frances Lewis, PhD, MN, University of Washington
Jean Mandelblatt, MD, MPH, Georgetown University Medical Center
Al Marcus, MD, AMC Cancer Research Center
Ross D. Martin, MD, MHA, Pfizer Human Health
Mary McCabe, RN, MA, Memorial Sloan-Kettering Cancer Center
Lee Newcomer, MD, UnitedHealth Group
Kevin Oeffinger, MD, Memorial Sloan-Kettering Cancer Center
Loria Pollack, MD, Centers for Disease Control and Prevention
David Poplack, MD, Texas Children's Cancer Center
Peter Raich, MD, Denver Health Medical Center
John Rainey, MD, Louisiana Oncology Associates
Eddie Reed, MD, Centers for Disease Control and Prevention
Julia Rowland, PhD, National Cancer Institute Office of Cancer
    Survivorship
Carolyn D. Runowicz, MD, University of Connecticut Health Center
Sheila Santacroce, APRN, PhD, Yale University School of Nursing
Aziza Shad, MD, Georgetown University Medical Center
Lawrence N. Shulman, MD, Dana-Farber Cancer Institute
Charles L. Shapiro, MD, Arthur G. James Cancer Hospital and Richard
    J. Solove Research Institute

Kenneth G. Schellhase, MD, Medical College of Wisconsin
Neil Schlackman, MD, National Coalition for Cancer Survivorship
Deborah Schrag, MD, Memorial Sloan-Kettering Cancer Center
Kathryn M. Smolinski, MSW, Association of Oncology Social Work
Ellen Stovall, National Coalition for Cancer Survivorship
James Talcott, MD, Massachusetts General Hospital
Ed Wagner, MD, Group Health Cooperative
Lari Wenzel, PhD, University of California at Irvine

Appendix C

Excerpt
From Cancer Patient to Cancer Survivor: Lost in Transition

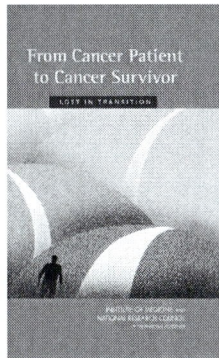

PROVIDING A CARE PLAN FOR SURVIVORSHIP

A strategy is needed for the ongoing clinical care of cancer survivors. There are many opportunities for improving care—psychosocial distress can be assessed and support provided; cancer recurrences and second cancers may be caught early and treated; bothersome symptoms can be effectively managed; preventable conditions such as osteoporosis may be avoided; and potentially lethal late effects such as heart failure averted.

Recommendation 2: Patients completing primary treatment should be provided with a comprehensive care summary and follow-up plan that is clearly and effectively explained. This "Survivorship Care Plan" should be written by the principal provider(s) that coordinated oncology treatment. This service should be reimbursed by third-party payors of health care.

Such a care plan would summarize critical information needed for the survivor's long-term care:

- Cancer type, treatments received, and their potential consequences;
- Specific information about the timing and content of recommended follow-up;
- Recommendations regarding preventive practices and how to maintain health and well-being;
- Information on legal protections regarding employment and access to health insurance; and
- The availability of psychosocial services in the community.

These content areas, adapted from those recommended by the President's Cancer Panel (President's Cancer Panel, 2004), are elaborated upon in Box 3-16.

The content of the survivorship care plan could be reviewed with a patient during a formal discharge consultation. Clinicians would likely have discussed some aspects of the survivorship care plan before or during treatment, for example, short- and long-term treatment effects and their implications for work and quality of life.[1] However, during acute treatment, much time is spent dealing with the acute toxicities of treatment that little emphasis is given to the post-treatment care plan. A substantial amount of information needs to be communicated during this consultation and then documented in an end-of-treatment consultation note. Appropriate reimbursement should be provided for such a visit, given the complexity and importance of the consultation.

The member of the oncology treating team who would be responsible for this visit could vary depending on the exact course of treatment. The responsibility could be assigned either to the oncology specialist coordinating care or to the provider responsible for the last component of treatment. Oncology nurses could play a key role. The survivorship care plan may need revision as new knowledge concerning late effects and interventions to ameliorate them, genetic disorders, and surveillance methods is identified. Cancer survivors can help to ensure that the plan is followed. The consultation at the conclusion of primary treatment could serve as a teaching event for survivors and their family members and provide opportunities to discuss with clinicians their prognosis, concerns, lifestyle issues, and follow-up schedules. The plan could be used by survivors subsequently to raise questions with doctors and prompt appropriate care during follow-up visits.

---

[1]Providing a survivorship care plan may prove difficult for those individuals who cease treatment prematurely and do not return for the remainder of their care. Primary care physicians involved in subsequent care of such patients may need to contact oncology providers to obtain a survivorship care plan.

BOX 3-16
Survivorship Care Plan

Upon discharge from cancer treatment, including treatment of recurrences, every patient should be given a record of all care received and important disease characteristics. This should include, at a minimum:

1. Diagnostic tests performed and results.
2. Tumor characteristics (e.g., site[s], stage and grade, hormone receptor status, marker information).
3. Dates of treatment initiation and completion.
4. Surgery, chemotherapy, radiotherapy, transplant, hormonal therapy, or gene or other therapies provided, including agents used, treatment regimen, total dosage, identifying number and title of clinical trials (if any), indicators of treatment response, and toxicities experienced during treatment.
5. Psychosocial, nutritional, and other supportive services provided.
6. Full contact information on treating institutions and key individual providers.
7. Identification of a key point of contact and coordinator of continuing care.

Upon discharge from cancer treatment, every patient and his/her primary health care provider should receive a written follow-up care plan incorporating available evidence-based standards of care. This should include, at a minimum:

1. The likely course of recovery from treatment toxicities, as well as the need for ongoing health maintenance/adjuvant therapy.
2. A description of recommended cancer screening and other periodic testing and examinations, and the schedule on which they should be performed (and who should provide them).
3. Information on possible late and long-term effects of treatment and symptoms of such effects.
4. Information on possible signs of recurrence and second tumors.
5. Information on the possible effects of cancer on marital/partner relationship, sexual functioning, work, and parenting, and the potential future need for psychosocial support.
6. Information on the potential insurance, employment, and financial consequences of cancer and, as necessary, referral to counseling, legal aid, and financial assistance.
7. Specific recommendations for healthy behaviors (e.g., diet, exercise, healthy weight, sunscreen use, immunizations, smoking cessation, osteoporosis prevention). When appropriate, recommendations that first-degree relatives be informed about their increased risk and the need for cancer screening (e.g., breast cancer, colorectal cancer, prostate cancer).
8. As appropriate, information on genetic counseling and testing to identify high-risk individuals who could benefit from more comprehensive cancer surveillance, chemoprevention, or risk-reducing surgery.
9. As appropriate, information on known effective chemoprevention strategies for secondary prevention (e.g., tamoxifen in women at high risk for breast cancer; aspirin for colorectal cancer prevention).
10. Referrals to specific follow-up care providers (e.g., rehabilitation, fertility, psychology), support groups, and/or the patient's primary care provider.
11. A listing of cancer-related resources and information (e.g., Internet-based sources and telephone listings for major cancer support organizations).

SOURCE: Adapted from the President's Cancer Panel (2004).

Agencies that accredit health plans and other providers could build compliance with the recommended consultation into their evaluation criteria (see
discussion of quality measures in chapter 4). With 61 percent of cancer
survivors aged 65 and older, the Medicare program could play a key role in
ensuring that the survivorship care plan is written, communicated, and
reimbursed. A formal assessment of survivorship care planning should be
undertaken to assess its value.

Survivorship care plans have been recommended by the President's
Cancer Panel and by the IOM committee; however, the implementation of
such plans has not yet been formally evaluated. Despite the lack of evidence
to support the use of survivorship care plans, the committee concluded that
some elements of care simply make sense—that is, they have strong face
validity and can reasonably be assumed to improve care unless and until
evidence accumulates to the contrary. Having an agreed upon care plan
that outlines goals of care falls into this "common sense" area. Health
services research should be undertaken to assess the impact and costs associated with survivorship care plans and to evaluate their acceptance by both
cancer survivors and health care providers.

Appendix D

Commissioned Background Papers

Appendix D.1

The Cancer Treatment Plan and Summary: Re-Engineering the Culture of Documentation to Facilitate High Quality Cancer Care

Deborah Schrag, MD, MPH *

Molla Donaldson, DrPH * *

Abstract:

Cancer chemotherapy is typically administered over many days, sometimes in the hospital and sometimes in office settings. It is notoriously difficult, and often impossible, to recreate cancer treatment histories from medical records. This impedes communication between and among health care systems, physicians, and patients as they traverse the spectrum of cancer care. Medical record keeping does not include preparation of synoptic overviews when patients transition from one therapy to another. For these reasons, it can be difficult for patients and physicians to assemble an accurate understanding of individual chemotherapy treatments as well as the overall trajectory of a patient's cancer care. The availability of new and better drugs for treating cancer means that patients are living longer, receiving more treatment, and managing the consequences of these therapies. In turn, living longer means that cancer patients' medical records become thicker and it becomes even more challenging and time-consuming to create a history from those written records. In addition, like society as a whole, cancer patients are increasingly mobile, seeking care at multiple settings and interacting with a variety of health care and allied professionals. In conjunction with the

*Health Outcomes Research Group, Memorial Sloan-Kettering Cancer Center
* *American Society of Clinical Oncology

*National Coalition for Cancer Survivorship(NCCS) and other pa-
tient advocacy groups, the American Society of Clinical Oncology
(ASCO), the major professional organization representing medical
oncologists, is developing strategies to encourage medical oncologists
to prepare synoptic documents that provide an overview of care at
key transition points. The goal is two-pronged: to create a synoptic
document which can not only be used by other providers to quickly
recreate patient medical histories, but also to serve as a springboard
for discussion with patients at key transition points. This background
paper first outlines the rationale for developing cancer treatment
plans and summaries as a strategy to improve the quality of cancer
care and then describes progress to date towards achieving this goal.*

I. Overview

Cancer care in the 21st century is exceedingly complex. As cancer
patients live longer and the range of chemotherapy treatment options ex-
pands, patients are ever more likely to receive care from multiple physicians, across diverse delivery systems, over periods of many years. Both the
longer periods of survival and the multiplicity of providers make it especially challenging for oncologists to assemble all the information that is
necessary to understand a patient's cancer treatment history. It is not just
that obtaining the actual physical records is problematic—although it can
be—rather, the more common challenge is obtaining a coherent summation
of myriad relevant events from a series of chronologically organized records.
Without a summary available to them, patients who have experienced a
series of complex treatments have great difficulty becoming partners in
their own care after completion of curative treatment.

Cancer survivors typically receive care from both oncology and nononcology providers and eventually transition back to the "regular" health
care system, where their care is usually provided by clinicians with no
special oncology training. Cancer survivors report that their providers are
sometimes uncertain about what, if any, special care might be required
given their cancer history.

To understand the cancer history, patients and their noncancer physicians face a choice between requesting entire oncology records (on the one
hand) or a few key documents (on the other). The drawback of obtaining
entire records from multiple settings is that they are time-consuming to
review and inefficient to transmit and store. Furthermore, only a small
fraction of the contents of those records is likely to be relevant for ongoing
care. However, the drawback of asking for select key documents is that
detail may be missing. Medical oncology treatment can be viewed as a story
which begins with a detailed chapter (the new visit note) and unfolds over

time in a series of follow-up chapters in office notes, chemotherapy flow sheets, surgical, radiation, imaging and laboratory reports, referrals, and possibly hospital discharge summaries. What both patients and providers often need, however, is a brief summary of this story. At present, there is no standard for preparing a "treatment summary," and it is not part of the culture of routine oncology practice.

Cancer quality-of-care research has highlighted the importance of care coordination for cancer patients. One strategy for improving coordination is to change the culture of medical records documentation so that preparation of synoptic treatment summaries becomes routine. The goal of this background paper is to: (1) describe the current practice of medical records documentation with a special focus on oncology; (2) discuss the rationale for a treatment summary; (3) address challenges for implementation and; (4) identify key components of these summaries with illustrations from sample templates developed in conjunction with the American Society of Clinical Oncology (ASCO).

This background paper focuses on the overall goal of changing the culture of medical records documentation to include treatment summaries for all patients, but highlights aspects of care that have special relevance for survivors. The "transition to survivorship" care plan is simply a special type of chemotherapy treatment summary that requires special attention to issues of long-term follow-up such as fertility, management of late- and long-term effects of cancer, and screening recommendations. The objective of ASCO and the National Coalition for Cancer Survivorship's (NCCS) treatment plan/treatment summary initiative is to ensure that synopses of care are provided for *all* cancer patients, including long-term survivors. Successful implementation of this initiative will require the collaboration of multiple stakeholders.

Medical oncologists are usually the providers who coordinate care for cancer patients receiving multimodality treatment. For this reason, this background paper emphasizes preparation of treatment plans and summaries by medical oncologists. Moreover, medical oncology treatments are especially challenging to track in medical records because, in contrast to surgery and radiation, they unfold over lengthy time intervals. However, it is important to emphasize that the preparation of treatment summaries is relevant for other cancer providers and indeed, for all health care providers who deliver care to persons with complex chronic conditions.

II. Background and Rationale:
Why Cancer Treatment Summaries Are Necessary

The development of a treatment summary can help achieve three objectives related to improving the quality of cancer care:[1] (1) to improve coor-

---

BOX D.1-1
Objectives of Adoption of Oncology Treatment Summaries

Adoption of a treatment summary could improve three interrelated aspects of cancer care delivery:
1) **Care Coordination:** between providers.
2) **Communication:** between patients and providers.
3) **Efficiency:** document tracking, recordkeeping for patients, providers, systems, and research.

Care Coordination is especially important because:
- Cancer survival has improved.
- Cancer treatment is increasingly complex.
- Society is increasingly mobile and patients transition across practice sites.
- Unexpected events—hurricanes and other disasters—happen.
- More fragmentation occurs as care teams include many subspecialized members.

Communication is especially important because:
- It is a prerequisite for shared decision making.
- More complex treatments and preference-sensitive options now exist.
- Patients desire it.

Efficiency is especially important because:
- It limits time spent reviewing/obtaining/providing medical records.
- It facilitates tracking of processes and outcomes of care for quality improvement initiatives.
- It facilitates document storage, retrieval, copying, and transmission.
- It facilitates tracking of care for public health and research data collection—e.g., cancer registries.

---

dination of care as patients transition among various health care providers; (2) to improve communication between patients and physicians; and (3) to improve the efficiency of cancer care delivery by streamlining documentation for clinicians and clinical support staff. Box D.1-1 describes three components of care—care coordination, communication, and efficiency—that could be improved by changing the culture of oncology practice to include treatment summaries.

The Need for Treatment Summaries—Insights from Quality of Care Research

A series of influential reports by the Institute of Medicine (IOM) called attention to systemic problems in the general health care delivery system and recommended several strategies to improve the quality of health care.[2-4] With the release in 1999 of the IOM report *Ensuring Quality Cancer Care* and subsequent work of the National Cancer Policy Board, it has become clear that in the United States, many cancer patients, even those with adequate health insurance, do not receive the most effective available treatments in a timely fashion.[2-4] Since these reports' publication, the quality of cancer care has remained in the national spotlight. Major efforts to measure, understand, and improve the quality of cancer care have also been undertaken. In particular, the NCI and ASCO have conducted large-scale studies to characterize the state of cancer treatment and more recently to develop "Navigator" programs to prevent patients from becoming lost in the web of a complex system.[5,6] Starting in 1998, ASCO and the Susan G. Komen Foundation sponsored the National Initiative on Cancer Care Quality (NICCQ). Researchers from Harvard University and the RAND Corporation reviewed medical records and interviewed patients diagnosed with breast and colorectal cancer in five U.S. cities in order to characterize the quality of their care.[6] This study underscored how difficult and time-consuming it was for highly trained researchers to locate patient data and accurately determine the treatments patients had received in order to assess whether those patients had received appropriate adjuvant chemotherapy. Even after Institutional Review Board (IRB) approval to review these records was received, many barriers to ascertaining chemotherapy use from medical record review remained. First, patients were seen by many physicians and sometimes by more than one medical oncologist. Second, most oncologists practice alone or in small-group settings and usually have paper records. Third, even when researchers were able to access oncology records, information about chemotherapy use was not easy to abstract because of highly variable patterns of documentation. Although many oncologists use flow sheets to record their use of chemotherapy, the organization and style of these documents varies considerably. Although these records may be relatively easy for oncologists to understand, they are less comprehensible to other clinicians because they include many oncology abbreviations and details of concern only to the treating oncologist, such as the white blood cell count after each dose of therapy. Information about treatment in medical oncology charts is usually recorded in an event-by-event chronological format; as a result, researchers often had to sift through many pages of notes to obtain key information about a patient's treatment. It was even more difficult to glean from medical records whether patients had completed prescribed courses of treatment, the reasons for treatment discontinuation, and the planned next steps. Fourth, even determining diagnosis was challenging. Although initial consultation notes usually record an initial diagnosis, records often contain incomplete information because the diagnosis may evolve as more information is obtained.

The Harvard-RAND researchers presented their work to an advisory group of ASCO members interested in quality of care, representatives from the Susan G. Komen Breast Cancer Foundation, and other advocacy groups such as the NCCS. In a discussion of "lessons" learned from this large scale observational study, the utility of a chemotherapy treatment summary was recognized as a logical and potentially effective quality improvement tool. The emerging idea of an oncology treatment summary coincided with national initiatives by the NCCS, ASCO, the Lance Armstrong Foundation, the National Cancer Institute (NCI), the American Cancer Society, and the IOM to improve the care of cancer survivors.

The need for a treatment summary was also evident in other research initiatives, including the NCI's Cancer Care Outcomes Research and Surveillance Consortium (CanCORS),[5] in research from the Cancer Research Network, an affiliation of large HMOs,[5] as well as large interview studies highlighting problems with care coordination as especially prevalent in cancer.

The treatment summary was also recognized as a potentially valuable tool to address problems with communication between patients and providers. In a recent population-based study of 1,067 colorectal cancer patients from Northern California, cancer patients completed surveys modified from the Picker Institute to report on their access to care, symptom control, psychosocial support, health information, treatment-specific information, confidence in providers and coordination of care. They identified access to information, psychosocial support, and care coordination as the three most deficient aspects of their care.[7] Black, Hispanic and other non-English speaking patients reported significantly more problems than white English speakers, and this was especially pronounced in the domains of communication and coordination of care. Despite health information being readily available in multiple media formats, this and other research indicates that patients are dissatisfied with communication with their physicians. This is in part because patients value having health information that is filtered by a trusted and knowledgeable source, synthesized and custom-tailored to their individual circumstances.

Coordination of Care Among Oncologists and Other Health Care Professionals

Coordination of care involves facilitating patients' access to practitioners whose expertise may improve their health outcomes or experience. These providers must have key clinical information at hand to formulate recommendations and then function collaboratively as a team to deliver care. Some practices are multispecialty and multidisciplinary, though even in these settings coordination can be a challenge. In other cases, cancer care involves providers who practice in different locations, health systems, and specialties. Coordination is generally improved when one provider—typically the medical oncologist, but sometimes the surgeon or the primary care physician—assumes responsibility for orchestrating and overseeing all aspects of care. This critical coordination function helps to ensure that health care providers work together to provide care. This role may extend well beyond making referrals. The coordinating physician must be actively engaged to ensure that neither essential pieces of information, nor the patient himself or herself, gets lost within the complex system. The coordinating physician must also ensure that other practitioners' expertise is obtained to address frequently overlooked needs, such as psychosocial distress.

Not all providers involved in a patient's care need or want the entire oncology record. A cardiologist, for example, needs to know how much doxorubicin a patient has received, and a dentist must know what precautions are needed for a patient with a MediPort in place or when there is a history of low platelets. However, synoptic treatment plans and summaries are not simply intended to make care safer and more effective for cancer patients in nononcology settings; they can also help oncologists with coordination. When communicating with other oncologists and between oncologists and their colleagues in closely related fields like surgery and radiation oncology, every oncologist has confronted the onerous task of reading through reams of office notes and flow sheets to ascertain what chemotherapy was delivered, why it was delivered, and how it was tolerated.

Communication of the Treatment Plan and Summary, and the Post-Treatment Plan Between Medical Oncologists and Patients

Oncologists have complex communication responsibilities when talking with patients. They must explain the patient's diagnosis, prognosis, and therapeutic options in a comprehensible way, and listen to and incorporate patient preferences while formulating a treatment plan. Documenting treatment plans can serve as a valuable springboard for discussion about current and future chemotherapy. That is, systematic review of the information with the patient may help him or her understand the purpose of treatment, and to structure conversations about treatment decisions. Providing patients with a copy of the treatment plan may also empower them to begin conversations with family members and other health care practitioners, as well as their oncologist. Creating documents that patients can review at a later time also addresses the widely recognized phenomenon that patients remember only a small proportion of the information provided during an office visit. A physical (or access to an electronic) record enables patients to review the key content in a more relaxed setting at a place and time when information may be more easily absorbed and shared with others.

After a course of chemotherapy is complete, the summary and plan for follow-up, including surveillance for recurrence and late effects may serve as a valuable foundation for discussion. Providing patients with a document empowers them to communicate effectively with other providers. whether or not they understand every sentence in the document. This may be especially important for non-English speaking patients

Practice Efficiency: Minimize the Administrative Burden for Administrators and Staff

Information about medical oncology treatment is not recorded in a single place or in a standardized format in health care records. As a result, when multiple oncologists are involved in a patient's care, they typically request a patient's entire record and thus create a workload that burdens office staff and physicians. A chemotherapy treatment plan outlining the planned regimen and a subsequent treatment summary describing how treatment was tolerated and the outcomes of care could streamline communication among oncologists and between oncologists and other key cancer-care providers, such as surgeons and radiation oncologists.

Facilitate Quality of Care Monitoring and Improvement

In order to evaluate the quality of cancer care, it is not necessary to know the number of milligrams of every treatment dose. Neither is it necessary to know the specifics of every dose delay or reduction. The inclusion of chemotherapy treatment summaries in medical charts would have greatly simplified the work of the NICCQ investigators by reducing the need to sift through pages of records that were not relevant to assessing quality.

More generally, quality of care monitoring also involves ensuring patients' safety, both individually and as a member of a group receiving similar chemotherapeutic agents. For example, it is critical to identify harmful effects of chemotherapy drugs that emerge after these drugs have received FDA approval (sometimes called, "after market" monitoring). Treatment summaries that track and aggregate the toxicities that patients experience could greatly facilitate monitoring such unexpected effects, especially if the treatment summary is developed in electronic form with flexible reporting capability.

III. The Culture of Medical Records Keeping by Physicians

Physicians are required to keep medical records that describe health care delivery. These records serve multiple purposes. They enable the individual physician to recall his or her thoughts and plans from one visit to the next. Documentation also provides key information to other health care providers working with the oncologist as well as clinicians at other sites. Documentation fulfills a legal function by creating a permanent record of health care.

Although some new electronic systems are changing the *status quo*, medical records are almost always organized chronologically by events, such as visits. The abstraction necessary to create a synopsis is challenging, time-consuming and requires physician input. However, electronic systems can be structured to facilitate this activity by populating specific fields of key relevance such as diagnostic information; for example, site, histology and stage. When care evolves over time, these records become progressively denser and more difficult to review. It is common practice to focus on the most recent history, and for this reason key information may become buried in a thick stack of documents. Consider the challenge for an emergency room (ER) physician evaluating a dehydrated patient with longstanding metastatic breast cancer. The ER physician can easily determine what operations have been performed by searching the record for operative and pathology reports. Episodes of radiation are summarized. Hospitalizations are described with a discharge summary. However, re-creating the trajectory of the cancer care history requires review of medical oncology notes to determine the drugs given and the context of treatment. Although this information is available, it is often spread across multiple visit notes, flow sheets, and treatment administration records. It can be sufficiently difficult to reconstruct a cancer history from a medical record that a physician in the ER may avoid the chart altogether and instead try to obtain this history directly from the patient. When patients are careful historians and attentive to important detail, this strategy works reasonably well. However, when patients are too ill to provide history, lack informed caregivers, or have language barriers, they may not be able to provide important information.

In addition, records include detail that may not be helpful, even to treating oncologists. A key example is documentation for the purpose of billing. In the mid-1990s, the Health Care Financing Administration (HCFA, now the Centers for Medicare and Medicaid Services or CMS) developed a detailed set of rules delineating documentation standards for billing Medicare. These rules specified the number of items in the physical exam (for example three aspects of the respiratory system) and the number of body systems that need to be included in a systems review in order to bill for complex "evaluation and management" visits. These requirements led to burgeoning detail in medical records and widespread use of templates with detailed physical exams and reviews of systems to support reimbursement. However, this information often has minimal value for either patients or providers. Physicians developed standardized templates as workarounds to circumvent the repetitive and onerous task of documentation. Although these billing templates may provide a reasonably accurate assessment of a patient's status at a point in time, they are notoriously poor for conveying the larger picture of a patient's overall trajectory for a chronic disease such as cancer. Nor does this documentation provide useful information for quality reporting or practice improvement. Unlike HFCA rules for reimbursement, the purpose of the treatment plan/treatment summary initiative is to infuse meaning into medical recordkeeping.

Some medical events are straightforward to describe because they involve a particular date or procedure. When physicians want to know which surgical treatment a cancer patient has had, they know to ask for two critical documents: the operative report and the pathology report. Although these documents do not provide a summary of postoperative complications, they set forth—in a fairly standardized format—the reason for performing the operation, the procedure planned and actually performed, and any immediate complications.

In radiation oncology, the concept of a radiation treatment summary is widely accepted. When meeting with a patient who reports prior radiation at an outside hospital, physicians know to ask for this summary document. In most circumstances, they neither need nor want more detail than is included in this summary: typically the reason for radiation, the area radiated, the treatment planned, and the treatment actually delivered. Radiation oncologists may use different templates for this summary, some providing more or less accompanying narrative detail. However, the culture of radiation oncology is that all providers prepare some version of this key document.

In contrast to radiation and surgery, which constitute discrete episodes of care, a chemotherapy regimen has less clear boundaries. A regimen may be given once or over a period of years, and the amount of information that needs to be summarized may vary significantly. In some cases, patients may be given a three-drug regimen, develop an allergy to one drug, and have a component of the initial regimen discontinued or an alternative drug substituted. Patients may embark on long-term maintenance therapy with hormones. They sometimes temporarily stop treatment to relieve symptoms, to take a needed break from medication, or to attend to personal obligations. In this fashion, the boundaries of a chemotherapy regimen may become indistinct. Nevertheless, it is possible to provide some guidelines regarding what is meant by a "chemotherapy regimen" for those who will complete treatment summaries.

Oncologists share with other clinicians the challenge of complementing the chronological longitudinal approach to recordkeeping with succinct synopses. Treatment summaries are also recognized as important in the management of complex chronic care conditions such as mental illness with psychosis, diabetes, inflammatory bowel disease, and multiple sclerosis. Progress towards developing and implementing treatment summaries in these areas has been slower.

On the other hand, other health care professionals do create summary documents that provide overviews for lengthy episodes of health care that do not occur on a single date. For example, obstetricians have overviews that detail antepartum, pre-, intra- and postpartum care on a single page. These summaries are invaluable when a woman presents for a second pregnancy because the obstetrician can quickly determine a woman's level of obstetrical risk. Similarly, pediatricians have summary documents that record a child's immunization record, growth and development, and major childhood illnesses. These documents work well because most obstetrical and pediatric care adheres to a similar routine. Pediatric oncology offers another example. In pediatric oncology the Children's Oncology Group (COG) has drafted a treatment summary template for survivors of childhood cancer. In comparison, there are as of yet no accepted oncology-specific prototypes for adult oncology. Several promising initiatives are underway, however, to implement the recommendation of both the President's Cancer Panel and the IOM Committee on Cancer Survivorship. These efforts are focused on developing a care plan, treatment summary, and follow-up plan for patients finishing their primary treatment. With input from key stakeholders, ASCO has developed and has begun pilot testing a chemotherapy treatment summary. Certain cancer centers have developed their own treatment summaries (e.g., Memorial Sloan-Kettering Cancer Center, The Massey Cancer Center) and survivorship care plans (UCLA, Memorial Sloan-Kettering). These interrelated and complementary efforts have not yet converged on a single well-accepted standard. What is clear, however, is that the concept and goal is universally recognized and considered valuable by both patients and providers. The challenge is to develop consensus regarding the intended target audience for the summaries, how these documents should be structured, what they should contain, at what level of detail, and the timing for their completion. The objective of the ASCO initiative is to develop treatment plans in stages, beginning with core elements of a treatment plan and summary for other clinicians and for patients. Later stages will include cancer-specific versions, patient-oriented versions, and electronic versions that can be used as templates by electronic oncology record vendors. There is no expectation that we will arrive at a single document that will work in all circumstances. However, providing practitioners with a variety of templates that can be customized for particular practice needs and patient populations is a starting point.

IV. What Are the Key Elements in a Chemotherapy Treatment Plan and Treatment Summary?

Chemotherapy Treatment Plan

A chemotherapy *treatment plan* is a one-page document. It should include:

- Diagnosis: cancer site, histology and stage;
- Goals of therapy, anticipated benefits;
- Name of the regimen, the component drugs in the regimen, and the starting dosages;
- Duration of treatment and number of planned cycles;
- Strategy for assessing response;
- Side effects and precautions*;
- Assessment of risks and benefits; and alternatives.

Ideally, the document should be reviewed with the patient and his or her family member when a treatment is started. Because patients are often overwhelmed by information at the time of diagnosis and have difficulty assimilating information after receiving bad news, having a written treatment plan that could be referred to later by patients, family members, and potentially by other physicians, is a logical and sensible strategy. This is particularly relevant for non-English speakers and low-income patients, whose cancer care is often fragmented across providers or rotating trainees.

Chemotherapy Treatment Summary

A chemotherapy *treatment summary* is a succinct, ideally one-page document prepared at the end of a course of treatment or when a patient completes adjuvant therapy when a regimen is discontinued because of toxicity. The summary might be appended to the treatment plan. The treatment summary should include:

- The duration of treatment or the number of treatments planned and the number actually delivered;
- Whether any drugs were dropped from the regimen;

---

*The treatment summary is not designed to review every side effect of every agent since this information can be better provided on "chemotherapy fact cards" and through provision of other educational materials about what to anticipate during treatment. It is critical to emphasize that these are synopses, not comprehensive overviews.

- Any major toxicity and hospitalization resulting from treatment complications such as febrile neutropenia;
- Response to treatment (based on radiographic, biochemical, or clinical criteria, or combinations of these criteria;
- The reason treatment was discontinued;
- Planned next steps (e.g. hospice care, an alternative regimen, expectant management, posttreatment surveillance etc.);
- Who is responsible for performing follow-up and any other special monitoring.

Survivorship Care Plan

When cancer patients transition from active treatment to surveillance, and then from close surveillance to long-term survivorship, it is important to generate both a summary document that specifies any ongoing problems for that patient and schedules for follow-up evaluations and procedures.

Figure D.1-1 illustrates a draft ASCO treatment summary for a patient with stage III colon cancer. It was completed at the end of adjuvant therapy. This document is synoptic; that is, it does not include all details about the care provided. Although it is intended to be shared with patients, it includes enough detail for other treating health practitioners. These documents are not meant to replicate the medical record. The treatment plan/summary should include no more detail than two sides of a sheet of paper. This is consistent with most operative reports, hospital discharge summaries, pathology reports, pediatric records of growth and immunization, and other key synopses that are well-accepted in health care. The goal of the ASCO treatment summary initiative is to obtain consensus among oncology professionals about key elements. For now, it focuses on care coordination and traditional medical issues rather than on psychological well-being or secondary prevention such as tobacco use, nutrition, or exercise, though these are nonetheless recognized as very important.

V. Challenges for Implementation of Cancer Treatment Plans and Summaries

Changing the professional culture of medical oncology to include preparation of treatment plans and treatment summaries will be extremely challenging. Previous pilot work conducted by ASCO with volunteer physician practices indicates that although physicians think that treatment plans and summaries are important and worthwhile, the main obstacle to preparing them is limited time given their busy and demanding practices. Demonstrating that this mode of documentation can ultimately save rather than add time—particularly with development of electronic versions that are easy to

Adjuvant/Neoadjuvant Chemotherapy Treatment Summary

Patient Name:	Jennifer Smith
Patient ID#	1234567
Initial Diagnosis Date: October 2, 2005	
Start Date for This Treatment Course: 12/3/05	
End Date for this Treatment Course: 04/26/06	

1. Context of Treatment

Cancer Site: Cecal   Type/Histology:Adenoca   Molecular Features: MSI+

Stage at Initial Diagnosis: T3N2 IIIC   Performance Status at Start: ECOG 0

Reason for Treatment (Circle):   Adjuvant : YES   Neoadjuvant: NO

Treatment Combined with Radiation? (Circle) **No**   Yes

Recent Surgery for this cancer?   Emergent Right hemicolectomy Dr. Weiser 11/14/05

Important Comorbid Conditions? Type I diabetes, Pregnant at diagnosis, desires fertility

2. About This Regimen: Name: FOLFOX6   # of cycles: 12 Duration: 24 weeks

Drug Names: (Dose, Route)	Frequency	Dose Reduction	# of cycles given
5FU 400mg/m2 IV	Q2 wks	No	12
Leucovorin 400mg/m2	Q2 wks	Stopped Allergy	2
Oxaliplatin 85mg/m2	Q2 weeks	Yes	7
5FU 1200mg/m2 IVCI	Q2 weeks	Yes	12

3. How was treatment tolerated?

	No	Yes	Details
Any Grade 3-4 toxicity?		X	Neuropathy from oxaliplatin, Vomiting, Mucositis
Hospitalized for toxicity?		X	Dehydration and mucositis also from diabetes
Unusual problems with any drug?		X	Anaphylaxis to 2nd dose of leucovorin
Special supportive care measures?		X	Aprepitant for nausea and vomiting
Any persistent toxicities?		X	Resolving neuropathy
Were planned # of cycles given?		X	Oxaliplatin stopped early for neuropathy
Evidence of disease at end?	X		Normal CEA and CT scan at end

4. Next Steps:

What are planned next steps?	Yes	No	Details
Surgery	X		Ileostomy closure, August
Radiation		X	
Chemotherapy (eg hormones)		X	
Other therapy		X	May need hormone replacement
Post-treatment surveillance	X		As per standard guideline, but annual colonoscopy
Oncology Visits	X		Every 3 months for 1 year, then every 6 for 4 years
Lab Testing	X		CEA every 3 months
Radiology Evaluation(s)	X		CT of chest/abdomen/pelvis annually
Other Evaluations/Referrals	X		Mediport removal after surgery Colonoscopy in 11/06

FIGURE D.1-1 Draft treatment summary.

5. Care Coordination: Key Information for Other Providers

Treatment Consequences	Yes	No	Details
Persistent effects of treatment?	X		Persistent neuropathy—consider neurontin if not better in 3 months, also diabetic
Anticipated late effects?	X		May enter early menopause
Special precautions for future care?	X		SEVERE LEUCOVORIN ALLERGY
Special screening recommendation?	X		Annual uterine ultrasound, close eval for gyn bleeding
Psychosocial concerns?		X	No acute issues, post-treatment anxiety is common, social work referral made,
Reminders for oncology care:	X		Absolute contraindication to leucovorin, nausea responds to aprepitant
Reminders for general care:	X		Strong family history of early onset CC

Other Providers Name/Role	Contact Information
Dr. Weiser/Colorectal Surgery	212-639-6898
Beth Sferazza RN Stoma care Nurse	212-639-6578 for ?s and issues related to ostomy function
Dr. Jamison/PCP in NJ	203-123-4567
Carole Krueger-Social Work	212-456-3456
Dr. Offit/genetics	212-639-4567 Will evaluate with family members in the fall.
Dr. Kelly/Gyn/Reproductive Endo	201-567-1234
Dr. Salk/ Diabetologist	212-456-8956

Who to see, what to look for	Comments
Who will follow for late side effects, possible recurrence?	Dr. Schrag Will perform bloodwork and routine CEA and will add Hgb A1C and send to Dr. Salk.
Who will follow and perform routine health care maintenance?	Dr. Jamison-PCP Dr. Kelly, pap smear, routine GYN care
What symptoms are of concern?	Persistent tiredness, numbness and tingling of hands, blood in stool, change in bowel habits, unintentional weight loss, depressed mood.

Narrative Summary: Ms. Smith had a very rough time with her adjuvant chemotherapy course. She ultimately completed 7 cycles of FOLFOX and 5 of 5FU alone. She has a severe allergy to leucovorin and must never receive this agent. She also has persistent neuropathy from the oxaliplatin but it is gradually subsiding without pharmacologic intervention. Her coping skills have been remarkable and she has met with our social worker who has identified local cancer support resources in New Jersey. A post-treatment scan including a PET scan reveals no evidence of recurrent disease. Her CEA is 3. We have reviewed plans for post-treatment surveillance. We have decided to leave her Mediport until after her ileostomy closure in early August. We have made a follow-up in 3 months for routine surveillance, but she knows to call me sooner if the neuropathy does not continue to gradually subside from week to week. She will have routine follow-up are with Dr. Salk for her diabetes and Dr. Jamison for routine health needs but I will continue to see her every 3 months through 2007 and then every 6 as well as when she is hospitalized in August.

MD Signature _____

Date reviewed with patient_____

Cc: Drs. Weiser, Kelly, Salk, Jamison.

complete—will be necessary for their widespread adoption as a part of routine practice. Reimbursement for completing the summaries and liability issues are secondary concerns. Overall, a profound cultural shift will be required to change entrenched practice patterns.

Who Is the Primary Target Audience?

This section addresses some of the most frequent questions and concerns that have been raised by oncologists, primary care physicians, active patients, and survivors during the early development phases of the ASCO initiative.

The target audience for treatment plans and summaries includes both patients and health care providers; however, it is a challenge to address both audiences effectively with the same document. ASCO's early versions of a summary (Figure D.1-1) are geared more towards health care providers than patients. Although technical, rather than lay language is used to convey material succinctly, the goal is for oncologists to use these summaries as a springboard for discussion with patients. A treatment plan/summary prepared for the patient would look somewhat different but could constitute the next phase of development.

For any version, the core elements would be consistent but the language and terminology would vary based on who the primary user will be. If it is the patient, then the summary should use Standard English and avoid medical terminology. If nononcology health care providers are the intended recipients, medical terminology without the use of oncology-specific abbreviations and jargon is appropriate. If other oncologists are the intended audience, details including regimen names and oncology-specific abbreviations are appropriate and helpful.

It is neither feasible nor practical to have separate documents geared towards distinct audiences because of the time and workload required to prepare these documents. At present, the goal is to develop a version that is relatively free of oncology-specific jargon and therefore suitable for nononcology medical providers. Ideally, preparation of these documents will trigger conversations between patients and physicians that clarify meaning and any unfamiliar terms. To some extent, the level of the detail and tone of the document should also vary based on the disease context. For example, patients with advanced metastatic cancer are cared for by oncology professionals or palliative care professionals who are familiar with cancer-related terms and abbreviations. A patient with chronic myelogenous leukemia, metastatic breast, ovarian, or prostate cancer may be followed for many years and across many sites of care. However, a primary oncologist is likely to remain involved in management. In these situations, it is reasonable to anticipate that the summary will be reviewed most frequently by other oncologists. In contrast, when patients complete treatment for early stage disease such as adjuvant or primary therapy (and pass through the customary subsequent period of close surveillance) they will transition to a nononcologist, likely their primary care physician. In this case, the target audience will be a nononcology health care professional and the context of care should influence the detail oncologists provide.

The ASCO draft summaries are intended to be used by patients and providers of all types, but they focus primarily on use by nononcologist physicians, based on the presumption that they are the group most likely to need to know the details of prior treatment. ASCO's rationale for this is that the primary goal of the treatment summary is to facilitate coordination of care for patients as they navigate through a complex fragmented health care system. Patients themselves should be encouraged not only to keep but also to provide a copy of their treatment summary and plan for follow up to future health care provider. Because of the documents' more general medical language, many patients will understand their details with little difficulty. Some patients will use these summary documents as the basis of discussion.

When Should a Summary Be Prepared?

There are many situations in oncology where it makes sense to prepare a summary: for example, at the end of a course of adjuvant therapy, or at the completion of primary curative therapy. There are other situations where it is less clear. For patients with chronic diseases like low-grade lymphoma, the duration of one treatment may be many months. It is not possible to define the precise time interval of various treatments. In general, whenever there is a substantial change in treatment or a regimen is completed, a summary should be prepared. Specific time points, such as those developed by the National Comprehensive Cancer Network, can be built into guidelines.[8] However, these determinations will also involve judgment on the part of individual physicians.

What Is the Right Platform—Paper or Computer?

The optimal strategy for development of treatment summaries is to integrate them as components of electronic health record systems. If these documents are three-dimensional with branching logic, drop-down menus, and checklists, they will be able to capture more important detail more succinctly and efficiently. ASCO is committed to developing electronic versions that can be downloaded, used, and modified.

However, many oncology practices still rely entirely on paper for recordkeeping and of the few oncology practices that have true electronic medical records, many use systems that are hard to adapt. Therefore, development must proceed on several fronts simultaneously: paper versions that can be completed by pen, templates for telephone dictation, and electronic versions. Priority should be given to developing an electronic version, given its greater capabilities. Health information technology vendors are competing to develop oncology products, and achieving consensus on the core elements of summary documents will advance their timely incorporation into electronic health record systems.

Static or Living Document?

Treatment summaries will need to be updated as screening recommendations change, as recurrences that warrant additional testing arise, and as new evidence on late effects emerge. For patients with metastatic disease, an old treatment plan and summary will be superseded by a new one. For patients who have completed therapy, recommendations for screening or follow-up may change. However, because the goal is not to replace the medical record, which provides a longitudinal comprehensive record of care, even a summary that is not updated is still likely to be valuable.

Some physicians are concerned about their liability exposure: for example, if a screening recommendation changes but a form is not updated. A solution may be to date the documents and make it clear to patients that recommendations included in summaries may become outdated. Such concerns, however, should not impede the ultimate goal of having useful summaries that can be shared.

Can This Activity Be Reimbursed?

Preparation of a treatment summary and reviewing the material with a patient is considered complex coordination of care and can be submitted for payment using level four or level five codes for evaluation and management. There is no reason to expect that insurers would not reimburse providers for this service; however, it is not clear that preparation of the summary would be a reimbursed service if it did not include face-to-face interaction with the patient.

Should There Be One or Several Versions of the Treatment Plan/Summary?

Developing a template that works for all situations in oncology is a challenge. ASCO's goal is to make sample templates freely available to encourage its membership to prepare these documents, review them with patients, and adapt and improve them. Pilot experience suggests that the information that is needed on a summary for patients with metastatic disease who transition from one treatment to the next is quite different from what is needed for patients who have completed adjuvant or primary curative therapy. For this reason, at least two templates are needed: one for patients following a course of adjuvant/neoadjuvant therapy, and one for patients with advanced disease. These synoptic documents will be most useful if they are tailored to the specific disease. If these templates are available in modifiable format, oncologists will be able to customize and adapt them to suit their own specific purposes based on the types of patients they see. ASCO can create a repository to serve as a clearinghouse for sharing these documents as different versions are developed. The goal is to create a source for open-access to nonproprietary templates that include core elements and standard vocabularies for those elements (e.g., staging). Adaptations based on extent and type of disease could build on these core elements.

How Can Implementation Be Encouraged?

Few patients currently receive a treatment plan or summary. Ensuring that all cancer patients receive these summaries will require fundamental change in how oncologists deliver care. Changing deeply embedded practice and documentation patterns, however, will not be easy. Even with its strong influence, ASCO may not be able to accomplish this without support and encouragement from other stakeholders. For adoption of treatment plans and summaries on a widespread basis, implementation will need to proceed along several fronts. Patient advocacy groups like NCCS can encourage patients to ask for these documents. Other organizations such as the American Board of Internal Medicine and the National Committee for Quality Assurance can include this aspect of oncology care in their provider evaluations. Improvements in care could be made by adopting as a standard measure of quality patients' receipt of treatment plans and summaries and through initiatives designed to reengineer the culture of medical record-keeping.

Electronic medical record vendors can embed treatment plan and summary templates in their systems. Payors could facilitate their adoption by explicitly reimbursing providers for the work of developing treatment plans and summaries and posttreatment planning and reviewing them with patients.

Coordinating care and communicating with patients about their treatments may be the most valued services oncologists provide and should be encouraged. Currently, oncologists are not well compensated for developing mutually agreed-upon treatment plans or posttreatment surveillance plans following completion of adjuvant therapy, for engaging in discussions regarding whether or not to administer chemotherapy, or for implementing an end-of-life care plan.

Altering traditions and entrenched systems requires great effort. However, it is imperative to align the reimbursement system with services that can foster patient-centered high quality care. In collaboration with major health care payers, particularly the Centers for Medicare and Medicaid Services, policymakers must work to modify the current reimbursement system to ensure that providers are appropriately compensated for these essential cognitive services that are highly valued by patients rather than rewarded for spending inordinate amounts of time complying with billing rules mandating documentation of detailed physical exams and reviews of systems that do not improve care.

Can Nononcology Professionals Prepare These Summaries?

Some hospitals rely on nononcology professionals to prepare discharge summaries. This is particularly the case when these discharge summaries are focused on maximizing reimbursement. However, because the goal of this treatment planning/summary effort is to foster dialogue between oncologists and their patients, oncologists should engage directly in this process. Some aspects of the plan or summary could be completed by support staff or nurses in the hospital or oncology practice. In fully electronic environments, the formulary and pharmacy records of treatments given could populate fields in a treatment plan and treatment summary Both oncology physicians and oncology nurses can, and should, review the treatment summary with their patients. Ultimately the treatment summary is not a valuable activity if it is purely an administrative or secretarial chore.

VI. Conclusion

Increasingly, problems relating to coordination and communication have been recognized as hampering the delivery of high quality cancer care. The goal of the treatment plan and summary is to achieve meaningful improvement in cancer care delivery and the patient experience. Changing the culture of documentation is intended to facilitate improved dialogue between patients and their health care providers. With some behavior change and restructuring of documentation requirements, it should be possible to foster better coordination and communication and more readily track cancer treatment histories in medical records. This initiative will depend upon standardized forms, ideally in electronic formats that are made freely available. As a first step, pilot work will be necessary to develop templates that work across diverse practice sites and in diverse clinical situations. The transition to survivorship for patients who have completed

curative therapy or adjuvant/neoadjuvant treatment is a logical and important starting place because of the large and increasing numbers of cancer
patients who are making this transition. Patients, payors, and providers
must all engage in this process. If a critical mass of providers engages in this
effort, a "tipping point" will be reached such that all providers will begin to
participate in this process to conform to the standards of their peers. Professional organizations like ASCO, in partnership with patient advocacy organizations, can facilitate this process by developing consensus regarding
what key elements these documents should include and by ensuring that
reimbursement is linked to documentation that is accessible and useful to
patients and physicians. Changing the professional culture and accepted
practices of documentation and aligning incentives to support this effort
should promote better communication and coordination. As a result, we
can achieve meaningful improvement in the quality of cancer care.

REFERENCES

1. Schrag D. Communication and coordination: the keys to quality. *J Clin Oncol.* Sep 20 2005;23(27):6452-6455.
2. Institute of Medicine. *To Err Is Human: Building a Safer Health System.* Washington, D.C.: National Academy Press; 2000.
3. Institute of Medicine. *Crossing the Quality Chasm: A New Health System for the 21st Century.* Washington, D.C.: National Academy Press; 2001.
4. Institute of Medicine. *1st Annual Crossing the Quality Chasm Summit: A Focus on Communities.* Washington, D.C.: The National Academies Press; 2004.
5. Ayanian JZ, Chrischilles EA, Fletcher RH, et al. Understanding cancer treatment and outcomes: the Cancer Care Outcomes Research and Surveillance Consortium. *J Clin Oncol.* Aug 1 2004;22(15):2992-2996.
6. Malin JL, Schneider EC, Epstein AM, Adams J, Emanuel EJ, Kahn KL. Results of the National Initiative for Cancer Care Quality: how can we improve the quality of cancer care in the United States? *J Clin Oncol.* Feb 1 2006;24(4):626-634.
7. Ayanian JZ, Zaslavsky AM, Guadagnoli E, et al. Patients' perceptions of quality of care for colorectal cancer by race, ethnicity, and language. *J Clin Oncol.* Sep 20 2005;23(27):6576-6586.
8. National Comprehensive Cancer Network. National Comprehensive Cancer Network. http://www.nccn.org/. Accessed May 24, 2006.

Appendix D.2

Recommendations for Health Behavior and Wellness Following Primary Treatment for Cancer

Lee W. Jones, PhD*
Wendy Demark-Wahnefried, PhD, RD, LDN**

Introduction

Every 23 seconds, an American is diagnosed with cancer.[1] Given advances in early detection and treatment, 64% of those diagnosed with this disease can expect to be alive in 5 years.[1] These individuals will join the ever-expanding numbers of cancer survivors who now number over 10 million and constitute 3-4% of the U.S. population.[2,3] While these numbers are encouraging, it is important to acknowledge that the impact of cancer is significant and associated with several long-term health and psychosocial sequelae.[2-15] Indeed, cancer survivors constitute a vulnerable population who have distinct health care needs.[7,16] Data clearly show that compared to general age- and race-matched populations, cancer survivors are at greater risk for developing second malignancies and other diseases, such as cardiovascular disease (CVD), diabetes, and osteoporosis.[2-16] An early comparison by Brown et al.[6] of over 1.2 million patient records obtained from the SEER database with those obtained from the National Center for Health Statistics found a significantly higher noncancer relative hazards ratio for cancer patients of 1.37 and concluded that "the evidence that cancer patients die of noncancer causes at a higher rate than persons in the general population is overwhelming." Data collected over the past decade confirm these findings.[2-4,8,17] These competing causes of death and comorbid conditions are believed to result from cancer treatment, genetic predisposition, and/or common lifestyle factors.[2,4,13-15]

---

*Department of Surgery, Duke University Medical Center
**Department of Surgery and School of Nursing, Duke University Medical Center

Hewitt et al.[10] also report that cancer survivors have almost a two-fold increase in having at least one functional limitation, and in the presence of another comorbid condition the odds ratio increases to 5.06 (95%CI 4.47-5.72). These findings have been confirmed by other studies in diverse populations of cancer survivors.[18-23] From an economic perspective, an analysis by Chirikos et al.[24] indicated that "the economic consequence of functional impairment exacts an enormous toll each year on cancer survivors, their families and the American economy at large"[24], findings confirmed by others.[25-28]

Based on these national trends, cancer survivorship is fast emerging as a public health concern and has been set as a national priority.[2-5,8,13] In a recent Institute of Medicine (IOM) report entitled "From Cancer Patient to Cancer Survivor: Lost in Transition,"[29] the numerous health issues of cancer survivors were summarized, and the potential benefits of lifestyle modifications were briefly reviewed. From this report, recommendations were put forth to guide health care providers, patient advocates, and other stakeholders in an effort to improve the health and well-being of this rapidly expanding and high-risk population—a population that heretofore "has been relatively neglected in terms of advocacy, education, clinical practice and research."[29] The goal of this paper is to review these recommendations in light of more recent advances, with the following topic areas addressed: (1) strength of evidence for recommendations in areas of weight management, diet, exercise, smoking cessation, as well as other areas, such as alcohol and sunscreen use, complementary and alternative therapies, management of osteoporosis, and immunizations; (2) perceived needs of cancer survivors for health information and preferred channels of delivery; and (3) resources available to providers and patients regarding healthful lifestyle practices. To this end, gaps in the IOM report were identified and in addition, an updated search of literature published within the past 2 years was performed using CancerLit, PubMed, and Medline databases and employing search terms of cancer survivor(s) or neoplasms/survivor cross-referenced with MeSH terms of lifestyle, health behavior, cardiovascular training, rehabilitation, physical fitness, physical activity, exercise, body weight, obesity, weight loss, diet, nutrition, complementary therapies, dietary supplements, tobacco, smoking cessation, alcohol drinking, sunprotective agents, osteoporosis, immunization and intervention studies. Relevant articles were then hand-searched for pertinent previously published papers.

Health Promotion Concerns for Cancer Survivors

Weight Management

Positive and negative energy balance are dual concerns in cancer populations. For some groups of survivors, such as those diagnosed with select respiratory, gastrointestinal or childhood cancers, or those living with advanced-staged disease, anorexia and cachexia may be problems that persist after primary treatment.[30-32] For these survivors, continued supportive care therapies including dietary counseling and the potential use of pharmacotherapy (e.g., megestrol acetate) and/or nutritional support may be critical for recovery and may enhance the ability to eat and to maintain adequate nutritional stores[30,31,33] that are important for improved functional status and well-being.[34] Physical activity also may help to increase appetite, relieve constipation, and improve quality of life in these survivors.[35] As noted in the IOM report,[29] as critical as anorexia and cachexia are to cancer care, for the majority of cancer survivors, obesity and overweight are problems that are far more prevalent.[35-37] Obesity is a well-established risk factor for cancers of the breast (postmenopausal), colon, kidney (renal cell), esophagus (adenocarcinoma), and endometrium;[38,39] thus a high proportion of cancer survivors are overweight or obese at the time of diagnosis. Furthermore, increased premorbid body weight has been associated with cancer mortality for cancers of the breast, esophagus, colon and rectum, cervix, uterus, liver, gallbladder, stomach, pancreas, prostate, kidney, non-Hodgkin's lymphoma and multiple myeloma, as well as all cancers combined.[40-42] Finally, additional weight gain is common during or after treatment for various cancers, and may exacerbate risk for functional decline, comorbidity and perhaps even cancer recurrence and cancer-related death.[43-45] While studies exploring the relationship of post-diagnosis weight gain and survival have been somewhat inconsistent,[45-50] the most recent published study by Kroenke and colleagues,[45] the largest to date (N=5,204), suggests that breast cancer survivors who increased their BMI by 0.5 to 2 units were found to have a relative risk (RR) of recurrence of 1.40 (95% CI: 1.02-1.92) and those who gained more than 2.0 BMI units had a RR of 1.53 (95% CI: 1.54-2.34); both groups also experienced significantly higher all-cause mortality. In addition, several studies have reported that increased body weight post-diagnosis negatively impacts quality of life.[37,44,51] This accumulating evidence of adverse effects of obesity in cancer survivors, plus evidence indicating that obesity has negative consequences for overall health and physical function make the pursuit of weight management a priority for cancer survivors,[35,37,52-55]—a priority that is substantiated through viable physiologic mechanisms,[55-57] as well as concern that the health issues of this population are overlaid upon the pandemic of overweight and obesity currently existing in this nation.[41,58]

Despite the demonstrated adverse effects of obesity in cancer survivors, only five reported studies have examined weight management in cancer populations and all were conducted among women with breast cancer. Two of these studies were performed largely on survivors who had completed active treatment, and found that individualized dietary counseling provided by a dietitian was effective in promoting weight loss.[59,60] The more recent study by Djuric and colleagues[60] found that counseling by a dietitian was most effective if combined with a structured Weight Watchers® program which included exercise with weight change at 12 months being +.85 ± 6.0 kg vs. −8.0 ± 5.5 kg or −9.4 ± 8.6 kg in the control versus dietitian or dietitian plus Weight Watchers® program, respectively. Multiple behavior interventions that utilize a comprehensive approach to energy balance, and that include both diet and exercise components may have the potential to be more effective than interventions relying on either component alone.[61] In their evaluation of a diet and exercise intervention among early stage breast cancer patients which was begun during the time of treatment and extended throughout the year following diagnosis, Goodwin et al. found that exercise was the strongest predictor of weight loss.[62,211,212] Given evidence that sarcopenic obesity (gain of adipose tissue at the expense of lean body mass) is a documented side effect of both chemotherapy and hormonal therapy,[63-67] exercise, especially strength training exercise, may be of particular importance for cancer survivors since it is considered the cornerstone of treatment for this condition.[68] To date, however, only one study has reported the physiologic effects of resistance training exercise in cancer survivors, a pilot study by McKenzie and Kalda[69] where preliminary data suggest that arm exercises among breast cancer patients are safe and not associated with increased risk of lymphedema, but where no outcomes exist regarding body composition.[69]

As noted in the IOM report[29] and the research of others,[70] cancer survivors also may have particular problems with self-esteem and depression that may undermine the ultimate success of weight management programs. More research is needed to develop interventions that not only address the unique physiological needs of this population, but also their distinct psychological issues as well. Until more is known, guidelines established for weight management in general populations should be applied to cancer survivors, and include not only dietary and exercise components, but also behavior therapy.[71] With research indicating that 70% of cancer survivors are overweight or obese, there is a definite need to develop effective weight management interventions for this needy population.[52]

Nutrition and Diet

Energy Restriction

As noted in the previous section, accumulating evidence suggests that weight management should be the uppermost nutritional priority for cancer survivors. Thus, for the majority of cancer survivors who are overweight, energy-restricted diets are recommended. [35,52,54,55] Moderate energy deficits of up to 1,000 calories/day can be achieved by concomitantly increasing energy expenditure (via exercise) and reducing energy intake. Energy restriction can be achieved by reducing the energy density of the diet by substituting low-energy density foods (e.g., water-rich vegetables, fruits, cooked whole grains, soups) for foods that are higher in calories.[72] This "volumetric approach" can enhance satiety and reduce feelings of hunger and deprivation that often serve to undermine energy-restricted diets. An additional strategy is limiting portion sizes of energy dense foods.[73-77] Newly issued dietary guidelines for cancer survivors will emphasize energy balance and by and large endorse dietary recommendations that have been established for the primary prevention of cancer and other chronic diseases.[28,35,52,78,79]

Balancing Fat, Protein, and Carbohydrate Intake

Protein, carbohydrate, and fat all contribute energy (calories) in the diet, and each of these dietary constituents is available from a wide variety of foods. Making informed choices about foods that provide these macronutrients can ensure variety and nutrient adequacy. In general, the choice of foods and their proportions within an overall diet (dietary pattern) may be more important than absolute amounts.[35,37,58] Given that cancer survivors are at high risk for other chronic diseases, the recommended amounts and type of fat, protein, and carbohydrate to reduce these disease risks also are germane.[35] A 2005 study by Kroenke et al. of 2,619 breast cancer survivors participating in the Nurse's Health study suggests that those who report a prudent diet (e.g., high proportional intakes of fruits, vegetables, whole grains, and low-fat dairy products) had significantly lower mortality from non-breast cancer causes compared to those who reported a Western-type diet (e.g., high proportional intakes of meat, refined grains, high-fat dairy products, and desserts).[79]

Fat

To date, 14 studies examining the relationship between fat intake and survival after the diagnosis of breast cancer have been reported, and the results are notably inconsistent.[80] In prostate cancer, only one study has explored the association between fat intake and survival and found that saturated fat intake (but not total fat) was associated with worse survival.[81] One recently completed study (Women's Intervention Nutrition Study [WINS]) and one ongoing study (Women's Healthy Eating and Living study [WHEL]), were designed to test whether a reduction in fat intake can reduce risk for recurrence and increase overall survival in women who were diagnosed with early stage breast cancer.[82,83] Preliminary results from the WINS study suggest that women assigned to the low-fat diet arm (< 15% energy from fat) exhibited a 24% reduction in risk for recurrence; with subset analyses suggesting that this effect was even greater among women with ER-disease (i.e., 42%).[82] The main results from the WHEL Study are anticipated by 2008; however to date, the low fat, high fruit and vegetable intervention has been found to significantly reduce estradiol levels.[84] It should be noted that four other randomized controlled trials have been reported among cancer survivors that were aimed at determining the efficacy of individualized counseling, group classes or volunteer-led programs in reducing fat intake. All of these programs were effective in promoting dietary change, and three of the four studies resulted in significant weight loss.[85-88]

Some types of fat, such as monounsaturates, are associated with reduced risk for heart disease and possibly cancer, whereas others, such as saturated fats, are associated with increased risks.[58,89] Some studies have suggested that omega-3 fatty acids may have specific benefits for cancer survivors.[89] However, in light of a recent systematic review by MacLean et al. [90] which found little support for any protective association between omega-3 fatty acids and cancer risk, more research is required. That said, consuming foods that are rich in omega-3 fatty acids, such as fish and walnuts, should be encouraged because of the strong relationship between omega 3 intake and reduced risk for cardiovascular disease (CVD) and overall mortality.[90-92] Currently, the recommended level of fat in the diet is 20-35% of energy, with saturated fat intake limited to <10% and trans fatty acids limited to <3% of total energy intake.[58]

Protein

To date, few studies have examined the relationship between protein intake and cancer specific outcomes in humans. One study, however, found that, increased intakes of red meat, bacon and liver were associated with recurrence among early-stage breast cancer survivors.[93] Given these data, as well as strong evidence that red meat and processed meat are associated with increased primary risk for colorectal cancer, survivors are encouraged to limit their consumption of these foods.[35,89] Protein intakes of roughly 0.8 g/kg of body weight are recommended with 10-35% of energy coming from protein.[94]

Carbohydrates

As with protein, little research has been undertaken with regard to carbohydrates (starches, sugars and fiber) and cancer survival, though fiber has been explored extensively with regard to recurrence of precancerous lesions (e.g., colorectal adenomas),[95,96] where it's role may be influenced by gender and is still unclear. Given that glycemic control is a newly emerging area of interest in relation to cancer, more research is anticipated in this area in the next few years.[97] Given a lack of definitive data, survivors are encouraged to follow dietary guidelines established for the prevention of chronic diseases that endorse intakes of carbohydrates ranging from 45-65% of total energy intake and fiber intakes of 14 g. per 1,000 kcal.[58] Carbohydrates should come primarily from nutrient-dense food sources, such as vegetables, whole fruits, and whole grains—low-energy density foods that promote satiety, and weight control, while enhancing nutrient adequacy.[35,58,75] Refined carbohydrates and sugars are discouraged given their relative lack of nutritional benefit and their contribution to energy intake.[35,58,91]

Vegetables and Fruits

Given high concentrations of various phytochemicals, anti-oxidants, and fiber, vegetables and fruits have been promoted not only among healthy populations for the prevention of cancer, but also among cancer survivors.[35,75,89] In the 10 observational studies that have examined the relationship between intakes of vegetables and fruit (or nutrients indicative of those foods) and risk for cancer recurrence, the evidence has been mixed. Half of the studies have observed a significant protective effect of fruits or vegetables in general, or specific items or families of items, such as tomato sauce or cruciferae, and the other half found no associations.[35] However, plasma carotenoids (a marker of vegetable and fruit intake) have been associated with greater likelihood of recurrence-free survival in one observational study.[98] Results of the WHEL study, which not only promotes a low fat diet, but also daily minimum intakes of five vegetable and three fruit servings, 16 oz. of vegetable juice, and 30 g of dietary fiber should be helpful in assessing the impact of a high vegetable and fruit diet among survivors.[83,99] In the meantime, cancer survivors are encouraged to consume amounts consistent with guidelines established for survivors and the U.S. Dietary Guidelines, i.e., at least five daily servings, with an ultimate goal of at least seven (for women) to nine (for men) daily servings.[35,58,91]

Specific Foods or Dietary Regimens

While various functional foods and dietary regimens have been identified as being potentially helpful in hindering progressive or recurrent disease among cancer survivors, to date, there is little consensus or results from randomized controlled trials, to support the use of specific foods, such as soy or regimens, such as macrobiotic diets. Guidelines therefore call for a varied diet that is based on principles of moderation.[35,89]

Exercise

In recent years, several research groups have started to examine the potential effects of exercise as a supportive care intervention that may compliment existing anticancer therapies and address a multitude of concerns associated with cancer and its treatment. The Institute of Medicine report on exercise behavior for cancer survivors was primarily based on the 2004 Agency for Healthcare Research and Quality (AHRQ) evidence review.[61] In the interim, four other systematic reviews have been published and summarize current evidence on exercise and adult cancer survivors.[100-103] In total, these five reviews identified 16 independent research investigations that examined the role of exercise in cancer survivors following the completion of primary therapy. To summarize, most studies were conducted in breast cancer survivors with fewer studies in colorectal, non-Hodgkin's lymphoma, or mixed cancer populations. All studies either tested the effects of endurance or mixed (endurance combined with progressive resistance training) exercise training programs prescribed at a moderate-vigorous intensity (50-75% of baseline exercise capacity), 3 or more days per week, for 10 to 60 minutes per exercise session. The length of the exercise programs lasted from 2 to 15 weeks. Major outcomes of these reports were varied and included cardiorespiratory fitness, strength, quality of life, pain, immune parameters, and depression. Overall, these reports conclude that exercise interventions following completion of primary treatment were associated with consistent and positive effects on the following outcomes: (1) vigor and vitality; (2) cardiorespiratory fitness; (3) quality of life; (4) depression; (5) anxiety; and (6) fatigue.[61,101-103] Despite these positive findings, all four reviews concluded that the current putative literature provides *promising preliminary* evidence of the potential role of exercise in this setting and that additional large-scale, well-controlled intervention studies are required.[61,101-103]

In this updated review, we have examined eight additional independent studies[104-111] that have been published during the past year and evaluate them against the back-drop of published reviews and reports. Similar to the studies reviewed in the IOM (AHRQ) report and the three prior systematic reviews, these recent studies continue to predominantly focus on breast cancer[104-106,108,110,111] with one study each in lung[109] and mixed cancer patients.[107] Most studies tested the effects of a combined endurance and progressive resistance training program,[104-111] two used endurance only,[110,111] and one used resistance training only.[105] The intervention length ranged from 2 to 12 months, and study endpoints were varied and included cardiorespiratory fitness, quality of life indices, lymphedema, body composition, and metabolic hormone profile. Overall, the results of these eight recent studies support previous findings; significant benefits of exercise on several identified study endpoints are presented in Table D.2-1.

These findings corroborate the conclusions of the 2004 AHRQ report and the other systematic reviews suggesting that exercise is associated with a moderately positive effect on cardiorespiratory fitness and quality of life.[61,101-103] Exercise also was generally associated with a small positive effect on other outcomes of interest, such as fatigue, anxiety, and depression. Importantly, no study reported any exercise-related adverse events. However, additional large-scale, well-controlled intervention studies in other cancer populations, as well as breast cancer survivors, are required that provide a comprehensive examination of safety issues.

Since the IOM report, two recent landmark studies have been reported that examined the association between physical activity and cancer recurrence and overall survival in persons diagnosed with breast[112] and colon cancer.[113] In the first study, Holmes and colleagues examined the association between self-reported physical activity levels and breast cancer recurrence and mortality in a cohort of 2,987 female nurses participating in the Nurses Health Study who had been diagnosed with early-stage breast cancer.[112] Results indicated that women who engaged in 9 or more metabolic equivalent (MET) hours per week (equivalent to brisk walking for 1 hour, 5 days/wk) had an unadjusted absolute mortality risk reduction of 6% at 10 years compared with women who engaged in less than 3 MET hours per week (equivalent to walking at an average pace for 1 hour).[112] In the second study, Meyerhardt et al.[113] examined the influence of self-reported physical activity on outcome in 816 patients with colon cancer. After adjustment for medical and demographic variables, preliminary results indicated that men and women who engaged in more than 25 MET-hours of physical activity per week had a hazards ratio for disease-free survival of 0.65 (95% CI, 0.38-1.11; p for trend = 0.02) compared with patients who reported low levels of physical activity.[113] These are the first reports to examine the association between exercise behavior and cancer recurrence and survival. Overall, these results significantly strengthen the evidence supporting the role of exercise for cancer survivors following the completion of primary treatment. Large-scale randomized controlled trials are now required to confirm these exciting and important findings.

Although much work remains to be done, the current literature provides sufficient evidence that exercise is a safe and well-tolerated supportive intervention that physicians can recommend to their patients following the completion of primary therapy. Clearly, as in other clinical and nonclinical populations, cancer survivors should obtain physician/oncologist clearance before embarking on any exercise intervention or program. This may be particularly important in cancer survivors who may be at high risk for late-occurring toxicity secondary to treatment. For example, anthracycline-based chemotherapy regimens and left-sided chest radiotherapy are associated with acute and late-occurring cardiac toxicity,[114-117] whereas conventional anticancer therapies are associated with several progressive disorders such as endothelial dysfunction,[118] and weight gain.[63,119] Either one or a combination of these disorders increases patients' risk of CVD. Thus, appropriate CVD and cardiac screening procedures are recommended prior to the initiation of an exercise program. One additional long-term concern in breast cancer survivors initiating an exercise program is lymphedema. Although few studies have examined this question, the current evidence suggests that upper body exercise does not induce or exacerbate lymphedema.[61] However, as stated in the IOM report, further research is required on this topic to formulate appropriate exercise prescriptions for women with or at risk for lymphedema;[61] it is important to note that a gap in research still remains, since there have been no published studies in the interim. Until more evidence is available, current recommendations of the American Cancer Society, the Centers for Disease Control, and the American College of Sports Medicine are advised: engage in at least moderate activity for 30 minutes or more on 5 or more days per week (see Table D.2-2).[35,89]

Smoking Cessation

As noted in the IOM report, nearly one-third of all cancers are caused by smoking; thus, there is a high likelihood of tobacco use among survivors, especially those who have been diagnosed with smoking-related malignancies, i.e., lung, head and neck, cervix, bladder, kidney, pancreas, and myeloid leukemia.[120,121] Persistent tobacco use postdiagnosis also is associated with poorer outcomes, including increased complications of treatment, progressive disease, second primaries, and increased comorbidity.[122,123] Thus, while smoking cessation plays a substantial role in prevention and primary care, it is perhaps even more critical for cancer survivors to quit smoking.[124] Fortunately, many survivors respond to the "teachable moment" that a cancer diagnosis provides,[125] and high quit rates are noted (~50%) among survivors with smoking-related tumors.[78,126] Unfortunately, many survivors are unable to remain smoke-free, with approximately one-third of smokers continuing to smoke after their cancer diagnosis.[78] Recent data from the National Health Interview Survey also suggest that current smoking rates may be especially high in younger cancer survivors (ages 18-40) than in the general population,[127] though subsequent controlled analyses on data with longer follow-up suggest that these differences may not be as discrepant as previously thought.[128]

Given evidence that combined interventions that utilize behavioral

TABLE D.2-1 Exercise Studies Following the Completion of Primary Therapy (authors in alphabetical order)

Authors, Year	Site	Sample	Age	Design	Exercise Intervention
Damush et al.[111]	Breast	34 survivors an average of 3 yr post treatment	59.6	Pre-Post	Oncologist-referred self-management program to increase physical activity
Lane et al.[104]	Breast	16 dragon boat participants with no history lymphedema	52.4	Pre-Post	Resistance and endurance exercise training program with dragon boat training
Ohira et al.[105]	Breast	86 survivors an average of 2 yr post diagnosis	Exercise (53) Control (53)	RCT	Progressive resistance exercise training program
Pinto et al. [106]	Breast	86 survivors an average of 2 yr post diagnosis	Exercise (53) Control (53)	RCT	Home-based physical activity intervention program
Thorsen et al.[107]	Mixed	139 lymphoma, breast, gyneco- logic, or testicu- lar survivors an average of 1 month post treatment	Exercise (39) Control (39)	RCT	Home-based endurance and resistance exercise training program
Cheema et al.[108]	Breast	34 dragon-boat survivors an average of 5 yr post treatment	57.7	Pre-Post	Combined supervised resistance and endurance exercise training program
Spruit et al. [109]	Lung	10 survivors an average of 3 months post treatment	65.5	Pre-post	Combined supervised resistance and endurance exercise training program
Wilson et al. [110]	Breast	24 African- American survivors an average of 3 month post treatment	55	Pre-post	Theory-based community-based walking program

ABBREVIATIONS: IGF-II, Insulin-like growth factor II; METs, metabolic equivalent; QOL, quality of life; RCT, randomized controlled trial; RPE, rate of perceived exertion; VO_{2peak}, Peak Oxygen Consumption $(mL.kg.min^{-1})$.

Duration	Frequency/ Intensity	Results
6 months	3×/wk 1-hr sessions for 3 weeks and telephone support	Statistically significant ↑ in self-reported physical activity, physical fitness, perceived barriers to exercise, and QOL
5 months	3×/wk resistance (8-12 repetitions of 6 different exercises) and 3×/wk endurance (60% of maximum heart rate) exercise training. Dragon boat training 2×/wk for 90 min	Statistically significant ↑ in upper extremity strength and volume over the course of the intervention. Changes consistent on both arms
6 months	2×/wk 1-hr supervised sessions for 13 weeks followed by 2×/wk home-based sessions for 13 weeks	Statistically significant ↑ overall QOL, upper and lower body strength, ↓ body fat and IGF-II. Changes in strength were correlated with changes in some psychosocial outcomes
3 months (follow-up at 6 and 9 months)	5×/wk for 12 weeks at 55% to 65% of maximum heart rate	Statistically significant ↑ total and moderate physical activity minutes and physical fitness. Exercise group reported ↑ vigor and ↓ fatigue
14 weeks	Minimum of 2 sessions/wk at 60% to 70% of maximum heart rate	Exercise had greater increase in cardiorespiratory fitness and fatigue in comparison with control group
2 months	2×/wk resistance (8-12 repetitions of 10 different exercises) and 3×/wk endurance (65% to 85% of maximum heart rate) exercise training sessions	Statistically significant ↑ in body composition, upper and lower body strength, aerobic endurance and overall QOL
2 months	Daily cycle ergometry, treadmill walking, weight training and gymnastics at a moderate intensity	Statistically significant ↑ in peak and endurance exercise capacity. No improvements in pulmonary function
2 months (follow-up at 3 months)	8 weekly 75 minute large and small physical activity counseling sessions	Statistically significant ↑ in number of steps & exercise beliefs. Significant ↓ body mass index & body weight

TABLE D.2-2 Exercise Prescription Guidelines for Cancer Survivors after Completion of Primary Treatment

Low Intensity (Light Effort) Endurance Exercise
- 20–39% of $HR_{reserve}$; 40–50% VO_{2peak}; RPE of 10–11; 2–4 METs
- 45–60 minutes per day (total exercise minutes can be accumulated by performing short bouts of light intensity endurance exercise throughout the day)
- 5–7 days of week
- Gardening, carrying groceries, raking lawn

Moderate Intensity (Moderate Effort) Endurance Exercise
- 40–59% of $HR_{reserve}$; 60–75% VO_{2peak}; RPE of 12–13; 4–6 METs
- 20–60 minutes per day (total exercise minutes can be accumulated by performing short bouts of moderate intensity endurance exercise throughout the day)
- 3–5 days of week
- Brisk walking, ($\geq$ 2.5–4.0 mph), swimming, cycling

Vigorous Intensity (Strenuous Effort) Endurance Exercise
- 60–84% of $HR_{reserve}$; $\geq$ 75% $VO2_{peak}$; RPE of 14–16; 6–8 METs
- 20–45 minutes per day (total exercise minutes can be accumulated by performing short bouts of vigorous intensity endurance exercise throughout the day)
- 3–5 days of week
- Jogging ($\geq$ 5.0mph), vigorous swimming, vigorous cycling

Progressive Resistance Exercise (Weight-Bearing)
- 1–2 sets (each of 8–12 repetitions) of 8–10 different resistance large-muscle group exercises at moderate intensity
- 2–3 nonconsecutive days of week

Flexibility/Stretching Exercise (Weight-Bearing)
- Gentle reaching, bending and stretching of the large muscle groups
- Hold each stretch for 20–30 seconds; perform each stretch at least twice
- 3–7 days per week

CALCULATIONS: $HR_{reserve}$ = maximal heart rate (HR_{max}) minus resting heart rate (HR_{rest}). Multiply $HR_{reserve}$ by .20 to .84 to obtain target heart rate for desired intensity of exercise.
SOURCE: Adapted from Courneya[208], Brown et al.,[35] and Warburton et al.[209,210].

counseling along with pharmacotherapy are effective, definitive guidelines exist for providing care as it relates to smoking cessation.[29] The 5-A approach endorsed by the U.S. Preventive Services Task Force provides a concrete framework for health care providers to deliver appropriate care regarding smoking cessation and is a featured element within the IOM report.[29,129] Despite this extant framework, the barriers to longstanding smoking cessation success are substantial and findings from intervention trials have been mixed; the IOM report provides a solid overview of studies conducted up until 2005 and notes the significance of smoking cessation within the survivor population and the numerous barriers that exist.[29] Fortunately, the early trials of Gritz et al.[130] as well as the most recent trial of Emmons et al.[131] provide success stories that can guide future treatment, research, and practice. The randomized controlled trial by Emmons et al.[131] tested a peer telephone counseling intervention with tailored materials against standardized self-help materials (both with optional nicotine replacement) among 796 currently smoking adult childhood cancer survivors. They found that quit rates were significantly higher in the counseling group compared to the self-help group at both the 8-month (16.8% vs. 8.5%; $p < .01$) and 12-month follow-up (15% vs. 9%; $p < .01$).[131] This home-based intervention also was found to be cost-effective. This recent positive trial not only is important for its contribution to smoking cessation research, but it also paves the way more generally for future health promotion programs by testing innovative strategies that are well accepted and more readily disseminable to survivor populations who often are hard to reach. As noted in the IOM report,[29] opportunities also exist for interventions that incorporate social or familial support as a key element. An ongoing trial that is currently testing the efficacy of such a family-based intervention is entitled "Family Ties" (CA92622) and results are anticipated within the next 2 years. As in areas of diet and exercise, more research is necessary to determine interventions that are optimally effective and promote permanent smoking cessation—acknowledging that continued tobacco-use may be particularly resistant in cancer survivors. It is also worth noting that smokers may represent a prime population not only for smoking cessation efforts, but also for multiple risk factor interventions, since findings of Butterfield et al.[132] suggest that the majority (63%) of cancer survivors who smoke also are likely to engage in at least two to three other unhealthful lifestyle behaviors, such as sedentary behavior, high red meat consumption, and excessive alcohol use.

Other Areas (Alcohol and Sunscreen-Use, Complementary and Alternative Therapies, Osteoporosis Prevention, and Immunizations)

Alcohol Use

Alcohol, like tobacco, is an addictive substance, with the use of both being highly correlated and associated with higher risk of similar cancers, such as kidney and head and neck cancers. Given these similarities, a need for multiple behavior interventions that integrate both smoking cessation with alcohol abstinence,[133,134] particularly in high-risk populations (e.g., veterans) are needed.[133] To date, the only intervention undertaken that has addressed both behaviors has been in 64 adolescent cancer survivors and from the perspective of preventing high risk behaviors rather than actively intervening in those who have longstanding addictions.[135] This intervention by Hollen et al.[135] was effective in modifying attitudes and behaviors short-term (1-month follow-up), but not long term (6-month follow-up).

In considering alcohol as an independent risk factor, data suggest that head and neck patients who continue to drink at least 15 servings of alcohol per week have roughly a four-fold increased risk of developing a second primary tumor compared to those who abstain.[136] Morbidity due to other causes such as pulmonary and cardiovascular disease, as well as alcohol-related conditions, also is significantly higher among survivors who continue to drink.[137] In contrast, current evidence does not suggest that continued alcohol-use increases risk of recurrence or all-cause mortality among breast cancer survivors, even though alcohol-use is associated with the development of mammary carcinoma.[37] Differences in dose and the reduced prevalence of alcoholism within this population may explain the lack of an association. Indeed, recent analyses of the 2000 National Health Interview Survey, suggest that overall cancer survivors do not drink any more than those in the general population, though moderate-to-heavy drinking is noted more frequently among select groups, such as survivors of head, neck and lung cancers (24.1%), as well as prostate cancer (22.3%).[127,128] Like smoking, however, alcohol-use diminishes significantly with age,[127,128] and "risky-use" (> 2 drinks per day for men and >1 drink/day in women) is noted among only 4.1% of cancer survivors who are age 65 and older. The low prevalence of risky drinking among the majority of cancer survivors, plus established findings indicating that light-to-moderate alcohol-use is protective against CVD are taken into account in diet and physical activity recommendations established by the American Cancer Society.[35,89] These recommendations parallel those purported in the U.S. Dietary Guidelines,[58] and the American Heart Association,[138] i.e., those who choose to drink alcohol, should do so sensibly (up to 2 drinks/day for men and up to 1 drink/day for women) and should not be taking medications or have conditions for which alcohol is contraindicated.

Complementary and Alternative Medicine:

As noted in the IOM report, the use of complementary and alternative medicine (CAM) is prevalent both in the general population and particularly among cancer survivors.[29] Common categories of CAM include specific dietary or exercise regimens (e.g. the Gonzales diet, Reiki, yoga, etc), dietary and herbal supplements, acupuncture, massage and psychological or mind-body therapies (e.g. imagery, journaling, support groups). A recent paper by Hann et al.[139] suggests that up to two-thirds of adult cancer

TABLE D.2-3 Patient Guidelines for Complementary and Alternative Medicine

- Take charge of your health by being an informed consumer. Find out what scientific studies have been done on the safety and effectiveness of the CAM treatment in which you are interested.

- Decisions about medical care and treatment should be made in consultation with a health care provider and based on the condition and needs of each person. Discuss information on CAM with your health care provider before making any decisions about treatment or care.

- If you use any CAM therapy, inform your primary health care provider. This is for your safety and so your health care provider can develop a comprehensive treatment plan.

- If you use a CAM therapy provided by a practitioner, such as acupuncture, choose the practitioner with care. Check with your insurer to see if the services will be covered. (To learn more about selecting a CAM practitioner, see our fact sheet, "Selecting a Complementary and Alternative Medicine Practitioner.")

survivors use some form of CAM therapy, with 69% reporting a belief that it will prevent recurrence and 25% stating that it will offer cure. A 2005 review by Monti and Yang,[140] reports that CAM-use fulfills psychosocial needs that are inadequately addressed by the conventional biomedical system, and as the IOM report suggests, survivors may derive potential benefit for managing select side effects, as well as reducing pain and anxiety. Therefore physicians are encouraged to recommend select CAM therapies, such as support groups, massage, and relaxation therapy that appear safe for cancer survivors. However, given the paucity of evidence on the biological agents (e.g., chelation therapy, restrictive dietary regimens or dietary supplements), current guidelines do not endorse the use of these products or regimens.[35,89,141] Instead, patients are encouraged to access reliable sources of information, such as the National Center for Complementary and Alternative Medicine (http://nccam.nih.gov) and to follow key points when considering CAM therapies (see Table D.2-3). Open dialogues with physicians and other health care providers play an integral role in this process, especially given the potential for deleterious interactions between various CAM therapies and prescribed treatments. However, as noted in the IOM review,[29] patients are often reluctant to divulge such information. Thus, physicians are encouraged to initiate and maintain open communication regarding CAM.[29,139-141]

Sun-Protective Behaviors:

Skin cancer is the most common form of cancer in the United States.[1] In 2006, it is expected that more than one million men and women will be diagnosed with one of three forms of skin cancer – basal cell carcinoma, squamous cell carcinoma, or melanoma. High levels of exposure to UV radiation increase the risk of all three types of skin cancer, and approximately 65% to 90% of melanomas are caused by UV exposure. As such, risk of skin cancer can be substantially reduced by adopting sun-protective behaviors (i.e., sunscreen-use, wearing clothing, seeking shade) that limit exposure to sunlight – the primary source of UV radiation.[142]

Given the central role of radiation-induced DNA damage in the etiologies of both melanoma and basal cell carcinoma, cancer survivors who have previously received locoregional radiotherapy, particularly childhood and hematopoietic cell transplantation cancer survivors, are at increased risk for certain forms of melanoma and basal cell skin cancers.[143-146] In these reports, nonmelanoma cancer development occurred after a considerable latency period (10 to 20 years after radiation) suggesting that younger patients (particularly children) may have a greater inherent sensitivity to radiation.[147] Given this evidence, cancer survivors, particularly those who have received radiation at a young age (i.e., childhood cancer survivors, hematopoietic cell transplant survivors) should be closely monitored for skin cancers. Physicians are encouraged to perform regular examinations during patient follow-up visits as well as recommend sun-protective behaviors demonstrated to reduce skin cancer incidence.

Despite convincing evidence that sun protective behaviors can reduce the primary incidence of benign and malignant skin lesions, only one study has attempted to increase these behaviors in cancer survivors. In this study, 200 patient-caregiver dyads were given an education-based, sun-protective intervention at 2 and 6 months following skin cancer surgery. Results indicated that both patients and caregivers reported higher sun-protective knowledge, intentions, and behavior at 1 year postsurgery.[148] Although more research in cancer survivors is required, the extensive available literature documenting the benefits of these behaviors on the primary prevention of skin cancer provides sufficient evidence for physicians to recommend sun protective behaviors as part of comprehensive cancer care in these high risk patients. It is important to note, however that a controversy currently exists regarding the pros and cons of sunlight exposure in other cancers, most notably lung, prostate and colorectal cancers. The findings of Giovannuci et al.[149] and others[150-151] suggest that modest sunlight exposure may be protective, not only for the primary risk of cancer, but also in survival.[149-151] These data call into question current guidelines and underscore the need for further research.

Osteoporosis Prevention

Osteoporosis is a common disease in healthy adults over the age of 50 years, with one in three women and one in four men being affected world-wide;[152] it is a condition for which diet and physical activity play important roles. Epidemiologic findings suggest that bone density may be biomarker of cancer risk, with lower bone density being a risk factor for colorectal cancer and increased bone density being positively associated with uterine and post-menopausal breast cancer.[153-157] Even though lower bone density may be protective for breast cancer in older women, clinical studies suggest that osteoporosis is still a prevalent health problem even in these survivors; data of Twiss et al.[158] indicate that 80% of older breast cancer patients have t-scores less than −1 and thus have clinically confirmed osteopenia or frank osteoporosis at the time of their initial appointment.[158] Thus, substantial proportions of colorectal and breast cancer patients may have suboptimal bone density at the time of diagnosis.

In addition, various cancer therapies, such as gonadotropin-releasing hormone agonists (hormone therapy), glucocorticoids, certain chemotherapeutics (e.g., methotrexate, cyclophosphamide, doxorubicin), radiation therapy, and thyroid-stimulating hormone suppressive therapy all enhance bone turnover and act to further compromise bone integrity.[159,160] As such, osteo-penia, osteoporosis, and increased rates of fracture have been noted in a wide spectrum of cancer survivors, including breast, prostate, testicular, thyroid, gastric, and central nervous system cancers, as well as non-Hodgkin's lymphoma and various hematologic malignancies.[160-163]

Osteoporosis is a well-documented problem not only among older adult survivors, but also among young adult survivors of childhood cancers.[27,164-167] The goals of patient care are early recognition of those patients at high risk for osteoporosis and to prevent fractures in patients with documented bone deterioration. The American Society of Clinical Oncology (ASCO) has outlined a management strategy to promote bone health that includes baseline bone density assessment with continued monitoring and treatment based on bone density results.[168] As reviewed by Chlebowski,[159] these guidelines focus largely on pharmacologic means (e.g., pamidronate, zoledronic acid) and selective estrogen-receptor modulators (e.g., raloxifene) to improve bone density and reduce risk of fracture. Lifestyle interventions are also postulated to play an important role in addressing this issue. In healthy adults, current recommendations for osteoporosis prevention and treatment include dietary and lifestyle changes (e.g., weight-bearing exercise, consumption of adequate amounts of calcium (800-1,500 mg/day depending on age range and gender) and adequate amounts of vitamin D (400-600 iu/day), as well as reduction of ancillary risk factors found to affect intake, calcium absorption, or bone turnover, such as smoking, caffeine, alcohol, sodium, and excessive protein consumption).[169] Potential improvements on bone mineral density of lifestyle interventions are yet to be tested specifically among cancer survivors.[170] To date, the only research that has been reported is a pilot study by Waltman and colleagues[171] who examined the effects of a 12-month multicomponent program of progressive resistance training, alendronate, calcium, and vitamin D on preventing osteoporosis in 21 postmenopausal breast cancer survivors who had completed primary treatment. All participants experienced a significant increase in bone mineral density (BMD) of the spine and hip. Clearly, preliminary data from this study combined with the demonstrated effects of combined regimens of exercise, diet and pharmacologic agents on BMD in healthy adults provides strong suggestive evidence for future larger randomized trials to investigate the effects of multicomponent interventions that include exercise and diet on skeletal health in cancer survivors; until then the guidelines established by ASCO appear the most germane.[168]

Immunizations

Infections are responsible for more than half a million cancer cases worldwide each year. Of the numerous infections that have been associated with increased cancer risk, the human papillomavirus (HPV) is the most commonly recognized. The association between HPV and malignancies of the lower anogential tract, particularly the cervix, is well established.[172] In the United States, comprehensive cervical cancer screening programs (the papanicolaou [pap] test) has dramatically decreased the risk of cervical cancer.[172]

Although the role of vaccinations in the prevention of certain forms of cancer and other diseases is an established part of clinical practice, the role of these therapies in persons who have been diagnosed with cancer remains largely unknown.[173] Individuals diagnosed with cancer are often immuno-compromised as a result of treatment (e.g., chemotherapy, high-dose steroids) or the disease itself (hematologic malignances are immunosuppressive). Thus, it appears logical that immunizations may play a beneficial role in cancer survivors who may be susceptible to bacterial, viral, and fungal infections. However, there is concern that cancer patients may be unable to provide a protective response to immunizations and, paradoxically, immunizations may even increase the risk of clinical infection.[173]

A recent systematic review examined the available published evidence on the role of immunizations in cancer patients who had not undergone bone marrow transplantation.[173] The authors reviewed the efficacy and safety of vaccination against nine preventable diseases (i.e., haemophilus influenzae type b, hepatitis B, influenza, measles, meningococcal meningitis, poliomyelitis, 23-valent polysaccharide pneumococcus, tetanus, and varicella) that are associated with considerable morbidity and mortality among cancer survivors. After the completion of primary treatments, the influenza vaccine response in patients with solid tumors was similar to that of healthy adults and side effects were mild. Overall, influenza vaccinations appear to be safe and well-tolerated by cancer patients both during and following primary treatments and may confer some protection against influenza-related morbidity and mortality. Fewer studies have examined the efficacy of measles vaccinations in cancer survivors because of the risks involved with vaccinating immunocompromised individuals with live vaccines. Therefore, the Centers for Disease Control and Prevention recommends that cancer patients undergoing chemotherapy should not receive measles vaccinations. In patients who have completed primary treatment, there are currently insufficient data to support measles vaccinations or vaccinations against the other preventable diseases listed. As a general rule, any patient considering vaccination should obtain physician clearance and wait at least 4 weeks after the completion of primary treatment.[173]

Perceived Needs for Health Promotion and Preferences for Delivery Among Cancer Survivors

Health Beliefs

Surveys conducted among cancer survivors over the past two to three decades have produced consistent findings regarding survivors' attributions of the cause of their disease. The most frequently reported reasons (attributions) are heredity, environmental pollutants, occupation, stress, and tobacco use.[174-179] These findings were confirmed in a recent population-based study by Wold et al.,[180] who found attributions of cause for the following nonmodifiable and modifiable risk factors (reported as the percentage response of breast, prostate, and colorectal cancer survivors [N=670]): family history (83%); smoking (79%); environmental pollutants (69%); occupational exposures (59%); stress (56%); various dietary factors (47-51%); obesity (45%); and lack of exercise (28%). The authors concluded that public health organizations and providers need to educate survivors, as well as their healthy counterparts, on modifiable risk factors associated with the primary prevention of cancer and related morbidity.

Therefore, while most survivors attribute their cancer diagnosis to factors beyond their control (with the exception of tobacco use), relatively few credit dietary factors and obesity, and less than one-third attribute, lack of exercise. Despite these attributions, other surveys among survivor populations suggest high levels of interest in diet (54%) and exercise (51%) interventions, as well as comparable levels of interest in smoking cessation programs (60%), among adult cancer survivors who currently smoke, with this interest in behavioral change attributed to a desire to "prevent recurrence."[181] These findings are remarkably similar in pediatric cancer survivor populations (with even higher levels of interest noted among their parents).[36] Van Weert et al.[182] recently reported even higher levels of interest (80%) in multiple behavior interventions. Thus, the cancer diagnosis may signal a notable "about-face" in terms of health beliefs and may be an opportune time or a "teachable moment" for undertaking health behavior change.

Behavior Change Postdiagnosis

To date, published findings exist on 30 studies that have explored persistent lifestyle practices (those that extend beyond the initial treatment year) among cancer survivors; a majority of these studies were systematically reviewed by Demark-Wahnefried et al.[52] The preponderance of earlier research suggested that the practice of healthy lifestyle behaviors was higher among cancer survivors than in the population at large; however, many of these studies relied on modest-sized convenience samples and were limited in terms of length of follow-up and heterogeneity of cancer type.[52] Three recent reports emanating from much larger datasets and assessing behaviors in longer-term survivors indicate that few health behavior differences exist between cancer survivors and healthy populations or noncancer controls.[43,127,128]

Two of these studies relied on data collected from survivors of several different cancers and who were nested within a national sample that included both cancer cases and controls, thus yielding data that are less likely to be influenced by responder bias.[127,128] Analyses by Coups and Ostroff[127] and Bellizzi et al.[128] on health behaviors of cancer cases compared to age- and race-matched controls participating in the National Health Initiative Survey-2000 indicate that while cancer survivors are 9% (95% CI, 1.03-1.16) more likely to adhere to physical activity guidelines, for the most part their health behaviors parallel those of the general population—a population marked by inactivity, overweight or obesity, suboptimal fruit, vegetable, and fiber consumption, and high intakes of fat.[58,129,130] Similar results were found in another study that exclusively tracked lifestyle behaviors in a cohort of women (N=2,321) with early-stage breast cancer.[43] Thus, findings of these larger, more recent studies are in direct contrast to prior findings—differences that may be attributable to more heterogeneous samples of survivors who were followed for longer periods of time. These recent data provide us with a paradigm shift and the potential realization that although many cancer patients report healthful lifestyle changes after diagnosis, these changes may not generalize to all populations of cancer survivors or may be temporary. Given higher rates of comorbidity within this population and evidence that diet, exercise, and tobacco use affect risk for other cancers and other chronic diseases, these recent data support a need for lifestyle interventions that target this vulnerable population, and perhaps with greater need than previously thought.[2,3,5-7,11-13,16,17,21,22, 27,29,45,79,129,130]

When Is the Best Time to Intervene?

Few data exist as to when cancer survivors may be most receptive to health behavior interventions. An early study of 988 breast and prostate cancer survivors,[181] suggests that most (57%) reported a preference for diet, exercise, and/or smoking cessation information "at diagnosis or soon thereafter" and that a significant decrease ($p=.003$) was noted as time elapsed from diagnosis. These results are supported by unpublished data that show response rates among elderly cancer survivors to a home-based diet and exercise intervention are 34.3% among those within 18 months of diagnosis, as compared to 13.9% among those who are 5 or more years out.[183] Factors such as age and gender also may affect interest and uptake of lifestyle interventions. For example, McBride et al.[184] found that interest levels for lifestyle interventions may be sustained over time among women, but not in men, since the psychological impact of disease diminishes significantly with time from diagnosis among male, but not in female survivors.

Timing of interventions also is dependent upon the targeted behavior (diet, exercise, smoking cessation, etc); the channel of delivery (clinic- or home-based), treatments received (e.g., surgery, radiation, chemotherapy), side effects (fatigue, pain, nausea, etc.), and desired outcomes (short-term symptom management or overall long-term health). Furthermore, issues such as time, transportation, child care, and patients' willingness to undertake new lifestyle behaviors may undermine the success of health promotion efforts and require careful consideration regarding timing, content, delivery channel, and patient selection. Also important is the realization that several strategic iterations may be necessary in order to create an intervention that not only has proven efficacy, but that also is well accepted and generalizable to the patient population at large.

Preferred Channels for Delivery

As with intervention timing, there are relatively few studies that have explored preferences with regard to intervention delivery channel and even fewer that have compared the relative efficacy of different methods. In one study of 307 cancer survivors, Jones et al.[185] found that 85% of cancer survivors preferred face-to-face exercise counseling for a one-session class. Other researchers have found that distance and accompanying issues of time and transportation pose significant barriers for in-person programs, especially among older cancer survivors (61% of cancer survivors are comprised of those 65 years of age or older).[181,186-188] Such barriers also are present among survivors of more rarely occurring cancers who often have to travel great distances to receive specialized care in appropriate clinical settings, i.e., childhood survivors.[36] In a recent review of exercise interventions, van der Bij et al.[189] leveled criticism that most health promotion interventions and programs "never reach the people who would benefit most from them." Given the relative prevalence of cancer within the American population, as compared to more common health disorders such as CVD and diabetes, there is an enhanced need to develop interventions that, if not initially—then ultimately are disseminable to populations of cancer survivors at large. In two separate survey studies among breast and prostate cancer survivors (N=988, mean age 63 + 11 years) and childhood cancer survivors (N=209; mean age 20 + 6 years), Demark-Wahnefried and colleagues[36,181] found that distance medicine-based or home-based programs were significantly favored over clinic-based venues with the proportions of survivors (breast and prostate versus childhood cancer) reporting "extremely high" to "high" levels of interest in the following delivery channels: mailed interventions (53%/59%); computer-based interventions (CD-ROM or internet) (not assessed/45-47%); and telephone counseling (23%/10%). The surprising result that mailed interventions garnered higher preference scores than computer-based formats among younger cancer survivors also is supported by the findings of Im and Chee,[190] who found that cancer survivors report several barriers to computer-based programs. Also worthy to note are the recent findings of a review by Rutten et al.[191] who found that cancer survivors were twice as likely to report reliance on print materials as sources of health information rather than the internet or other media sources.[191] It is currently unknown whether these results are apt to change over time or whether there is a definite hardset preference for print materials over computer-based venues. Given that cancer is a disease associated with aging and that receptivity for computer-based formats is even lower in older populations, it is safe to say that although web-based programs offer future promise; full penetrance of such programs, especially among the most underserved populations of cancer survivors, is currently questionable.[52]

To date, the preponderance of reported health promotion efforts among cancer survivors have utilized clinic-based interventions and 11 studies have employed hybrid programs that rely on both clinic-based sessions and telephone counseling.[60,99,187,192-195] Far fewer studies have tested interventions that were delivered exclusively via home-based approaches. As referred to previously, the recent successful smoking cessation trial of Emmons et al.[131] which tested the efficacy of a telephone counseling and mailed material-based intervention is a foundational effort in this arena. In another study of 86 sedentary breast cancer survivors, Pinto et al.[106] found that women randomized to a 12-week telephone counseling-print material intervention, as compared to an attention control, experienced significantly greater improvements in fitness and vigor, and reduced fatigue, though no significant differences were noted in weight status or percent body fat. To date, there have been no reported findings of interventions that have been delivered exclusively through mailed or computer-based approaches, though favorable results of the Fresh Start Trial, a diet and exercise intervention delivered exclusively via series of sequentially-tailored mailed print materials, will be released at this year's ASCO meeting. By-in-large most health promotion interventions among cancer survivors have reported favorable findings with only one study by Segal et al.[196] comparing relatively efficacy between interventions delivered via clinic-based versus clinic-based plus telephone counseling formats. In their trial of 123 early stage breast cancer survivors, they found that physical functioning increased by 5.7 points in the mixed delivery group and 2.2 points in the clinic-based program, as compared a decrease of 4.1 points in the control group (p=.04), though no significant differences between groups were found in aerobic capacity.[196] More research obviously is needed to determine optimal approaches, not only with regard to delivery channel, but also to such factors as timing and pairing of behavioral components.

The Role of the Oncologist in Health Promotion

A consistent and well-known factor in promoting behavior change is the recommendation of the health care provider.[197-201] Currently, however only about 20% of oncology care physicians appear to offer guidance regarding healthful lifestyle change,[181,202] and report barriers, such as competing treatment or health concerns, time constraints, or uncertainty regarding the delivery of appropriate health behavior messages.[203-205] Creative strategies are needed to most efficiently harness the motivational power of the physician without unduly taxing resource-use. As an example, a recent randomized controlled trial (N=450) by Jones et al.[206] showed that breast cancer patients who received an oncologist's recommendation to exercise reported a mean increase of 3.4 MET hours per week, as compared to those not receiving a similar message (p=.011), furthermore, the physician's recommendation was found to directly affect perceived behavioral control associated with behavioral change.[207] Therefore, oncologists can play a key role in catalyzing behavior changes that have the potential for improving the overall long term health of their patients, and can rely on nurses and allied health personnel, as well as health behavior researchers to most efficiently and effectively promote behavior change.

Resources Available to Providers and Patients for Health Promotion

With the increasing recognition of the growing population of cancer survivors and the unique needs of this growing population, a wide range of evidence-based resources are now available. These resources not only educate oncology care providers about the unique issues facing today's cancer survivors, but also serve to educate survivors themselves about optimal health behaviors following a cancer diagnosis and completion of primary treatments. In Table D.2-4, a list of recommended resources are provided that offer comprehensive information on cancer survivorship issues reviewed in this report. A list of specialized resources also are provided that offer more in-depth information about select areas of health promotion (e.g., exercise, healthy weight, etc.). These resources may offer information that is cancer-specific, as well as providing more general assistance.

Summary

In a recent review of the benefits of various lifestyle factors (i.e., diet, exercise, smoking cessation, alcohol abstinence and sunscreen use), Kuhn and colleagues,[204] provided a rather grim assessment of the value of behavioral interventions among cancer patients. To be sure, little is known regarding the direct impact of postdiagnosis behavioral change on cancer-related progression, recurrence, or survival. In addition, there also are comparatively few data that support the role of behavior change on other health outcomes and comorbidity. Indeed, much more research is necessary, not only to determine proof of concept (i.e., that behavior change can make an impact on cancer-specific outcomes and overall health), but also to arrive at interventions that are well accepted and that reach cancer survivors who are most vulnerable. Data, however, are beginning to accumulate that show benefit. In the interim, oncology care providers can assist their patients by endorsing existing health guidelines and encouraging their patients to take active roles in pursuing general preventive health strategies.

TABLE D.2-4 Selected Resources Available to Oncology Providers and Patients Regarding Healthy Behaviors/Wellness

Health Behavior/Wellness	Organization	Contact Information	Recommended Publication/Brochure/Website
General Survivorship Issues	American Cancer Society	http:www.cancer.org; 1-800-ACS-2345	*General Information, as well as specific information on diet, exercise, smoking cessation, and sunscreen use*
	American Institute for Cancer Research	http://www.aicr.org; 1-800-843-8114	*General information, as well as specific information on diet, supplements, and exercise*
	Cancer Information Service	http://cis.nci.nih.gov; 1-800-4-CANCER	*General information, as well as specific information on smoking cessation*
	The Centers of Disease Control	1-800-CDC-INFO (1-800-232-4636); cdcinfo@cdc.gov; http://www.cdc.gov/cancer/survivorship/	*A National Action Plan for Cancer Survivorship: Advancing Public Health Strategies* (in conjunction with the Lance Armstrong Foundation)
	The Lance Armstrong Foundation, **LIVESTRONG**™	1-866-235-7205; http://www.livestrong.org	*LIVESTRONG*™ *Survivorship Notebook*
	National Cancer Center Office of Cancer Survivorship	http://cancercontrol.cancer.gov/ocs	*General information, as well as links to preventive care sites*

continued

TABLE D.2-4 Continued

Health Behavior/Wellness	Organization	Contact Information	Recommended Publication/Brochure/Website
	The National Coalition for Cancer Survivorship	877-NCCS-YES (877-622-7937); NCCS, 1010 Wayne Avenue, Suite 770, Silver Spring, MD, 20910; info@canceradvocacy.org; http://www.canceradvocacy.org/default.aspx	*Your Life After Cancer Treatment*
Weight Management	American Diabetes Association	1-800-DIABETES (1-800-342-2383); AskADA@diabetes.org; http://www.diabetes.org/weightloss-and-exercise/weightloss/portioncontrol.asp	*101 Weight Loss Tips for Preventing and Controlling Diabetes*
	American Heart Association	1-800-AHA-USA1 (1-800-242-8721); http://americanheart.org	*An Eating Plan for Healthy Americans* (http://americanheart.org/presenter.jhtml?identifier=1088)
	The Centers for Disease Control and Prevention	1-800-CDC-INFO (1-800-232-4636); cdcinfo@cdc.gov; http://www.cdc.gov/nccdphp/dnpa/obesity/	*Dietary Guidelines for Americans 2005* (http://www.healthierus.gov/dietaryguidelines)
	NAASO – The Obesity Society	http://www.obesityonline.org/site/index.cfm; http://www.naaso.org/information/practicalguide.asp	*Weight assessment, and diet, and exercise information.*
	National Heart Lung and Blood Institute	http://www.nhlbi.nih.gov/health/prof/heart/index.htm#obesity	*Weight assessment and diet and exercise information.*

Diet	American Dietetic Association	1-800-877-1600; http://eatright.org	*Step Up to Nutrition and Health*
	United States Department of Agriculture	1-888-7PYRAMID (1-888-779-7264); http://mypyramid.gov	http://mypyramid.gov/tips_resources/index.html
Exercise	American College of Sports Medicine	(317) 637-9200; http://www.acsm.org	*Current Comments* (a series of statements concerning sports medicine and exercise) http://www.acsm.org/AM/Template.cfm?Section=Current_Comments
	American Heart Association	1-800-AHA-USA1 (1-800-242-8721); http://americanheart.org	*How Can Physical Activity Become a Way of Life? Why Should I Be Physically Active?*
	The Centers for Disease Control and Prevention	1-800-CDC-INFO (1-800-232-4636); cdcinfo@cdc.gov; http://www.cdc.gov/nccdphp/dnpa/physical/	*Trials for Health: Increasing Opportunities for Physical Activity in the Community*
Smoking Cessation	The Centers for Disease Control and Prevention	1-800-CDC-INFO (1-800-232-4636); http://www.cdc.gov/tobacco; http://www.cdc.gov/tobacco/how2quit.htm.	*You can Quit Smoking: Consumer Guide* (http://www.cdc.gov/tobacco/quit/canquit.htm)
	National Cancer Institute	1-800-QUIT-NOW (1-800-784-8669); http://www.cancer.gov.	*Clearing the Air* (for all smokers) *Clear Horizons* (for smokers over age 50) *Forever Free* (for smokers who have recently quit) (all available at http://www.smokefree.gov/info.html)

continued

TABLE D.2-4 Continued

Health Behavior/Wellness	Organization	Contact Information	Recommended Publication/ Brochure/Website
Alcohol Use	The Centers for Disease Control and Prevention	1-800-CDC-INFO (1-800-232-4636); cdcinfo@cdc.gov; http://www.cdc.gov/alcohol/index.htm	Several links to government agencies and nonprofit organizations that address alcohol and health
	National Institute on Alcohol Abuse and Alcoholism	National Institute on Alcohol Abuse and Alcoholism (NIAAA), niaaaweb-r @exchange,nih.gov; http://www.niaaa.nih.gov	Several links to national alcohol data, NIAAA-sponsored websites, newsletters, etc.
Complementary and Alternative Medicine	National Cancer Institute	1-800-4-CANCER (1-800-422-6237); National Cancer Institute's Cancer Information Service; http://www.cancer.gov; http://www.cancer.gov/cancertopics/treatment/cam. Also see Office of Cancer Complementary and Alternative Medicine: http://www.cancer.gov/cam/	Links to several specific complementary and alternative medicine topics (http://www.cancer.gov/cancertopics/treatment/cam)
	National Center for Complementary and Alternative Medicine	1-888-644-6226; nccam.nih.gov; info @nccam.nih.gov	Links to several specific complementary and alternative medicine topics (http://nccam.nih.gov/health/)

Topic	Organization	Contact	Resources
Sun-Protective Behaviors	American Academy of Dermatology	866-503-SKIN (866-503-7546); http://www.aad.org	*Skin Cancer Updates* (several useful links on the latest skin cancer news) http://www.aad.org/public/News/DermInfo/DInfoSkinCancerUpdates.htm
	National Cancer Institute	1-800-4-CANCER (1-800-422-6237); National Cancer Institute's Cancer Information Service; http://www.cancer.gov; http://www.cancer.gov/cancer topics/types/skin	*What You Need to Know About Skin Cancer* http://www.cancer.gov/cancerinfo/wyntk/skin
	Skin Cancer Foundation	1-800-SKIN-490 (1-800-754-6490); http://www.skincancer.org	Links to several brochures and manuals about skin cancer; https://www.skincancer.org/catalog/index.php
Osteoporosis Prevention	The Centers for Disease Control and Prevention	1-800-CDC-INFO (1-800-232-4636); cdcinfo@cdc.gov; http://www.cdc.gov/nccdphp/dnpa/bonehealth	Links to several brochures and manuals about osteoporosis; http://www.cdc.gov/nccdphp/dnpa/bonehealth/osteoporosis_month.htm
	National Osteoporosis Foundation	202-223-2226; http://www.nof.org	Links to several brochures and manuals about osteoporosis; http://www.nof.org
Immunizations	The Centers for Disease Control and Prevention	1-800-CDC-INFO (1-800-232-4636); cdcinfo@cdc.gov; http://www.cdc.	Links to several brochures and manuals about the national immunization program; http://www.cdc.gov/nip/gov/nip/

REFERENCES

1. Jemal A, Siegel R, Ward E, et al: Cancer statistics, 2006. CA Cancer J Clin 56:106-30, 2006

2. Jemal A, Clegg LX, Ward E, et al: Annual report to the nation on the status of cancer, 1975-2001, with a special feature regarding survival. Cancer 101:3-27, 2004

3. Rowland J, Mariotto A, Aziz N, et al: Cancer Survivorship - United States. MMWR 53:526-529, 2004

4. Aziz NM: Cancer survivorship research: challenge and opportunity. J Nutr 132:3494S-3503S, 2002

5. Aziz NM, Rowland JH: Trends and advances in cancer survivorship research: challenge and opportunity. Semin Radiat Oncol 13:248-66, 2003

6. Brown BW, Brauner C, Minnotte MC: Noncancer deaths in white adult cancer patients. J Natl Cancer Inst 85:979-87, 1993

7. Day RW: Future need for more cancer research. J Am Diet Assoc 98:523, 1998

8. Edwards BK, Howe HL, Ries LA, et al: Annual report to the nation on the status of cancer, 1973-1999, featuring implications of age and aging on U.S. cancer burden. Cancer 94:2766-92, 2002

9. Ganz PA: Late effects of cancer and its treatment. Semin Oncol Nurs 17:241-8, 2001

10. Hewitt M, Rowland JH, Yancik R: Cancer survivors in the United States: age, health, and disability. J Gerontol A Biol Sci Med Sci 58:82-91, 2003

11. Leigh SA: The long-term cancer survivor: a challenge for nurse practitioners. Nurse Pract Forum 9:192-6, 1998

12. Li FP, Stovall EL: Long-term survivors of cancer. Cancer Epidemiol Biomarkers Prev 7:269-70, 1998

13. Meadows AT, Varricchio C, Crosson K, et al: Research issues in cancer survivorship: report of a workshop sponsored by the Office of Cancer Survivorship, National Cancer Institute. Cancer Epidemiol Biomarkers Prev 7:1145-51, 1998

14. Schultz PN, Beck ML, Stava C, et al: Cancer survivors. Work related issues. Aaohn J 50:220-6, 2002

15. Travis LB: Therapy-associated solid tumors. Acta Oncol 41:323-33, 2002

16. Nord C, Mykletun A, Thorsen L, et al: Self-reported health and use of health care services in long-term cancer survivors. Int J Cancer 114:307-16, 2005

17. Wingo PA, Ries LA, Parker SL, et al: Long-term cancer patient survival in the United States. Cancer Epidemiol Biomarkers Prev 7:271-82, 1998

18. Ashing-Giwa K, Ganz PA, Petersen L: Quality of life of African-American and white long term breast carcinoma survivors. Cancer 85:418-26, 1999

19. Baker F, Haffer SC, Denniston M: Health-related quality of life of cancer and noncancer patients in Medicare managed care. Cancer 97:674-81, 2003

20. Bradley CJ, Neumark D, Luo Z, et al: Employment outcomes of men treated for prostate cancer. J Natl Cancer Inst 97:958-65, 2005

21. Mandelblatt JS, Edge SB, Meropol NJ, et al: Predictors of long-term outcomes in older breast cancer survivors: perceptions versus patterns of care. J Clin Oncol 21:855-63, 2003

22. Silliman RA, Prout MN, Field T, et al: Risk factors for a decline in upper body function following treatment for early stage breast cancer. Breast Cancer Res Treat 54:25-30, 1999

23. Williams ME: Identifying the older person likely to require long-term care services. J Am Geriatr Soc 35:761-6, 1987

24. Chirikos TN, Russell-Jacobs A, Jacobsen PB: Functional impairment and the economic consequences of female breast cancer. Women Health 36:1-20, 2002

25. Chang S, Long SR, Kutikova L, et al: Estimating the cost of cancer: results on the basis of claims data analyses for cancer patients diagnosed with seven types of cancer during 1999 to 2000. J Clin Oncol 22:3524-30, 2004

26. Ramsey SD, Berry K, Etzioni R: Lifetime cancer-attributable cost of care for long term survivors of colorectal cancer. Am J Gastroenterol 97:440-5, 2002

27. Schultz PN, Beck ML, Stava C, et al: Health profiles in 5836 long-term cancer survivors. Int J Cancer 104:488-95, 2003

28. Yabroff KR, Lawrence WF, Clauser S, et al: Burden of illness in cancer survivors: findings from a population-based national sample. J Natl Cancer Inst 96:1322-30, 2004

29. Hewitt M, Greenfield S, Stovall EL: Institute of Medicine and National Research Council: From Cancer Patient to Cancer Survivors: Lost in Transition. Washington, DC, National Academies Press, 2006

30. Beckett DM: Rethinking nutritional support for persons with cancer cachexia: A call for research to evaluate the effects of nutaceuticals. Biological Research in Nursing, in press

31. Brown JK: A systematic review of the evidence on symptom management of cancer-related anorexia and cachexia. Oncol Nurs Forum 29:517-32, 2002

32. Meacham LR, Gurney JG, Mertens AC, et al: Body mass index in long-term adult survivors of childhood cancer: a report of the Childhood Cancer Survivor Study. Cancer 103:1730-9, 2005

33. Schattner MA, Willis HJ, Raykher A, et al: Long-term enteral nutrition facilitates optimization of body weight. JPEN J Parenter Enteral Nutr 29:198-203, 2005

34. Ravasco P, Monteiro-Grillo I, Vidal PM, et al: Dietary counseling improves patient outcomes: a prospective, randomized, controlled trial in colorectal cancer patients undergoing radiotherapy. J Clin Oncol 23:1431-8, 2005

35. Brown JK, Byers T, Doyle C, et al: Nutrition and physical activity during and after cancer treatment: An American Cancer Society guide for informed choices. CA Cancer J Clin, in press

36. Demark-Wahnefried W, Werner C, Clipp EC, et al: Survivors of childhood cancer and their guardians. Cancer 103:2171-80, 2005

37. Rock CL, Demark-Wahnefried W: Nutrition and survival after the diagnosis of breast cancer: a review of the evidence. J Clin Oncol 20:3302-16, 2002

38. Bergstrom A, Pisani P, Tenet V, et al: Overweight as an avoidable cause of cancer in Europe. Int J Cancer 91:421-30, 2001

39. Organization WH: International Agency for Research in Cancer Handbook of Cancer Prevention, 2002

40. Amling CL: The association between obesity and the progression of prostate and renal cell carcinoma. Urol Oncol 22:478-84, 2004

41. Calle EE, Rodriguez C, Walker-Thurmond K, et al: Overweight, obesity, and mortality from cancer in a prospectively studied cohort of U.S. adults. N Engl J Med 348:1625-38, 2003

42. Freedland SJ, Aronson WJ, Kane CJ, et al: Impact of obesity on biochemical control after radical prostatectomy for clinically localized prostate cancer: a report by the Shared Equal Access Regional Cancer Hospital database study group. J Clin Oncol 22:446-53, 2004

43. Caan B, Sternfeld B, Gunderson E, et al: Life After Cancer Epidemiology (LACE) Study: a cohort of early stage breast cancer survivors (United States). Cancer Causes Control 16:545-56, 2005

44. Herman DR, Ganz PA, Petersen L, et al: Obesity and cardiovascular risk factors in younger breast cancer survivors: The Cancer and Menopause Study (CAMS). Breast Cancer Res Treat 93:13-23, 2005

45. Kroenke CH, Chen WY, Rosner B, et al: Weight, weight gain, and survival after breast cancer diagnosis. J Clin Oncol 23:1370-8, 2005

46. Camoriano JK, Loprinzi CL, Ingle JN, et al: Weight change in women treated with adjuvant therapy or observed following mastectomy for node-positive breast cancer. J Clin Oncol 8:1327-34, 1990

47. Chlebowski RT, Weiner JM, Reynolds R, et al: Long-term survival following relapse after 5-FU but not CMF adjuvant breast cancer therapy. Breast Cancer Res Treat 7:23-30, 1986

48. Goodwin PJ, Panzarella T, Boyd NF: Weight gain in women with localized breast cancer—a descriptive study. Breast Cancer Res Treat 11:59-66, 1988

49. Heasman KZ, Sutherland HJ, Campbell JA, et al: Weight gain during adjuvant chemotherapy for breast cancer. Breast Cancer Res Treat 5:195-200, 1985

50. Levine EG, Raczynski JM, Carpenter JT: Weight gain with breast cancer adjuvant treatment. Cancer 67:1954-9, 1991

51. Courneya KS, Karvinen KH, Campbell KL, et al: Associations among exercise, body weight, and quality of life in a population-based sample of endometrial cancer survivors. Gynecol Oncol 97:422-30, 2005

52. Demark-Wahnefried W, Aziz NM, Rowland JH, et al: Riding the crest of the teachable moment: promoting long-term health after the diagnosis of cancer. J Clin Oncol 23:5814-30, 2005

53. Houston DK, Stevens J, Cai J, et al: Role of weight history on functional limitations and disability in late adulthood: the ARIC study. Obes Res 13:1793-802, 2005

54. Chlebowski RT, Aiello E, McTiernan A: Weight loss in breast cancer patient management. J Clin Oncol 20:1128-43, 2002

55. McTiernan A: Obesity and cancer: the risks, science, and potential management strategies. Oncology (Williston Park) 19:871-81; discussion 881-2, 885-6, 2005

56. Irwin ML, McTiernan A, Bernstein L, et al: Relationship of obesity and physical activity with C-peptide, leptin, and insulin-like growth factors in breast cancer survivors. Cancer Epidemiol Biomarkers Prev 14:2881-8, 2005

57. Calle EE, Kaaks R: Overweight, obesity and cancer: epidemiological evidence and proposed mechanisms. Nat Rev Cancer 4:579-91, 2004

58. Services USDohaH: Dietary Guidelines for Americans 2005, U.S. Department of Agriculture, 2005

59. de Waard F, Ramlau R, Mulders Y, et al: A feasibility study on weight reduction in obese postmenopausal breast cancer patients. Eur J Cancer Prev 2:233-8, 1993

60. Djuric Z, DiLaura NM, Jenkins I, et al: Combining weight-loss counseling with the weight watchers plan for obese breast cancer survivors. Obes Res 10:657-65, 2002

61. Quality AfHRa: Effectiveness of Behavioral Interventions to Modify Physical Activity Behaviors in General Populations and Cancer Patients and Survivors. Rockville, MD, U.S. Department of Health and Human Services (AHRQ Publ. No. 04-E027-2), 2004, pp 107-111

62. Goodwin P, Esplen MJ, Butler K, et al: Multidisciplinary weight management in locoregional breast cancer: results of a phase II study. Breast Cancer Res Treat 48:53-64, 1998

63. Demark-Wahnefried W, Peterson BL, Winer EP, et al: Changes in weight, body composition, and factors influencing energy balance among premenopausal breast cancer patients receiving adjuvant chemotherapy. J Clin Oncol 19:2381-9, 2001

64. Freedman RJ, Aziz N, Albanes D, et al: Weight and body composition changes during and after adjuvant chemotherapy in women with breast cancer. J Clin Endocrinol Metab 89:2248-53, 2004

65. Harvie MN, Howell A, Thatcher N, et al: Energy balance in patients with advanced NSCLC, metastatic melanoma and metastatic breast cancer receiving chemotherapy—a longitudinal study. Br J Cancer 92:673-80, 2005

66. Smith MR: Changes in body composition during hormonal therapy for prostate cancer. Clin Prostate Cancer 2:18-21, 2003

67. Warner JT, Evans WD, Webb DK, et al: Body composition of long-term survivors of acute lymphoblastic leukaemia. Med Pediatr Oncol 38:165-72, 2002

68. Heber D, Ingles S, Ashley JM, et al: Clinical detection of sarcopenic obesity by bioelectrical impedance analysis. Am J Clin Nutr 64:472S-477S, 1996

69. McKenzie DC, Kalda AL: Effect of upper extremity exercise on secondary lymphedema in breast cancer patients: a pilot study. J Clin Oncol 21:463-6, 2003

70. Jenkins I, Djuric Z, Darga L, et al: Relationship of psychiatric diagnosis and weight loss maintenance in obese breast cancer survivors. Obes Res 11:1369-75, 2003

71. Health NIo: The Practical Guide: Identification, Evaluation, and Treatment of Overweight and Obesity in Adults, 2000

72. Rolls BJ, Drewnowski A, Ledikwe JH: Changing the energy density of the diet as a strategy for weight management. J Am Diet Assoc 105:S98-103, 2005

73. Nestle M: Increasing portion sizes in American diets: more calories, more obesity. J Am Diet Assoc 103:39-40, 2003

74. Nielsen SJ, Popkin BM: Patterns and trends in food portion sizes, 1977-1998. Jama 289:450-3, 2003

75. Rolls BJ, Roe LS, Meengs JS: Reductions in portion size and energy density of foods are additive and lead to sustained decreases in energy intake. Am J Clin Nutr 83:11-7, 2006

76. Smiciklas-Wright H, Mitchell DC, Mickle SJ, et al: Foods commonly eaten in the United States, 1989-1991 and 1994-1996: are portion sizes changing? J Am Diet Assoc 103:41-7, 2003

77. Young LR, Nestle M: The contribution of expanding portion sizes to the US obesity epidemic. Am J Public Health 92:246-9, 2002

78. Demark-Wahnefried W, Pinto BM, Gritz ER: Promoting health and physical function among cancer survivors: Potential for prevention and questions that remain. J Clin Oncol, in press

79. Kroenke CH, Fung TT, Hu FB, et al: Dietary patterns and survival after breast cancer diagnosis. J Clin Oncol 23:9295-303, 2005

80. Rock CL: Diet and breast cancer: can dietary factors influence survival? J Mammary Gland Biol Neoplasia 8:119-32, 2003

81. Meyer F, Bairati I, Shadmani R, et al: Dietary fat and prostate cancer survival. Cancer Causes Control 10:245-51, 1999

82. Chlebowski RT, Blackburn GL, Elashoff RE, et al: Dietary fat reduction in postmenopausal women with primary breast cancer: Phase III Women's Intervention Nutrition Study (WINS). Proceedings of the American Society of Clinical Oncology 24, 2005

83. Pierce JP, Faerber S, Wright FA, et al: A randomized trial of the effect of a plant-based dietary pattern on additional breast cancer events and survival: the Women's Healthy Eating and Living (WHEL) Study. Control Clin Trials 23:728-56, 2002

84. Rock CL, Flatt SW, Thomson CA, et al: Effects of a high-fiber, low-fat diet intervention on serum concentrations of reproductive steroid hormones in women with a history of breast cancer. J Clin Oncol 22:2379-87, 2004

85. Hebert JR, Ebbeling CB, Olendzki BC, et al: Change in women's diet and body mass following intensive intervention for early-stage breast cancer. J Am Diet Assoc 101:421-31, 2001

86. Kristal AR, Shattuck AL, Bowen DJ, et al: Feasibility of using volunteer research staff to deliver and evaluate a low-fat dietary intervention: the American Cancer Society Breast Cancer Dietary Intervention Project. Cancer Epidemiol Biomarkers Prev 6:459-67, 1997

87. Nordevang E, Callmer E, Marmur A, et al: Dietary intervention in breast cancer patients: effects on food choice. Eur J Clin Nutr 46:387-96, 1992

88. Chlebowski RT, Rose D, Buzzard IM, et al: Adjuvant dietary fat intake reduction in postmenopausal breast cancer patient management. The Women's Intervention Nutrition Study (WINS). Breast Cancer Res Treat 20:73-84, 1992

89. Brown JK, Byers T, Doyle C, et al: Nutrition and physical activity during and after cancer treatment: an American Cancer Society guide for informed choices. CA Cancer J Clin 53:268-91, 2003

90. MacLean CH, Newberry SJ, Mojica WA, et al: Effects of omega-3 fatty acids on cancer risk: a systematic review. JAMA 295:403-15, 2006

91. Krauss RM, Eckel RH, Howard B, et al: Revision 2000: a statement for healthcare professionals from the Nutrition Committee of the American Heart Association. J Nutr 131:132-46, 2001

92. World Health Organization: Diet, Nutrition, and the Prevention of Chronic Diseases: Report of a Joint WHO/FAO EXpert Consultation. World Health Organization Technical Report Series 916, 2003

93. Hebert JR, Hurley TG, Ma Y: The effect of dietary exposures on recurrence and mortality in early stage breast cancer. Breast Cancer Res Treat 51:17-28, 1998

94. Institute of Medicine: Dietary Reference Intakes for Energy, Carbohydrates,, Fiber, Fat, Fatty Acids, Cholesterol, Protein, and Amino Acids. 2002

95. Asano T, McLeod RS: Dietary fibre for the prevention of colorectal adenomas and carcinomas. Cochrane Database Syst Rev:CD003430, 2002

96. Jacobs ET, Lanza E, Alberts DS, et al: Fiber, sex, and colorectal adenoma: results of a pooled analysis. Am J Clin Nutr 83:343-9, 2006

97. Krone CA, Ely JT: Controlling hyperglycemia as an adjunct to cancer therapy. Integr Cancer Ther 4:25-31, 2005

98. Rock CL, Flatt SW, Natarajan L, et al: Plasma carotenoids and recurrence-free survival in women with a history of breast cancer. J Clin Oncol 23:6631-8, 2005

99. Pierce JP, Newman VA, Flatt SW, et al: Telephone counseling intervention increases intakes of micronutrient- and phytochemical-rich vegetables, fruit and fiber in breast cancer survivors. J Nutr 134:452-8, 2004

100. Schmitz KH, Holtzman J, Courneya KS, et al: Controlled physical activity trials in cancer survivors: a systematic review and meta-analysis. Cancer Epidemiol Biomarkers Prev 14:1588-95, 2005

101. Knols R, Aaronson NK, Uebelhart D, et al: Physical exercise in cancer patients during and after medical treatment: a systematic review of randomized and controlled clinical trials. J Clin Oncol 23:3830-42, 2005

102. Conn VS, Hafdahl AR, Porock DC, et al: A meta-analysis of exercise interventions among people treated for cancer. Support Care Cancer, 2006

103. Galvao DA, Newton RU: Review of exercise intervention studies in cancer patients. J Clin Oncol 23:899-909, 2005

104. Lane K, Jespersen D, McKenzie DC: The effect of a whole body exercise programme and dragon boat training on arm volume and arm circumference in women treated for breast cancer. Eur J Cancer Care (Engl) 14:353-8, 2005

105. Ohira T, Schmitz KH, Ahmed RL, et al: Effects of weight training on quality of life in recent breast cancer survivors: the Weight Training for Breast Cancer Survivors (WTBS) study. Cancer, 2006

106. Pinto BM, Frierson GM, Rabin C, et al: Home-based physical activity intervention for breast cancer patients. J Clin Oncol 23:3577-87, 2005

107. Thorsen L, Skovlund E, Stromme SB, et al: Effectiveness of physical activity on cardio-respiratory fitness and health-related quality of life in young and middle-aged cancer patients shortly after chemotherapy. J Clin Oncol 23:2378-88, 2005

108. Cheema BS, Gaul CA: Full-body exercise training improves fitness and quality of life in survivors of breast cancer. J Strength Cond Res 20:14-21, 2006

109. Spruit MA, Janssen PP, Willemsen SC, et al: Exercise capacity before and after an 8-week multidisciplinary inpatient rehabilitation program in lung cancer patients: A pilot study. Lung Cancer 52:257-60, 2006

110. Wilson DB, Porter JS, Parker G, et al: Anthropometric changes using a walking intervention in African American breast cancer survivors: a pilot study. Prev Chronic Dis 2:A16, 2005

111. Damush TM, Perkins A, Miller K: The implementation of an oncologist referred, exercise self-management program for older breast cancer survivors. Psychooncology, 2005

112. Holmes MD, Chen WY, Feskanich D, et al: Physical activity and survival after breast cancer diagnosis. JAMA 293:2479-86, 2005

113. Meyerhardt JA, Heseltine D, Niedzwiecki D, et al: The impact of physical activity on patients with stage III colon cancer: Findings from Intergroup trial CALGB 89803. Proceedings of the American Society of Clinical Oncology, 2005

114. Henderson IC, Berry DA, Demetri GD, et al: Improved outcomes from adding sequential Paclitaxel but not from escalating Doxorubicin dose in an adjuvant chemotherapy regimen for patients with node-positive primary breast cancer. J Clin Oncol 21:976-83, 2003

115. Meinardi MT, van Veldhuisen DJ, Gietema JA, et al: Prospective evaluation of early cardiac damage induced by epirubicin-containing adjuvant chemotherapy and locoregional radiotherapy in breast cancer patients. J Clin Oncol 19:2746-53, 2001

116. Perez EA, Suman VJ, Davidson NE, et al: Effect of doxorubicin plus cyclophosphamide on left ventricular ejection fraction in patients with breast cancer in the North Central Cancer Treatment Group N9831 Intergroup Adjuvant Trial. J Clin Oncol 22:3700-4, 2004

117. Piccart MJ, Di Leo A, Beauduin M, et al: Phase III trial comparing two dose levels of epirubicin combined with cyclophosphamide with cyclophosphamide, methotrexate, and fluorouracil in node-positive breast cancer. J Clin Oncol 19:3103-10, 2001

118. Beckman JA, Thakore A, Kalinowski BH, et al: Radiation therapy impairs endothelium-dependent vasodilation in humans. J Am Coll Cardiol 37:761-5, 2001

119. Demark-Wahnefried W, Winer EP, Rimer BK: Why women gain weight with adjuvant chemotherapy for breast cancer. J Clin Oncol 11:1418-29, 1993

120. Cancer IAfRo: International Agency for Research on Cancer monographs on the evaluation of the carcinogenic risk of chemicals to humans. Lyon, France, International Agency for Research on Cancer Press, 2004

121. American Cancer Society: Cancer Prevention and Early Detection, 2006

122. Gritz ER, Dresler C, Sarna L: Smoking, the missing drug interaction in clinical trials: ignoring the obvious. Cancer Epidemiol Biomarkers Prev 14:2287-93, 2005

123. Lin K, Patel SG, Chu PY, et al: Second primary malignancy of the aerodigestive tract in patients treated for cancer of the oral cavity and larynx. Head Neck 27:1042-8, 2005

124. Gritz ER, Vidrine DJ, Lazev AB: Smoking cessation in cancer patients: Never too late to quit. In Given B, Given CW, Champion V, et al (eds): Evidence-Based Interventions in Oncology. New York, Springer Publishing Company, 2003, pp 107-140

125. McBride CM, Ostroff JS: Teachable moments for promoting smoking cessation: the context of cancer care and survivorship. Cancer Control 10:325-33, 2003

126. Gritz ER, Fingeret MC, Vidrine DJ, et al: Successes and failures of the teachable moment: smoking cessation in cancer patients. Cancer 106:17-27, 2006

127. Coups EJ, Ostroff JS: A population-based estimate of the prevalence of behavioral risk factors among adult cancer survivors and noncancer controls. Prev Med 40:702-11, 2005

128. Bellizzi KM, Rowland JH, Jeffery DD, et al: Health behaviors of cancer survivors: examining opportunities for cancer control intervention. J Clin Oncol 23:8884-93, 2005

129. Force USPST: Counseling to Prevent Tobacco Use and Tobacco-Related Disease: Recommendation Statement, 2003

130. Gritz ER, Carr CR, Rapkin D, et al: Predictors of long-term smoking cessation in head and neck cancer patients. Cancer Epidemiol Biomarkers Prev 2:261-70, 1993

131. Emmons KM, Puleo E, Park E, et al: Peer-delivered smoking counseling for childhood cancer survivors increases rate of cessation: the partnership for health study. J Clin Oncol 23:6516-23, 2005

132. Butterfield RM, Park ER, Puleo E, et al: Multiple risk behaviors among smokers in the childhood cancer survivors study cohort. Psychooncology 13:619-29, 2004

133. Lambert MT, Terrell JE, Copeland LA, et al: Cigarettes, alcohol, and depression: characterizing head and neck cancer survivors in two systems of care. Nicotine Tob Res 7:233-41, 2005

134. Pinto BM, Trunzo JJ: Health behaviors during and after a cancer diagnosis. Cancer 104:2614-23, 2005

135. Hollen PJ, Hobbie WL, Finley SM: Testing the effects of a decision-making and risk-reduction program for cancer-surviving adolescents. Oncol Nurs Forum 26:1475-86, 1999

136. Day GL, Blot WJ, Shore RE, et al: Second cancers following oral and pharyngeal cancers: role of tobacco and alcohol. J Natl Cancer Inst 86:131-7, 1994

137. Deleyiannis FW, Thomas DB, Vaughan TL, et al: Alcoholism: independent predictor of survival in patients with head and neck cancer. J Natl Cancer Inst 88:542-9, 1996

138. Association AH: American Heart Association Dietary Guidelines, 2006

139. Hann DM, Baker F, Roberts CS, et al: Use of complementary therapies among breast and prostate cancer patients during treatment: a multisite study. Integr Cancer Ther 4:294-300, 2005

140. Monti DA, Yang J: Complementary medicine in chronic cancer care. Semin Oncol 32:225-31, 2005

141. Rock E, DeMichele A: Nutritional approaches to late toxicities of adjuvant chemotherapy in breast cancer survivors. J Nutr 133:3785S-3793S, 2003

142. Saraiya M, Glanz K, Briss PA, et al: Interventions to prevent skin cancer by reducing exposure to ultraviolet radiation: a systematic review. Am J Prev Med 27:422-66, 2004

143. Leisenring W, Friedman DL, Flowers ME, et al: Nonmelanoma skin and mucosal cancers after hematopoietic cell transplantation. J Clin Oncol 24:1119-26, 2006

144. Euvrard S, Kanitakis J, Claudy A: Skin cancers after organ transplantation. N Engl J Med 348:1681-91, 2003

145. Bhatia S, Estrada-Batres L, Maryon T, et al: Second primary tumors in patients with cutaneous malignant melanoma. Cancer 86:2014-20, 1999

146. Baker KS, DeFor TE, Burns LJ, et al: New malignancies after blood or marrow stem-cell transplantation in children and adults: incidence and risk factors. J Clin Oncol 21:1352-8, 2003

147. Levi F, Moeckli R, Randimbison L, et al: Skin cancer in survivors of childhood and adolescent cancer. Eur J Cancer 42:656-659, 2006

148. Robinson JK, Rademaker AW: Skin cancer risk and sun protection learning by helpers of patients with nonmelanoma skin cancer. Prev Med 24:333-41, 1995

149. Giovannucci E, Liu Y, Rimm EB, et al: Prospective study of predictors of vitamin D status and cancer incidence and mortality in men. J Natl Cancer Inst 98:451-9, 2006

150. Gorham ED, Garland CF, Garland FC, et al: Vitamin D and prevention of colorectal cancer. J Steroid Biochem Mol Biol 97:179-94, 2005

151. Zhou W, Suk R, Liu G, et al: Vitamin D is associated with improved survival in early-stage non-small cell lung cancer patients. Cancer Epidemiol Biomarkers Prev 14:2303-9, 2005

152. Foundation IO: Osteoporosis in the European Community: a call to action - an audit of policy developments since 1998. Lyon, France, International Osteoporosis Foundation, 2003

153. Nelson RL, Turyk M, Kim J, et al: Bone mineral density and the subsequent risk of cancer in the NHANES I follow-up cohort. BMC Cancer 2:22, 2002

154. Buist DS, LaCroix AZ, Barlow WE, et al: Bone mineral density and endogenous hormones and risk of breast cancer in postmenopausal women (United States). Cancer Causes Control 12:213-22, 2001

155. Newcomb PA, Trentham-Dietz A, Egan KM, et al: Fracture history and risk of breast and endometrial cancer. Am J Epidemiol 153:1071-8, 2001

156. van der Klift M, de Laet CE, Coebergh JW, et al: Bone mineral density and the risk of breast cancer: the Rotterdam Study. Bone 32:211-6, 2003

157. Zmuda JM, Cauley JA, Ljung BM, et al: Bone mass and breast cancer risk in older women: differences by stage at diagnosis. J Natl Cancer Inst 93:930-6, 2001

158. Twiss JJ, Waltman N, Ott CD, et al: Bone mineral density in postmenopausal breast cancer survivors. J Am Acad Nurse Pract 13:276-84, 2001

159. Chlebowski RT: Bone health in women with early-stage breast cancer. Clin Breast Cancer 5 Suppl:S35-40, 2005

160. Mackey JR, Joy AA: Skeletal health in postmenopausal survivors of early breast cancer. Int J Cancer 114:1010-5, 2005

161. Smith MR: Therapy Insight: osteoporosis during hormone therapy for prostate cancer. Nat Clin Pract Urol 2:608-15; quiz 628, 2005

162. Greenspan SL, Coates P, Sereika SM, et al: Bone loss after initiation of androgen deprivation therapy in patients with prostate cancer. J Clin Endocrinol Metab 90:6410-7, 2005

163. Lee H, McGovern K, Finkelstein JS, et al: Changes in bone mineral density and body composition during initial and long-term gonadotropin-releasing hormone agonist treatment for prostate carcinoma. Cancer 104:1633-7, 2005

164. Arikoski P, Voutilainen R, Kroger H: Bone mineral density in long-term survivors of childhood cancer. J Pediatr Endocrinol Metab 16 (Suppl) 2:343-53, 2003

165. Baroncelli GI, Bertelloni S, Sodini F, et al: Osteoporosis in children and adolescents: etiology and management. Paediatr Drugs 7:295-323, 2005

166. Relling MV, Yang W, Das S, et al: Pharmacogenetic risk factors for osteonecrosis of the hip among children with leukemia. J Clin Oncol 22:3930-6, 2004

167. Kelly J, Damron T, Grant W, et al: Cross-sectional study of bone mineral density in adult survivors of solid pediatric cancers. J Pediatr Hematol Oncol 27:248-53, 2005

168. Hillner BE, Ingle JN, Chlebowski RT, et al: American Society of Clinical Oncology 2003 update on the role of bisphosphonates and bone health issues in women with breast cancer. J Clin Oncol 21:4042-57, 2003

169. Gass M, Dawson-Hughes B: Preventing osteoporosis-related fractures: an overview. Am J Med 119:S3-S11, 2006

170. Swenson KK, Henly SJ, Shapiro AC, et al: Interventions to prevent loss of bone mineral density in women receiving chemotherapy for breast cancer. Clin J Oncol Nurs 9:177-84, 2005

171. Waltman NL, Twiss JJ, Ott CD, et al: Testing an intervention for preventing osteoporosis in postmenopausal breast cancer survivors. J Nurs Scholarsh 35:333-8, 2003

172. Frazer IH, Cox JT, Mayeaux EJ, Jr., et al: Advances in prevention of cervical cancer and other human papillomavirus-related diseases. Pediatr Infect Dis J 25:S65-81, quiz S82, 2006

173. Arrowood JR, Hayney MS: Immunization recommendations for adults with cancer. Ann Pharmacother 36:1219-29, 2002

174. Faller H, Schilling S, Otteni M, et al: [Social support and social stress in tumor patients and their partners]. Z Psychosom Med Psychoanal 41:141-57, 1995

175. Linn MW, Linn BS, Harris R: Effects of counseling for late stage cancer patients. Cancer 49:1048-55, 1982

176. Linn MW, Linn BS, Stein SR: Beliefs about causes of cancer in cancer patients. Soc Sci Med 16:835-9, 1982

177. Maskarinec G, Gotay CC, Tatsumura Y, et al: Perceived cancer causes: use of complementary and alternative therapy. Cancer Pract 9:183-90, 2001

178. Stewart DE, Cheung AM, Duff S, et al: Attributions of cause and recurrence in long-term breast cancer survivors. Psychooncology 10:179-83, 2001

179. Stewart DE, Wong F, Duff S, et al: "What doesn't kill you makes you stronger": an ovarian cancer survivor survey. Gynecol Oncol 83:537-42, 2001

180. Wold KS, Byers T, Crane LA, et al: What do cancer survivors believe causes cancer? (United States). Cancer Causes Control 16:115-23, 2005

181. Demark-Wahnefried W, Peterson B, McBride C, et al: Current health behaviors and readiness to pursue life-style changes among men and women diagnosed with early stage prostate and breast carcinomas. Cancer 88:674-84, 2000

182. van Weert E, Hoekstra-Weebers J, Grol B, et al: A multidimensional cancer rehabilitation program for cancer survivors: effectiveness on health-related quality of life. J Psychosom Res 58:485-96, 2005

183. Demark-Wahnefried W: Unpublished data. 2006

184. McBride CM, Clipp E, Peterson BL, et al: Psychological impact of diagnosis and risk reduction among cancer survivors. Psychooncology 9:418-27, 2000

185. Jones LW, Courneya KS: Exercise counseling and programming preferences of cancer survivors. Cancer Pract 10:208-15, 2002

186. Glanz K: Behavioral research contributions and needs in cancer prevention and control: dietary change. Prev Med 26:S43-55, 1997

187. Pinto BM, Friedman R, Marcus BH, et al: Effects of a computer-based, telephone-counseling system on physical activity. Am J Prev Med 23:113-20, 2002

188. Rose MA: Health promotion and risk prevention: applications for cancer survivors. Oncol Nurs Forum 16:335-40, 1989

189. van der Bij AK, Laurant MG, Wensing M: Effectiveness of physical activity interventions for older adults: a review. Am J Prev Med 22:120-33, 2002

190. Im EO, Chee W: Issues in Internet survey research among cancer patients. Cancer Nurs 27:34-42; quiz 43-4, 2004

191. Rutten LJ, Arora NK, Bakos AD, et al: Information needs and sources of information among cancer patients: a systematic review of research (1980-2003). Patient Educ Couns 57:250-61, 2005

192. Courneya KS, Friedenreich CM, Quinney HA, et al: A randomized trial of exercise and quality of life in colorectal cancer survivors. Eur J Cancer Care (Engl) 12:347-57, 2003

193. Courneya KS, Friedenreich CM, Sela RA, et al: The group psychotherapy and home-based physical exercise (group-hope) trial in cancer survivors: physical fitness and quality of life outcomes. Psychooncology 12:357-74, 2003

194. Tyc VL, Rai SN, Lensing S, et al: Intervention to reduce intentions to use tobacco among pediatric cancer survivors. J Clin Oncol 21:1366-72, 2003

195. Wilson RW, Jacobsen PB, Fields KK: Pilot study of a home-based aerobic exercise program for sedentary cancer survivors treated with hematopoietic stem cell transplantation. Bone Marrow Transplant 35:721-7, 2005

196. Segal R, Evans W, Johnson D, et al: Structured exercise improves physical functioning in women with stages I and II breast cancer: results of a randomized controlled trial. J Clin Oncol 19:657-65, 2001

197. Mandelblatt J, Kanetsky PA: Effectiveness of interventions to enhance physician screening for breast cancer. J Fam Pract 40:162-71, 1995

198. Manne S, Fasanella N, Connors J, et al: Sun protection and skin surveillance practices among relatives of patients with malignant melanoma: prevalence and predictors. Prev Med 39:36-47, 2004

199. Rauscher GH, Hawley ST, Earp JA: Baseline predictors of initiation vs. maintenance of regular mammography use among rural women. Prev Med 40:822-30, 2005

200. Rimer BK: Improving the use of cancer screening for older women. Cancer 72:1084-7, 1993

201. Taylor V, Lessler D, Mertens K, et al: Colorectal cancer screening among African Americans: the importance of physician recommendation. J Natl Med Assoc 95:806-12, 2003

202. Jones LW, Courneya KS, Peddle C, et al: Oncologists' opinions towards recommending exercise to patients with cancer: a Canadian national survey. Support Care Cancer 13:929-37, 2005

203. Ahuja R, Weibel SB, Leone FT: Lung cancer: the oncologist's role in smoking cessation. Semin Oncol 30:94-103, 2003

204. Kuhn KG, Boesen E, Ross L, et al: Evaluation and outcome of behavioural changes in the rehabilitation of cancer patients: a review. Eur J Cancer 41:216-24, 2005

205. Yarnall KS, Pollak KI, Ostbye T, et al: Primary care: is there enough time for prevention? Am J Public Health 93:635-41, 2003

206. Jones LW, Courneya KS, Fairey AS, et al: Effects of an oncologist's recommendation to exercise on self-reported exercise behavior in newly diagnosed breast cancer survivors: a single-blind, randomized controlled trial. Ann Behav Med 28:105-13, 2004

207. Jones LW, Courneya KS, Fairey AS, et al: Does the theory of planned behavior mediate the effects of an oncologist's recommendation to exercise in newly diagnosed breast cancer survivors? Results from a randomized controlled trial. Health Psychol 24:189-97, 2005

208. Courneya KS: Exercise in cancer survivors: an overview of research. Med Sci Sports Exerc 35:1846-52, 2003

209. Warburton DE, Nicol CW, Bredin SS: Prescribing exercise as preventive therapy. CMAJ 174:961-74, 2006

210. Warburton DE, Nicol CW, Bredin SS: Health benefits of physical activity: the evidence. CMAJ 174:801-9, 2006

211. Demark-Wahnefried W, Kenyon A, Eberle P, et al: Preventing sarcopenic obesity among breast cancer patients who receive adjuvant chemotherapy: results of a feasibility study. Clin Exerc Physiol 4:44-9, 2002

212. Loprinzi CL, Athmann LM, Kardinal CG, et al: Randomized trial of dietician counseling to try to prevent weight gain associated with breast cancer adjuvant chemotherapy. Oncol 53:228-32, 1996

Appendix D.3

The Passport for Care

Improving the Lives of Childhood Cancer Survivors: Development of a Novel Internet Resource for Managing Long-Term Health Risks

David G. Poplack, MD, * Michael Fordis, MD,* * *
Marc E. Horowitz, MD, * Wendy Landier, RN, MSN, CPNP,
CPON,* + *Melissa M. Hudson, MD,* ++ *Smita Bhatia, MD,* +
Kevin C. Oeffinger, MD, # *Ann C. Mertens, PhD,* ##
and Quentin W. Smith, MS * *

1. Introduction to the Passport for Care (PFC)

The Institute of Medicine,[1] the President's Cancer Panel,[2] and the Centers for Disease Control and Prevention[3] have emphasized the importance of periodic evaluation and screening of cancer survivors for late effects of treatment for their cancers. The Children's Oncology Group (COG) recently released version 2 of a set of comprehensive, evidence-based, long-term follow-up guidelines for health care providers managing childhood cancer survivors.[4] While recognizing that the length and depth of the COG guidelines are important in order to provide clinically relevant, evidence-based recommendations and supporting health education materials, clinician time limitations and the effort required to identify the specific recommendations relevant to individual patients using the current paper-based

---

*Texas Children's Cancer Center, Baylor College of Medicine
* *Center for Collaborative and Interactive Technologies, Baylor College of Medicine
+City of Hope
++St. Jude Children's Research Hospital
#Memorial Sloan-Kettering Cancer Center
##University of Minnesota Medical School and Cancer Center

format of the guidelines have been identified as barriers to their clinical application. This report discusses the development of an online decision support tool, the PFC, which allows health care providers and childhood cancer survivors to quickly and accurately generate individualized exposure-based screening recommendations and patient educational materials according to the COG Long-Term Follow-Up Guidelines via a web-based, user-friendly interface.

The PFC includes an interface and database for recording summaries of survivor treatment exposures; a "Guidelines Generator" employing a logic layer with decision rules that link treatment exposures to periodic evaluations and screening recommendations; and back-end guideline administration and maintenance tools. When completed, the PFC will also provide the survivor ready access to individualized healthcare resources, an online survivor forum, and regular health screening information. It is designed for secure use by the childhood cancer survivor who, if they choose, can share information contained within the PFC with their physicians and other health care providers.

This background paper describes the rationale, process, and status of efforts to create this dynamic resource for survivors of childhood cancer and their health care providers. The PFC is designed to be easily modified to accommodate new and emerging findings regarding risks associated with cancer treatment exposures, and it offers a means of alerting survivors and professionals involved in their care regarding these findings.

In the ensuing pages, we provide a brief review of the current state of the knowledge regarding late effects of treatment for childhood cancer and the strategies for managing risks for late effects. We also describe the multidisciplinary collaborative effort involved in the creation, testing, refinement, and deployment of the PFC. Lastly, we provide a description of the current status of the PFC, discuss barriers and challenges to its development and implementation, and review the implications of the PFC as a potential model resource for follow-up of survivors of adult cancer and possibly other chronic diseases.

2. The Challenge Posed by Late Effects of Treatment for Childhood Cancer

2a. The Emergence of Cancer Survivorship as a National Priority. Within the last few years cancer survivorship has been recognized as a national public health priority by: (1) the Institute of Medicine (IOM) in their 2003 report *Childhood Cancer Survivorship: Improving Care and Quality of Life*;[1,5] (2) the Centers for Disease Control and Prevention (CDC) in its recently released *A National Action Plan for Cancer Survivorship: Advancing Public Health Strategies*;[3] and (3) the President's Cancer Panel in its 2003-2004 *Annual Report, Living Beyond Cancer: Finding a New Balance*.[2] Several themes emerged from the recommendations and strategies of all three documents: (1) There is a need to raise awareness among survivors themselves, family members, policy makers and the public about issues surrounding survivorship, including the long-term risk for late sequelae of cancer treatment; (2) survivors and providers need to be informed of the benefits of screening and periodic examinations as evidence and guidelines emerge regarding long-term follow-up; and (3) patient navigation systems and web-based tools need to be developed, tested, and maintained to facilitate optimum follow-up care of survivors.

2b. Challenges to Implementing Recommendations for Cancer Survivors. Cancer survivorship represents a prototypical serious chronic health problem. Recovery from cancer requires transitions from specialty care to primary care, with follow-up after treatment supported by evidenced-based guidelines for care.[2] Systematic follow-up studies of late effects in survivors of adult malignancies have been limited and comprehensive guidelines remain largely unavailable. However, the experience with long-term follow-up of childhood cancer survivors has provided sufficient evidence to link therapeutic exposures with potential late effects to inform guideline development. The pediatric oncology experience may provide a model for exploration of how guidelines for adult cancer follow-up care and management of other chronic conditions may be deployed and implemented.

2c. The Experience with Childhood, Adolescent, and Young Adult Cancer Care. Since the 1970's, the majority of children and adolescents with cancers have been treated in clinical trials sponsored by the National Cancer Institute. Professionals at institutions affiliated with the COG have, historically, treated over 90% of all children with cancer in the United States.[6] The affiliated institutions in the United States, Canada, Europe, and Australia, numbering 232 organizations as of May 2006,[7] offer innovative diagnostic and therapeutic interventions through 150 treatment protocols designed to improve clinical and functional outcomes for children and adolescents with cancer.[8]

The National Cancer Institute through its Surveillance Epidemiology and End Results (SEER) program has documented the success achieved in treatments of childhood, adolescent, and young adult cancer in recent years. Over the last quarter century, 5-year survival rates for the five age groupings used in tracking have increased as follows for childhood cancers of all sites: (1) ages 0-4: from 56.8% in 1974-1976 to 78.3% in 1995-2001; (2) ages 5-9: from 55.5% in 1974-1976 to 78.6% in 1995-2001; (3) ages 10-14: from 55.1% in 1974-1976 to 79.2% in 1995-2001; and (4) ages 15-19: from 63.8%% in 1974-1976 to 79.5% in 1995-2001.[9]

The population of childhood cancer survivors now numbers over 270,000.[1] Several reports have extrapolated from SEER data reported by Jemal and colleagues in estimating that roughly 1 in 570 individuals between 20 and 34 years of age is a long-term survivor of childhood cancer.[1,10-12] Whether or not improvements in survival continue at rates suggested by some researchers and epidemiologists, there are clear indicators of success in prolonging the lives of children with cancer through more effective treatment of the acute stages of disease. As a consequence, pediatric oncologists and others who have been involved in cancer care for children have recognized the obligation to examine the late sequelae of cancer and cancer treatment and to develop strategies to screen for and manage risks effectively.

2d. The Consequences of Treatment Success. The remarkable improvements in pediatric cancer survival rates have brought with them a new set of challenges for health care providers and for national, state, and local health care systems. Childhood cancer survivors commonly experience late effects of treatment.[13-24] Two-thirds or more of childhood cancer survivors are likely to experience at least one late effect,[13,16-20] and in 25-40% of long-term survivors, the late effects associated with treatment for cancer are likely to be severe or life threatening.[11,13-15,17,25] Late effects encompass a myriad of detrimental physical conditions providing evidence for the need for follow-up screening and early intervention These effects range from multiorgan and systems dysfunction or failure;[26-62] to subsequent malignancies.[21,48,63-71] In addition, chronic or subclinical changes persisting after cancer treatment may result in premature onset of common conditions associated with aging (e.g., diabetes mellitus, cardiovascular disease, hypertension, hyperlipidemia)[46-48,51,53,54,56-62,72] that place the long-term survivor at higher risk for chronic illness and premature death.

Treatment for childhood cancer can also affect normal growth, leading to reduced height[73-78] and increased risk for obesity.[79-82] The likelihood of growth problems associated with particular cancer treatments provides evidence for the need for regular screening in such patients and timely intervention to manage risks of abnormal stature and weight. Apart from physical manifestations of disease related to prior childhood cancer treatment, there is a large body of literature related to psychosocial effects of childhood cancer and its treatment on both survivors and family members.[83-103] These effects may be related to: stress and the trauma inflicted by cancer and its treatment on children and their families;[104-121] deficits in cognition and learning difficulties related to treatment;[92,122-130] and/or factors involving body image and self-concept in children and young adults who perceive themselves as being different from their peers.[97,131-135] The heightened risk for cognitive, behavioral, and interpersonal problems related to a prior cancer and cancer treatment experience requires vigilance on the part of care providers so that timely assessment and appropriate treatment services can be arranged, should symptoms of such problems appear.

2e. Complexity in Risk Assessment and Management. The difficulties that many health care providers experience in trying to gauge the types and levels of health risks associated with prior childhood cancer treatment were summarized succinctly by Landier and colleagues:

> . . . health care providers encountering childhood cancer survivors must be knowledgeable about potential cancer-related adverse effects in order to prescribe appropriate monitoring and to implement therapeutic interventions should health problems arise. Unfortunately, because of the relative rarity of childhood cancer, many health care providers lack familiarity with cancer-related health risks and risk-reduction methods relevant for this population. Moreover, the heterogeneous nature of pediatric malignancies, representing numerous histological subtypes with unique epidemiology, biology, and treatment regimens, further reduce the likelihood of primary care providers attaining proficiency in managing long-term childhood cancer survivors. At most, health care providers outside of academic centers may care for no more than a handful of survivors, usually each with different cancers, treatment exposures, and health risks, making delivery of appropriate care a daunting task. Consequently, primary care providers in the community setting are often unfamiliar with cancer-related health risks and uncomfortable with supervising the care of childhood cancer survivors.[136 pp.150-151]

2f. Survivors' Lack of Awareness of Health Risks and Effective Risk Management Strategies. Confounding the poor understanding of childhood cancer treatment-related health risks by many health professionals is the general lack of awareness of such risks by the survivors themselves. A limited number of studies have revealed significant knowledge deficits and misperceptions in survivors' understanding of their cancer diagnosis, treatment, and cancer-related health risks.[137-141] One study of adult survivors of childhood cancer diagnosed between 1945 and 1974 concluded that certain factors (e.g., younger age at treatment, nonwhite race, less intensive treatment, lower paternal education, diagnosis in the earlier years of the study) were associated with greater knowledge deficits among survivors.[137] In more recent studies, survivors demonstrated greater general knowledge about their cancer histories and associated health risks, but exhibited limited knowledge of specific treatment details, a key factor in coordinating long-term risk-based health care.[138,139,141] The knowledge deficits observed in two of these studies may be confounded by cultural and ethnic variations in attitudes regarding disclosure of the diagnosis of cancer, especially to very young children.[138,139] However, persistent knowledge deficits about cancer-related health risks in older survivors limit their participation in screening and risk-reducing interventions.[140]

Several studies indicate that survivors perceive themselves as more vulnerable to health problems than others not treated for cancer, requiring more attention by the provider in protecting his or her health.[135,142-147] However, health concerns do not consistently motivate engagement in protective behavioral practices or abstinence from risky behaviors.[143,147-149]

Examination of data on health service utilization from a large cohort of childhood cancer survivors confirmed that many of those who had treatments associated with higher risks failed to obtain follow-up screening as recommened.[150] Absence of recommended cancer-related medical visits within a 2-year period among survivors who should be screened based on known risks associated with specific treatments—including chest/mantle radiation therapy (RT), cumulative anthracycline dose ≥ 300 mg/m^2, bleomycin, etoposide or ifosfamide—was documented for nearly half of survivors surveyed in most cases. For those treated with chest/mantle RT, 47.9% did not report a cancer-related follow-up visit; for those treated with a ≥ 300 mg/m^2 cumulative anthracycline dose, the percentage not experiencing a cancer-related follow-up visit was 51.7%; for bleomycin treatment the percentage was 40.8%; and for high risk therapy, including any of the three just cited and/or treatment with etoposide or ifosfamide, the percentage was 50.7%.[150] The study authors concluded that, for most study participants, the likelihood of a cancer-related follow-up visit or a physical examination decreased at an age when the risks for potentially modifiable late effects from cancer were on the rise.[150]

3. Health System Factors Influencing the Delivery of Effective Follow-Up Services

3a. <u>Systems-Based Barriers to Effective Follow-Up.</u> Financial and health care systems barriers also influence follow-up care. One issue that has received considerable attention in the professional literature since the early 1990s relates to transition from pediatric to adult care.[151-164] There are well documented problems in the transition to adult care for young people with special health needs, including those previously treated for cancer. These problems include lack of needed treatment services (i.e., no place to refer young people when adult services are needed); provider unwillingness to take on young people with special needs; lack of comparability to services that had been available in the pediatric system; and lack of working knowledge among adult providers in managing the special needs of patients with conditions related to prior childhood diseases.[158,159,164]

Regarding procedural barriers, a major problem involves the transfer

of accurate, complete, and appropriate information from the pediatric oncology treatment setting to the adult primary care or adult oncology treatment setting. Effective follow-up of treatment-related health risks is contin-
gent on provision of a comprehensive medical summary to professionals
who will be involved in care of the younger or older adult who has a history
of treatment for childhood cancer.[165] The transfer of treatment risk-related
information to primary health care providers has been hampered by evolving cancer therapies and late effects profiles, as well as by the long latency
period needed to evaluate many health outcomes and the generally unknown risks of aging on treatment sequelae.[11]

The transfer is further hampered by the lack of uniform and/or compat-
ible information technology systems and electronic record distribution systems in U.S. health care. U.S. medical practices have been slow to adopt
information technologies that are increasingly important in health care
environments in which patients are likely to move geographically, change
health care providers either by choice or due to other factors (e.g., changes
in health care provider participation in specific third-party payer plans, loss
of health insurance coverage due to job changes), or otherwise alter their
health care seeking behaviors. Data suggest that, over a 12- to 24-month
period, between 15% and 25% of privately insured persons change their
health care provider due to changes in health plans.[166,167] Such changes
have the potential to disrupt the transfer of essential information (e.g.,
disease history, health risk data, and prior treatment exposures) to health
care providers who require the information in order to assist the patient in
making informed decisions about his or her care.

3b. Demands on Health Care Provider Time. Another systems-related issue
that impacts delivery of effective follow-up services to survivors of childhood cancer relates to demands placed on health care providers' time.
Expectations for comprehensive health screening and delivery of preventive
services by health care providers continue to grow. One recent study concluded that, in order for primary care providers to satisfy all the preventive
health care recommendations of the U.S. Preventive Services Task Force,
7.4 hours per working day would be devoted to preventive services—exclusive of any time spent in actual problem-based care.[168] Given the extra time
required in order to assess childhood cancer treatment-related risks, particularly in the absence of technology support in many settings, the potential for inadequate risk identification and management is high.

4. Childhood Cancer Survivors: A Model for Long-Term Follow-Up for Cancer Treatment

The survivors of childhood, adolescent, and young adult cancers represent a population that offers several important advantages for study of disease- and treatment-related factors that may increase risks for health problems later in life. Characteristics of this survivor group that lend themselves to modeling for health risk management include:

• The population is well characterized with initial exposures to treatment modalities documented by protocol;[1,4]

• Greater than 90% of children with cancer in the United States are treated within institutions that are members of the National Cancer Institute (NCI)-supported COG using therapeutic approaches that conform to COG-treatment protocols.[6]

• The late effects of cancer therapy have been and continue to be systematically investigated as part of the Childhood Cancer Survivor Study (CCSS), involving 20,346 childhood cancer survivors diagnosed between 1970 and 1986 and treated at 26 cancer centers in the U.S. and Canada.[169] Therefore, a large population of identifiable survivors is also readily available through the CCSS and long-term survivor clinics at select COG institutions for studies.[169] This population offers opportunities to test the effectiveness of interventions that can then be applied to the broader population of childhood, adolescent, and young adult cancer survivors, and ultimately extended to the total population of cancer survivors.

• Evidence-based guidelines for long-term follow-up have been developed by COG for survivors of childhood, adolescent, and young adult cancer.[4]

• The development and deployment of the PFC, an Internet-based decision support tool for both survivors and their health care providers is well underway. As recently reported, the PFC, a functional decision support system that includes automated capabilities to generate individualized screening and follow-up guidelines and resources, is entering the first phase of pilot testing in early 2007.[170] Progress toward development of the PFC is reviewed in the remainder of this chapter.

5. The Passport for Care

5a. <u>Purpose.</u> The PFC is an Internet-based decision support system being developed for use by patients and providers to guide long-term follow-up screening for late effects resulting from exposures for treatment of childhood cancer. The purposes of the PFC are to serve as a communication tool to bridge the transition in care from cancer treatment to long-term survivorship; to engage survivors and health care providers in an extended care relationship; and to engage and empower survivors in assuming control and direction for interventions to ensure health.

5b. <u>Description of PFC Features</u>. PFC features include a portable care summary of treatment exposures; individualized guidelines for care; alerts for guideline changes; individualized resources for the survivor and for the health care provider; survivor networks or virtual communities established through online forums; and opportunities to participate in survivor-related research. The PFC is being designed to contain separate online portals for survivors and health care providers; however survivors and providers will each have access to information across both portals. The survivor portal will contain information in presentation and language suitable for lay audiences. The health care provider portal will provide elements for subspecialty audiences of oncologists and for primary care providers.

The survivor will have options regarding which specific PFC components to share with various health care providers in either electronic or print formats. Also, the PFC will incorporate an audit function that will permit the survivor to review authorized access to the PFC. This latter function will enable the survivor to monitor PFC use by different providers, thereby facilitating tracking of communication among and between providers (e.g., oncologists, primary care providers, behavioral health specialists, others). Although not accessible by the survivor, the PFC will also contain tools for the guidelines developers to use to update or modify guidelines as recommended by the COG, review guidelines for standardization and consistency, and adjust guideline outputs.

In the pediatric arena, it is envisioned that the PFC will be an essential tool in reengineering the approach to care by preparing patients and/or family members for long-term survivorship. As treatment is completed, the details of the PFC are to be shared with the survivor and/or family members in preparation for participation. The discussion may be accompanied by reference to and review of specific steps that the patient and/or family member can take in monitoring for potential late effects and in intervening early if needed.

Discussion of PFC participation may serve several purposes. It provides an opportunity to communicate that a long-term follow-up plan is in place for the survivor, and it may diminish the sense of abandonment that some cancer survivors, both adults and children, describe with completion of acute treatment and discharge from care.[171, 172] PFC-related discussion may foster empowerment of the patient and may encourage establishment of extended partnerships with health care providers for purposes of health risk monitoring and intervention. Access to trusted and reliable resources for patient education and information may be facilitated via the PFC, laying the foundation for survivor-directed information seeking. Establishing a sense of independence and responsibility is important in building an effective health maintenance system that can be modified and updated to accommodate emerging risk-related research findings, as well as changing life circumstances specific to each patient.[1]

5c. <u>Overview of PFC Development, Structure and Elements</u>. The staged development of the PFC involves an iterative process informed by qualitative and quantitative research that includes focus groups and stakeholder interviews, prototype development, usability evaluation, clinic testing, and results-based improvement using an approach modified from that described by Mooney and Bligh.[173] Findings from qualitative data collection indicate that survivors want information that explains their previous treatments and risks for late effects; they want the ability to control their medical information; they want and need recommendations for their follow-up care and informational resources tailored to their specific cancer history; and they require summaries that can be shared with their personal health care providers in order to ensure that the provider is aware of risks associated with prior childhood cancer treatment. It is anticipated that research that will occur during the various stages of PFC development may identify additional needs of survivors and providers that the PFC can be modified to address.

5d. <u>The PFC: A Multi-Disciplinary Collaboration</u>. Led by faculty at the Texas Children's Cancer Center (TCCC) and the Center for Collaborative and Interactive Technologies at Baylor College of Medicine, the PFC has been developed in collaboration with representatives from the COG and the CCSS. The participants in the Working Group are noted in Table D.3-1. Input has also been obtained from members of a national steering committee and other stakeholders, including advocacy groups with particular interests in cancer survivorship and long-term follow-up care.

5e. <u>The Health Care Provider Portal</u>. The initial stage of PFC development has focused on creation of the "health care provider portal." A description of this portal is provided below.

As shown in Figure D.3-1, the health care provider portal has the following components:

- A summary of care including demographic data, diagnoses, and history of treatment exposures for each survivor;
- The COG Long-term Follow-up Guidelines for Survivors of Childhood, Adolescent, and Young Adult Cancers stored in a database;
- The decision rules linking treatment exposures to potential late effects and recommendations for screening and other resources;
- Web-based and print outputs providing individualized information regarding potential late effects, risk factors, and associated screening rec-

TABLE D.3-1 PFC Working Group Members and Organizational Affiliations (presented alphabetically by surname)

Smita Bhatia, MD City of Hope National Medical Center, Duarte, CA Chair, COG Late Effects Committee	Wendy Landier, RN, CPNP City of Hope National Medical Center, Duarte, CA Member, COG Nursing and Late Effects Committees
Sarah Bottomley, RN, MN, CPNP Texas Children's Cancer Center, Houston, TX	Ann Mertens, PhD University of Minnesota, Minneapolis, MN Investigator, Childhood Cancer Survivor Study
Michael Fordis, MD Center for Collaborative and Interactive Technologies Baylor College of Medicine, Houston, TX	Kevin Oeffinger, MD Memorial Sloan-Kettering, New York, NY Member, COG Late Effects Committee
Marc Horowitz, MD Texas Children's Cancer Center Baylor College of Medicine, Houston, TX	David Poplack, MD Texas Children's Cancer Center Baylor College of Medicine, Houston, TX
Melissa Hudson, MD St. Jude's Children's Research Hospital, Memphis, TN Member, COG Late Effects Committee	

ommendations (Figures D.3-2, D.3-3, and D.3-4; guidance for screening for other malignancies (Figure D.3-5); tailored survivor and health care provider education and information resources (Figure D.3-6); and evidence-based scoring of recommendations and references (Figure D.3-7); and

• Guideline editing and reviewing tools for use by guideline developers. The latter tool set has been used to assist with standardization of the latest version of the COG Long-Term Follow-up Guidelines for Survivors of Childhood, Adolescent, and Young Adult Cancers (Version 2.0—March 2006).[4] The PFC health care provider portal will serve as an electronic repository for the COG Long-Term Follow-Up Guidelines and as a tool to foster standardization of clinical services at the point of care.

5f. Internet-Based Deployment. Because of the distributed nature of anticipated users of the PFC, an Internet-based system was deemed most appropriate. An Internet-based approach offers the advantages of easy accessibility, interoperability, and public availability.

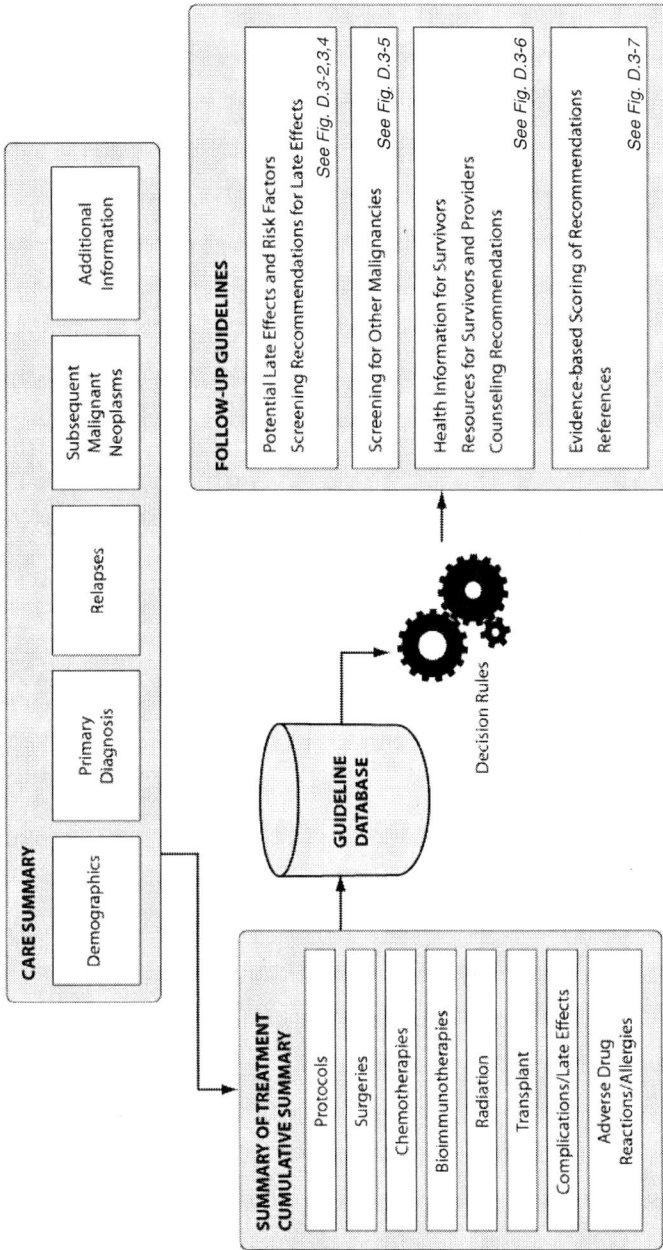

FIGURE D.3-1 The functional components of the PFC include a care summary containing demographics, primary diagnosis, relapses, subsequent malignant neoplasms, and additional information. These data are used to compile a cumulative summary of treatment. Screening recommendations and individualized resources are generated from the cumulative summary of treatment and the guideline database using a set of decision rules.

Passport *for* Care

Administration Section
Doug Alexander Logged In
Home | Help Desk | Log Out

Guidelines List | Cancer Screening | Care Summaries | + Add New Care Summary

Peter ALLTEST

Demographics | Primary Diagnosis | Relapses | TBRT | Additional Information | Cumulative Summary | Follow-Up Guidelines | Revision History

PERIODIC EVALUATIONS   CURRENTLY ACTIVE CHRONIC GVHD: ○ YES ● NO

Periodic Evaluations
PLE Risk Factors
Cancer Screening Guidelines
Initial Evaluation
Yearly Evaluation
Print Guidelines
Health Links
Evidence Based Scoring
References

This is a summary only. Please see complete guideline output under "Print Guidelines" for additional information for screening

History

EVALUATION	POTENTIAL LATE EFFECT	FREQUENCY	INFORMATION
General			
Assessment of nutritional status	1 Growth hormone deficiency	Yearly Every six months until growth is completed, then yearly.	Guideline References Health Links
Healthcare insurance and access	2A Limitations in healthcare and insurance access	Yearly	Guideline References Health Links
Heat intolerance, tachycardia, palpitations, weight loss, emotional lability, muscular weakness, hyperphagia	1 Hyperthyroidism	Yearly	Guideline References Health Links
Skin/Breast			
Galactorrhea	1 Hyperprolactinemia	Yearly	Guideline ...ences ...cks

Labs

EVALUATION	POTENTIAL LATE EFFECT	FREQUENCY	INFORMATION
8:00 a.m. serum cortisol	1 Central adrenal insufficiency	Yearly Yearly for at least 15 years after treatment and as clinically indicated.	Guideline References Health Links
ALT, AST, bilirubin	2A Hepatic dysfunction, Veno-occlusive disease (VOD)	Baseline and As Indicated Baseline at entry into long-term follow-up. Repeat as clinically indicated	Guideline References Health Links
	2A Hepatic dysfunction	as clinically indicated Baseline at entry into long-term follow-up. Repeat as clinically indicated	
	1 Hepatic toxicity	Baseline at entry into long term follow-up. Repeat as clinically indicated.	
BUN, Creatinine, Na, K, Cl, CO2, Ca, Mg, PO4	2A Renal toxicity	Baseline and As Indicated Baseline at entry into long-term follow-up. If abnormal, repeat as clinically indicated.	Guideline References Health Links
CBC/differential	1 Myelodysplasia; Acute myeloid leukemia	Yearly Yearly up to 10 years after transplant	Guideline References

FIGURE D.3-2 Periodic history, physical, diagnostic imaging, laboratory and other evaluations are displayed with the type of evaluation that should be performed, the potential late effect that is being evaluated, the frequency of recommended evaluations and links to important additional information such as the COG Healthlink (see Figure D.3-6), pertinent references and the full guideline (see Figure D.3-7).

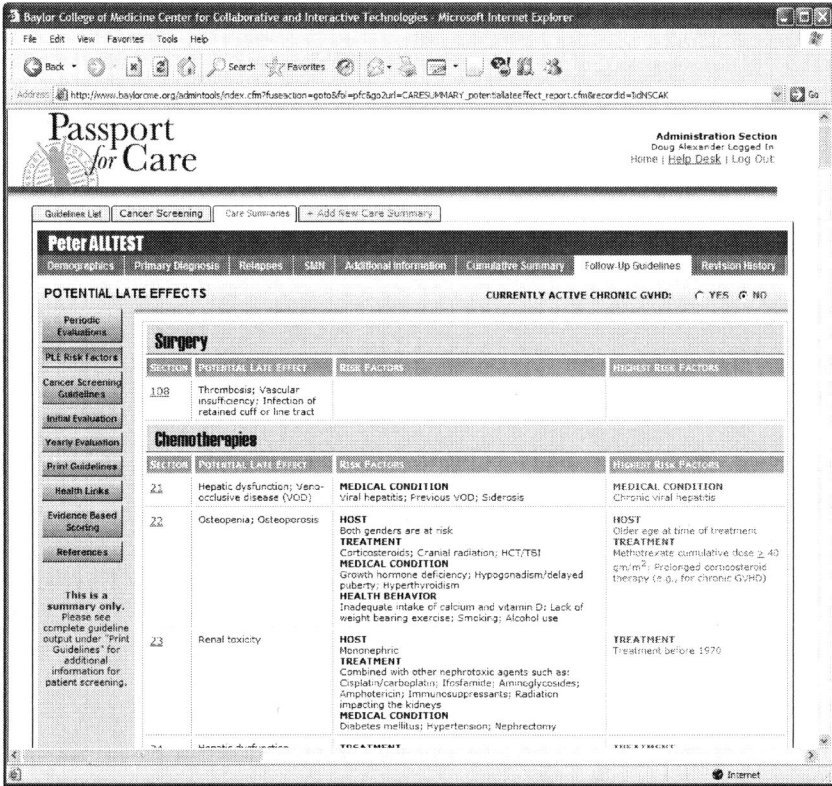

FIGURE D.3-3 This view of the guidelines allows the health care provider to view the risk factors for each of the potential late effect that the survivor is susceptible to.

5g. <u>COG LTFU Guidelines</u>. Comprehensive *Long-Term Follow-Up Guidelines for Survivors of Childhood, Adolescent, and Young Adult Cancers* have been developed by COG's Nursing Discipline and Late Effects Committee.[4,174] COG members have enthusiastically endorsed broader dissemination and use of the guidelines in helping childhood cancer survivors and other health professionals who provide care to survivors to recognize and manage health risks related to late effects of treatment. In the most recent version of the guidelines released to the public (version 2.0 issued in March 2006), potential late effects, risk factors, highest risk factors, recommended periodic evaluation and frequency, health protective counseling recommendations, considerations for further testing and interventions, and references are presented in tabular format corresponding to specific therapeutic agents.[4]

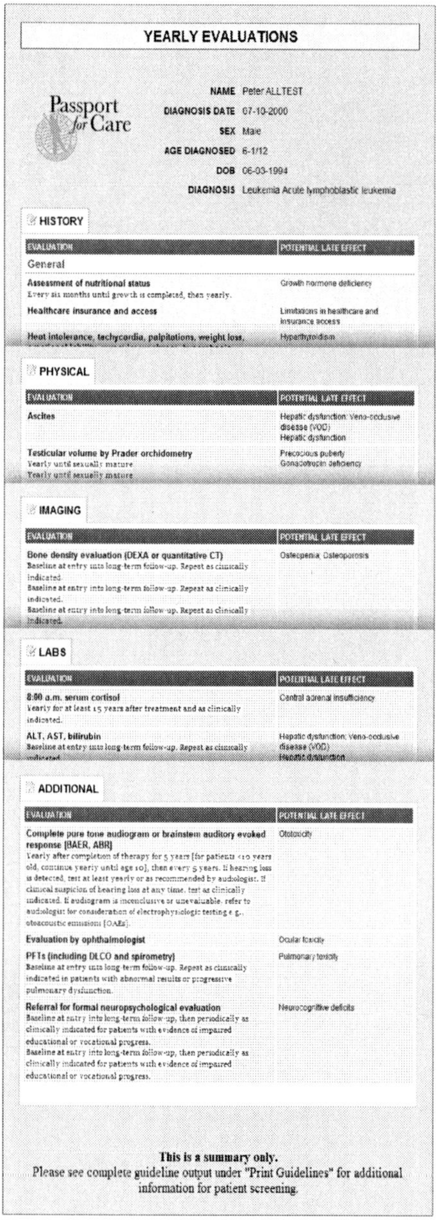

YEARLY EVALUATIONS

Passport for Care

NAME Peter ALLTEST
DIAGNOSIS DATE 07-10-2000
SEX Male
AGE DIAGNOSED 6-1/12
DOB 06-03-1994
DIAGNOSIS Leukemia Acute lymphoblastic leukemia

HISTORY

EVALUATION	POTENTIAL LATE EFFECT
General	
Assessment of nutritional status Every six months until growth is completed, then yearly.	Growth hormone deficiency
Healthcare insurance and access	Limitations in healthcare and insurance access
Heat intolerance, tachycardia, palpitations, weight loss,	Hyperthyroidism

PHYSICAL

EVALUATION	POTENTIAL LATE EFFECT
Ascites	Hepatic dysfunction: Veno-occlusive disease (VOD) Hepatic dysfunction
Testicular volume by Prader orchidometry Yearly until sexually mature Yearly until sexually mature	Precocious puberty Gonadotropin deficiency

IMAGING

EVALUATION	POTENTIAL LATE EFFECT
Bone density evaluation (DEXA or quantitative CT) Baseline at entry into long-term follow-up. Repeat as clinically indicated. Baseline at entry into long-term follow-up. Repeat as clinically indicated. Baseline at entry into long-term follow-up. Repeat as clinically indicated.	Osteopenia, Osteoporosis

LABS

EVALUATION	POTENTIAL LATE EFFECT
8:00 a.m. serum cortisol Yearly for at least 15 years after treatment and as clinically indicated.	Central adrenal insufficiency
ALT, AST, bilirubin Baseline at entry into long-term follow-up. Repeat as clinically	Hepatic dysfunction: Veno-occlusive disease (VOD) Hepatic dysfunction

ADDITIONAL

EVALUATION	POTENTIAL LATE EFFECT
Complete pure tone audiogram or brainstem auditory evoked response [BAER, ABR] Yearly after completion of therapy for 5 years [for patients <10 years old, continue yearly until age 10], then every 5 years. If hearing loss is detected, test at least yearly or as recommended by audiologist. If clinical suspicion of hearing loss at any time, test as clinically indicated. If audiogram is inconclusive or unevaluable, refer to audiologist for consideration of electrophysiologic testing e.g., otoacoustic emissions [OAEs].	Ototoxicity
Evaluation by ophthalmologist	Ocular toxicity
PFTs (including DLCO and spirometry) Baseline at entry into long-term follow-up. Repeat as clinically indicated in patients with abnormal results or progressive pulmonary dysfunction.	Pulmonary toxicity
Referral for formal neuropsychological evaluation Baseline at entry into long-term follow-up, then periodically as clinically indicated for patients with evidence of impaired educational or vocational progress. Baseline at entry into long-term follow-up, then periodically as clinically indicated for patients with evidence of impaired educational or vocational progress.	Neurocognitive deficits

This is a summary only.
Please see complete guideline output under "Print Guidelines" for additional information for patient screening.

FIGURE D.3-4 This summary of yearly evaluations with the corresponding potential late effects will allow the health care provider to quickly view what needs to be assessed on an annual basis.

Breast

At Risk Population	Over age 40; Family history of breast cancer in first degree relative; Early onset of menstruation; Late onset of menopause (age 55 or older); Older than 30 at birth of first child; Never pregnant; Obesity; Previous breast biopsy with atypical hyperplasia; Hormone replacement therapy
HIGHEST RISK	
Factors	Chest radiation with potential impact to the breast (see Section 68), including ≥20 Gy to the following fields: Mantle, Mini-Mantle, Mediastinal, Chest (thorax), Axilla; BRCA1, BRACA2, ATM mutation
Periodic Evaluation	[Physical] Breast self exam: Monthly, beginning at puberty. Clinical breast exam: Yearly, beginning at puberty until age 25, then every six months. [Screening] Mammogram: Yearly, beginning 8 years after radiation or at age 25, whichever occurs last.
Frequency	
Clinician Info Link	
STANDARD RISK	
Periodic Evaluation	ACS Recommendation: [Physical] Clinical breast exam: Every 3 years between ages 20-39, then yearly beginning at age 40. [Screening] Mammogram: Yearly, beginning at age 40.
Frequency	
Clinician Info Link	There is currently a deficiency in the literature regarding whether or not TBI is a risk factor for the development of breast cancer. Monitoring of patients who received TBI should be determined on an individual basis. Mammography is currently limited in its ability to evaluate premenopausal breasts. The role of MRI is evolving for screening of other populations at high risk for breast cancer (e.g., premenopausal known or likely carriers of gene mutation of known penetrance).
FURTHER INFORMATION	
Counseling	**Health Link** Breast Cancer (for patients at highest risk only) **Counseling** For patients at highest risk, counsel to perform breast self-examination monthly, beginning at puberty. For standard risk patients, provide general guidance regarding routine screening beginning at age 40 per current ACS guidelines. **Considerations for Further Testing and Intervention** Surgery and/or oncology consultation as cinically indicated.
Further Testing	

FIGURE D.3-5 Risk-adjusted recommendations for screening for subsequent malignancies are summarized.

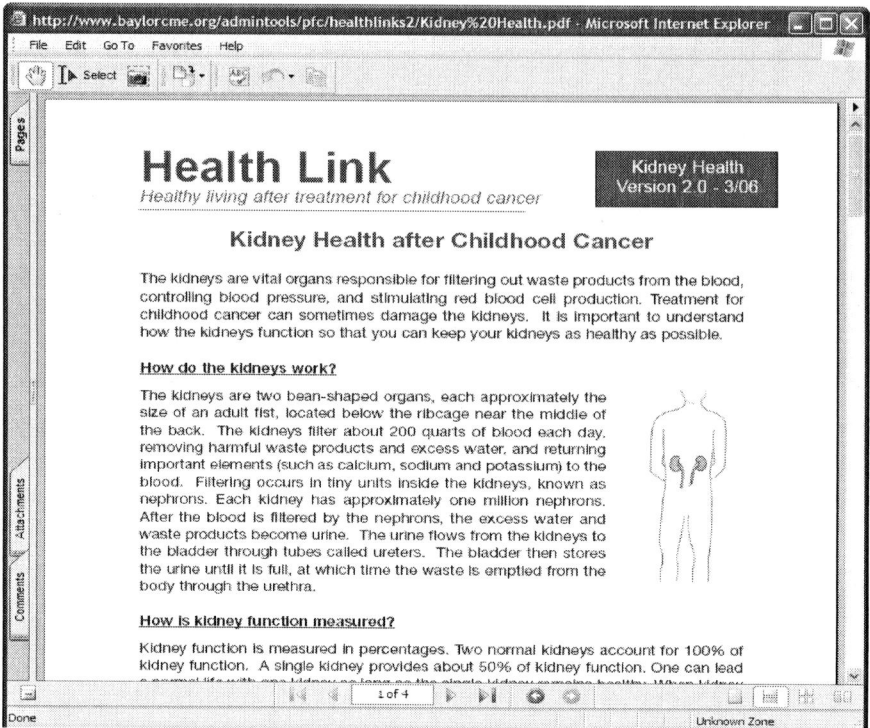

FIGURE D.3-6 The COG Healthlink information for survivors can be easily accessed by an online link to the COG website from the evaluations page (Figure D.3-2).

A summary of screening recommendations for common adult-onset cancers developing as subsequent malignancies in this population, directions regarding how to use the guidelines, a listing of references to relevant scientific literature, and a detailed topical index are included. An explanation of the levels of evidence related to each identified risk for a late effect is also presented. The scores assigned, according to a modified version of the National Comprehensive Cancer Network "Categories of Consensus,"[175] relate to the strength of association of the identified late effect with the specific therapeutic exposure based on current literature.[4] Each score is coupled with a recommendation for periodic health screening based on the collective clinical experience of the panel of experts who developed the guidelines. These scores enable users to judge the strength of the evidence associated with each late-effect risk and the recommendations accompanying it.

Therapeutic Agent(s)	#	Potential Late Effects	Risk Factors	Highest Risk Factors	Periodic Evaluation	Health Counseling/Further Considerations
Nephrectomy	114 (female)	**Renal toxicity** Proteinuria, Hyperfiltration; Renal insufficiency	**Treatment Factors** Combined with other nephrotoxic therapy such as Cisplatin; Carboplatin, Ifosfamide; Aminoglycosides; Amphotericin; Immunosuppressants; Methotrexate; Radiation impacting the kidneys		**PHYSICAL** **Blood pressure** (Yearly) **SCREENING** **BUN, Creatinine, Na, K, Cl, CO2, Ca, Mg, PO4** (Baseline at entry into long-term follow-up. If abnormal, repeat as clinically indicated.) **Urinalysis** (Yearly)	**Health Links** Single Kidney Health; See also Kidney Health **Counseling** Discuss contact sports, bicycle safety (e.g., avoiding handlebar injuries), and proper use of seatbelts (i.e., wearing lapbelts around hips, not waist). Counsel to use NSAIDS with caution. **Considerations for Further Testing and Intervention** Nephrology consultation for patients with hypertension, proteinuria, or progressive renal insufficiency. **SYSTEM = Urinary** **SCORE = 1**

> **SCORE 1: There is uniform consensus of the panel that: (1) there is high-level evidence linking the late effect with the therapeutic exposure and (2) the screening recommendation is appropriate based on the collective clinical experience of panel members.**

FIGURE D.3-7 The full guideline can be accessed by a link from the evaluations page (Figure D.3-2). The score of the strength of the evidence linking the potential late effect to the therapeutic exposure is presented.

However, because of the length of the guidelines and the detail contained in them, clinical utility of the paper-based version of the guidelines on a day-to-day basis in a busy clinical practice is limited. It is precisely for this reason that the PFC, with its ability to generate individualized follow-up recommendations, is anticipated to be attractive to the practicing clinician.

5h. Challenges in PFC Development and Its Adoption. PFC development has required addressing a number of challenges. A brief review of the barriers confronting PFC developers may prove informative for the broader initiatives addressing the needs of all 10 million adult cancer survivors in the United States.

(1) Impacts of Guideline Publication on Provider Behavior. Studies dating back nearly two decades have documented problems related to guideline adherence across different types of adult and childhood practice settings and disease states.[176-181] Feifer and colleagues summarized barriers to effective guideline implementation at the healthcare provider level (i.e., not knowing that guidelines exist, not being familiar with and/or agreeing with content, lacking time to apply guidelines in the clinical setting); the patient level (i.e., inconsistency with health beliefs, time and financial constraints, lack of trust in the guidelines); and systems level (i.e., not having the right information in the right place at the right time, resource constraints, patient volume).[181]

Despite the literature suggesting poor adherence to clinical guidelines in many practice settings, there is growing recognition of the attributes of clinical guidelines that improve the likelihood of their application in clinical settings. Studies have indicated that factors that enhance the likelihood of adherence to clinical guidelines include: engaging patients as partners;[182-185] using point-of-care reminders;[186-189] and employing population-based management techniques.[190-194] For these reasons the PFC was designed to include components that address the needs of both the survivors and their providers in a health care partnership providing resources tailored to survivor or provider needs and offering point-of-care or near point-of-care decision support individualized to the needs of the specific survivor.

(2) Guideline Development. The process of development of the comprehensive *Long-term Follow-up Guidelines for Survivors of Childhood, Adolescent, and Young Adult Cancers* has been well described and will not be reviewed here.[174] However, mention must be made of the public investment from the National Cancer Institute (NCI) in the CCSS that, along with other efforts, has proven essential for identifying and link-

ing therapeutic exposures to late effects. The NCI has also supported development of the COG Long-Term Follow-Up Guidelines under the U10 CA098543 grant. Similar initiatives are needed across the spectrum of adult cancers to accelerate development of an evidence base that can provide the foundation for guideline development. In this regard it is worth noting the approach that COG has taken in guideline development.

Even in the arena of pediatric cancer treatment and follow-up, a complete evidence base for development of screening guidelines is lacking. Therefore, COG experts made use of the literature linking late effects to treatment exposures and combined the available evidence with expert consensus. In doing so, COG guideline developers recognized that there are no randomized clinical trials available on which to base recommendations for periodic screening evaluations of childhood cancer survivors.[4] As a consequence, professionals involved in guideline development examined "… the strength of data from the literature linking a specific late effect with a therapeutic exposure, coupled with an assessment of the appropriateness of the screening recommendation based on the expert panel's collective clinical experience."[4,p. 4] Each guideline was then scored using a modified version of the National Comprehensive Cancer Network "Categories of Consensus" to communicate the levels of evidence and consensus to users.[175]

(3) <u>Care Summary Development</u>. Although modifications and refinements continue to be made, an end-of-treatment summary or care summary that permits data collection that can be used for clinical and research purposes has been developed by COG committees. While it is attractive to collect more data rather than less, caution should be exercised in this regard. For example, in the case of the PFC, generation of individualized guidelines requires only a limited subset of the information contained in the complete COG Care Summary dataset. Collection and archiving of the complete dataset could require commitment of time and money that, for some clinicians, may discourage participation and use. We are exploring approaches for streamlining data collection strategies in a manner that allows for use of the more limited dataset for the PFC, however, permits collection of the larger dataset (if preferred by the provider) and expansion of data collection as evidence evolves.

(4) <u>Accommodating Change</u>. Accommodating change in a project such as the PFC can, in itself, pose a barrier to effective implementation. Change can occur at many levels (e.g., survivor's treatment history, providers' roles in working with the survivor in long-term follow-up

care, the guidelines knowledge base and emergence of new findings with regard to risks and the recommendations for follow-up evaluation). While the COG Care Summary incorporated into the PFC is not designed to be a complete medical record, a careful effort was undertaken to permit capturing changes in treatment exposures that could influence follow-up guideline recommendations. In particular, the Care Summary accommodates treatments for relapses and subsequent malignancies. Relapses and subsequent malignancies that occur during care or follow-up at a COG institution could presumably be entered into the PFC database using personnel and approaches similar to those used in creating the initial Care Summary.

Should relapses or subsequent malignancies occur in adulthood under the care of an adult oncologist, staff less familiar with the PFC would need to become involved in updating the history of treatment exposures in the PFC. Training and support mechanisms, necessary to prepare health care providers and other clinical staff who will be involved in such activities, will be incorporated into the patient portal of the PFC under development. Contemplation of such developments invites consideration of whether guideline recommendations will need to accommodate the later exposures to treatments. With respect to changes in provider roles, the patient portal of the PFC is being designed to allow for capture of information on changes in healthcare providers and contact information on former and current providers, thereby facilitating timely contact with current providers, as well as providers involved earlier in care.

As data emerge regarding indications and recommendations for follow-up, the guidelines for long-term follow-up for potential late effects are anticipated to change. With paper-based or token-based (e.g., a smart card) systems, the recommendations accompanying the treatment history may become dated, if not obsolete, presenting a significant barrier to use. In contrast, an Internet-based deployment for the PFC offers the advantages that guidelines can be conveniently modified in one location with changes populating any recommendations subsequently produced. This is accomplished using administrative tools created and deployed for use by guideline developers and maintainers.

(5) Standardization and Interoperability. Use of proprietary software and systems can produce significant barriers to data sharing and interoperability. For example, one can envision: (1) the possible requirement to aggregate or exchange data with other electronic systems, including electronic medical records (EMRs), insurance or payer databases, or other clinical decision support systems; or (2) the need to develop reports or analyses based on any number of parameters (e.g.,

diagnoses, treatment exposures, procedures). As noted in recent reviews of clinical support systems, such tasks can be greatly facilitated by use of coded data, standard vocabularies, and messaging standards (e.g., Health Level Seven [HL7]).[195, 196] More broadly, support is coalescing around a new vision for nationwide health information using a decentralized "network of networks" facilitated by consensus regarding shared policies and common technical standards. *Connecting for Health Common Framework: Resources for Implementing Private and Secure Health Information Exchange* is an initiative underwritten by the Markle Foundation that involves a wide range of stakeholders with interests in health and health care information.[197] Monitoring of this initiative, which has advanced from the conceptual to the demonstration phase, will provide guidance in ensuring that the end result of efforts like the PFC are accessible to a wide range of audiences using varying hardware and software configurations to access summary data and other components of programs designed to foster effective long-term follow-up of care services.

(6) Integrating into Clinical Workflows. Technology, no matter how compelling, will remain unused if it does not serve the needs of the clinician or clinical staff, and if it does not integrate seamlessly into workflows of clinical service settings. For this reason, it is critical that stakeholders are involved in developmental efforts, providing input and feedback throughout the processes of prototype creation and iterative testing and improvement. Early stakeholder involvement ensures that the selection of technologies and applications meets provider needs and can be used within extant clinical environments. Stakeholder involvement must engage the full range of individuals who will be involved in application use and maintenance (e.g., individuals entering clinical data into the Care Summary, nurses and health care providers using the recommendations, guideline developers, and patients). Training and support procedures are also essential components of a deployment plan to ensure that integration into the clinic workflow can proceed smoothly.

(7) Protecting Patient Confidentiality and Privacy. Protecting the privacy of survivors and ensuring confidentiality is a paramount concern in designing any software application involving identifiable health information. Protection of privacy and confidentiality is also a legal requirement under the Health Insurance Portability and Accountability Act of 1996 (HIPAA).[198] Providing reliable and effective security for digital information requires a multimodal strategy involving access authorizations (e.g., passwords, user IDs, user tokens) and attribution

(e.g., audit logs), as well as application and data, transmission, network, and physical (i.e., hardware) security using various tools and strategies (e.g., data encryption, firewalls, virtual private networks [VPNs], locked rooms with key card or biometric access). Included in the technical specifications for the PFC is explicit information on strategies for ensuring that the program is secure and that the resulting program complies with federal mandates, including HIPAA requirements. In this regard, it is worth noting that the PFC has been designed with security: (1) at the browser level, involving digitally secured certificate access via a secure hypertext transfer protocol (HTTPS) connection and an encrypted identifier for each user; (2) at the application level through user authentication, log-in with user ID and password protection, verification through the database, assignment to a clinic and record set, and creation of an audit trail providing a log of who viewed specific data and when it was viewed; and (3) at the database level via encrypted storage files that are keyed at multiple levels within the encrypted application page. Deployment will also include additional network and physical security of the type described above. In addition to conforming to HIPAA requirements, further security will be assured through review and compliance with the requirements of the Baylor College of Medicine IT security and requirements of the Institutional Review Board (IRB). IRB approval will be secured prior to any personal information being gathered for storage and use via the PFC database. Informed consent will be required in order for survivors to participate in testing or later use of the PFC.

(8) <u>Development and Maintenance Costs</u>. While public funding is available for research and evaluation of extant tools, limited funding is available for the development of novel technological applications. Investigators interested in advancing the creation of new tools for managing chronic disease may find themselves seeking funding from private sources, including foundations, private individuals, and their own institutions. Even greater challenges may be faced by developers who, for legitimate scientific reasons, must focus initially on smaller audiences or specific subsets of larger patient populations, such as childhood cancer survivors. Public funding agencies interested in encouraging development of innovative decision-support tools for chronic disease, should consider reevaluating current requests for applications (RFAs) to accommodate the needs of pilot projects focusing on well-defined populations as long as sufficient data can be gathered to demonstrate the value of the particular innovative approaches.

(9) <u>Other Challenges</u>. There are other challenges to be met in designing and implementing projects like the PFC. Collaboration across disciplines is essential, and as experience with the PFC has demonstrated, engagement of clinical experts with informatics specialists at the earliest phases of guideline development can greatly accelerate the critical transition from print to electronic formats. Also, involvement of other experts in areas such as health communications, patient adherence, quality improvement, social psychology, health literacy, patient privacy and confidentiality, ethics, security, and interoperability standards may prove valuable in application development and in achievement of a successful outcome. Furthermore, resources, including funding, should be available to explore experimentally the efficacy and practicality of approaches for health care provider and patient behavioral change, including evolving continuing medical education and patient education approaches that may prove critical in improving professional and patient compliance and changes in health outcomes.

Finally, perhaps the most significant challenge to development of any tool like the PFC for any population of survivors is the assurance that the patient and guideline information will be updated and maintained in the future. Ensuring that the PFC or similar initiatives will be available to survivors throughout their lifetimes requires new models ensuring extended support. Consideration of models and strategies to provide for the longevity of the PFC are items under active discussion and exploration.

5i. <u>PFC Testing and Roll-out</u>. A fully operational version of the PFC is undergoing initial testing in preparation for early deployment and evaluation in the TCCC survivor clinic. Initial pilot testing will allow for assessment of the effectiveness of the automated guideline generator to determine if decision algorithms have been properly formulated and programmed, if data components are properly linked to respond effectively to risk-related queries, and if the responses to queries yield the correct information with regard to risk-based follow-up. Testing results will be used to modify and refine the PFC in preparation for subsequent testing in three additional COG clinics.

Once pilot testing has been completed, and the PFC has been revised and/or refined to ensure that it operates effectively it will be made available, in a staged manner to COG-affiliated institutions for initial field implementation. At this point, one portal will be operational—a portal for oncology health care providers for use in COG oncology clinics. Simultaneously, a second PFC portal, for survivors and primary care providers, will be developed and undergo testing and evaluation.

5j. <u>Survivors of Adult Cancer and the PFC</u>. It is attractive to consider applying a PFC-like approach to the care of adult survivors of cancer, however, it is important to recognize that follow-up of patients treated for cancer as adults poses unique challenges that differ from those encountered in the population of childhood cancer survivors.

Adult cancer patients are typically treated in the offices of private oncologists, rather than in academic medical centers, as are the majority of children with cancer. Furthermore, adult cancer care may reflect a greater diversity of approaches, with many patients not treated on standardized protocols. Follow-up studies of adult cancer survivors and the evidence base linking treatment exposures to potential late effects are limited. Comprehensive follow-up guidelines for survivors of most adult cancers have not been developed, and consensus regarding the development and use of an end-of-treatment summary is still evolving. It is important to note that the PFC is widely adaptable and may have far-ranging applications, including to the adult cancer survivor population, once comprehensive consensus-based guidelines for various adult cancers have been developed.

CONCLUSION

The substantial successes achieved in the treatment of childhood cancers over recent decades and the increased longevity of such patients has been accompanied by the additional need to address the late sequelae associated with cancer therapy. The Passport for Care (PFC) is a dynamic resource designed to provide survivor and provider education, resources, decision support, and health care recommendations tailored to the individual needs of the long term survivor of childhood cancer. Although the PFC targets a comparatively small population, the approach or elements of the approach is likely to be informative and/or serve as a model for applications designed to address the needs of the 10 million adult cancer survivors in the United States.

Successful development and deployment of such applications are anticipated to face a variety of challenges, including those relevant to scientific, clinical, health systems, logistical, interoperability, provider and patient adherence, security, guideline updating, long-term maintenance, and financial support issues. Strategies are available to address or begin to address a number of the potential barriers; however, significant hurdles do remain in the initial stages with respect to the provision of support to develop such model health care information tools and systems.

Finally, if such models prove successful and cost-effective in improving health outcomes, public health policy makers in partnership with other public and private stakeholders will need to develop policies and systems that can accommodate the long-term needs for maintaining decision support tools demonstrated to improve the lives of patients with chronic disease.

REFERENCES CITED

1. National Cancer Policy Board (U.S.), Weiner SL, Simone JV, Hewitt ME. *Childhood Cancer Survivorship: Improving Care and Quality Of Life.* Washington, D.C.: The National Academies Press; 2003.
2. Reuben S. *Living beyond cancer: finding a new balance.* Bethesda, MD.: U.S. Dept. of Health and Human Services, National Institutes of Health, National Cancer Institute; 2004.
3. Centers for Disease Control and Prevention. *A National Action Plan for Cancer Survivorship: Advancing Public Health Strategies.* Atlanta, GA: The Centers for Disease Control and Prevention and The Lance Armstrong Foundation; April 2004.
4. CureSearch: Children's Oncology Group. Long-term follow-up guidelines for survivors of childhood, adolescent, and young adult cancers, v 2.0. March 2006; 227. Available at: http://www.survivorshipguidelines.org/pdf/LTFUGuidelines.pdf. Accessed June 13, 2006.
5. National Cancer Policy Board (U.S.), Weiner SL, Simone JV. *Childhood cancer survivorship: improving care and quality of life.* Washington, D.C.: The National Academies Press; 2003.
6. American Cancer Society. Detailed guide: cancer in children. How are childhood cancers treated? *Cancer reference information* [January 4, 2005; http://www.cancer.org/docroot/CRI/content/CRI_2_4_4X_How_Are_Childhood_Cancers_Treated_7.asp. Accessed April 18, 2006.
7. Children's Oncology Group. Resource Directory: COG Institutions by Country http://www.curesearch.org/resources/cog.aspx. Accessed May 30, 2006.
8. National Cancer Institute. Care for children and adolescents with cancer: Questions and Cancers *National Cancer Institute FactSheet* [November 10, 2005; http://www.cancer.gov/PDF/FactSheet/fs1_21.pdf. Accessed April 17, 2006.
9. Ries L, Eisner M, Kosary C, et al. SEER Cancer Statistics Review, 1975-2002. *SEER Cancer Statistics Review* [2005; http://seer.cancer.gov/cgi-bin/csr/1975_2002/search.pl#results. Accessed April 8, 2006.
10. Jemal A, Murray T, Ward E, et al. Cancer statistics, 2005. *CA Cancer J Clin.* Jan-Feb 2005;55(1):10-30.
11. Hudson MM. A model for care across the cancer continuum. *Cancer.* Dec 1 2005; 104(11 Suppl):2638-2642.
12. Bhatia S, Meadows AT. Long-term follow-up of childhood cancer survivors: future directions for clinical care and research. *Pediatr Blood Cancer.* Feb 2006;46(2):143-148.
13. Garre ML, Gandus S, Cesana B, et al. Health status of long-term survivors after cancer in childhood. Results of an uniinstitutional study in Italy. *Am J Pediatr Hematol Oncol.* May 1994;16(2):143-152.
14. von der Weid N, Beck D, Calfisch U, Feldges A, Wyss M, Wagner H. Standardized assessment of late effects in long-term survivors of childhood cancer in Switzerland. Results of a Swiss Pediatric Oncology Group study. *Int J Pediatr Hematol Oncol.* 1996;3:483-490.
15. Stevens MC, Mahler H, Parkes S. The health status of adult survivors of cancer in childhood. *Eur J Cancer.* Apr 1998;34(5):694-698.

16. Crom DB, Chathaway DK, Tolley EA, Mulhern RK, Hudson MM. Health status and health-related quality of life in long-term adult survivors of pediatric solid tumors. *Int J Cancer Suppl.* 1999;12:25-31.
17. Oeffinger KC, Eshelman DA, Tomlinson GE, Buchanan GR, Foster BM. Grading of late effects in young adult survivors of childhood cancer followed in an ambulatory adult setting. *Cancer.* Apr 1 2000;88(7):1687-1695.
18. von der Weid N, Swiss Pediatric Oncology Group. Late effects in long-term survivors of ALL in childhood: Experiences from the SPOG late effects study. *Swiss Med Wkly.* April 2001;131(13-14):180-187.
19. Hudson MM, Mertens AC, Yasui Y, et al. Health status of adult long-term survivors of childhood cancer: a report from the Childhood Cancer Survivor Study. *JAMA.* Sep 24 2003;290(12):1583-1592.
20. Bhatia S. Cancer survivorship—pediatric issues. *Hematology (Am Soc Hematol Educ Program).* 2005;Prepublication release:507-515.
21. Bassal M, Mertens AC, Taylor L, et al. Risk of selected subsequent carcinomas in survivors of childhood cancer: a report from the Childhood Cancer Survivor Study. *J Clin Oncol.* Jan 20 2006;24(3):476-483.
22. Friedman DL, Freyer DR, Levitt GA. Models of care for survivors of childhood cancer. *Pediatr Blood Cancer.* Feb 2006;46(2):159-168.
23. Bottomley SJ, Kassner E. Late effects of childhood cancer therapy. *J Pediatr Nurs.* Apr 2003;18(2):126-133.
24. Pogany L, Barr R, Shaw A, Speechley K, Barrera M, Maunsell E. Health status in survivors of cancer in childhood and adolescence. *Qual Life Res.* 2006;15:143-157.
25. Lackner H, Benesch M, Schagerl S, Kerbl R, Schwinger W, Urban C. Prospective evaluation of late effects after childhood cancer therapy with a follow-up over 9 years. *Eur J Pediatr.* Oct 2000;159(10):750-758.
26. Shalet SM, Rosenstock JD, Beardwell CG, Pearson D, Jones PH. Thyroid dysfunction following external irradiation to the neck for Hodgkin's disease in childhood. *Clin Radiol.* Sep 1977;28(5):511-515.
27. Green DM, Brecher ML, Yakar D, et al. Thyroid function in pediatric patients after neck irradiation for Hodgkin disease. *Med Pediatr Oncol.* 1980;8(2):127-136.
28. Kaplan MM, Garnick MB, Gelber R, et al. Risk factors for thyroid abnormalities after neck irradiation for childhood cancer. *Am J Med.* Feb 1983;74(2):272-280.
29. Constine LS, Donaldson SS, McDougall IR, Cox RS, Link MP, Kaplan HS. Thyroid dysfunction after radiotherapy in children with Hodgkin's disease. *Cancer.* Feb 15 1984;53(4):878-883.
30. Devney RB, Sklar CA, Nesbit ME, Jr., et al. Serial thyroid function measurements in children with Hodgkin disease. *J Pediatr.* Aug 1984;105(2):223-227.
31. Fleming ID, Black TL, Thompson EI, Pratt C, Rao B, Hustu O. Thyroid dysfunction and neoplasia in children receiving neck irradiation for cancer. *Cancer.* Mar 15 1985; 55(6):1190-1194.
32. Oberfield SE, Allen JC, Pollack J, New MI, Levine LS. Long-term endocrine sequelae after treatment of medulloblastoma: prospective study of growth and thyroid function. *J Pediatr.* Feb 1986;108(2):219-223.
33. Katsanis E, Shapiro RS, Robison LL, et al. Thyroid dysfunction following bone marrow transplantation: long-term follow-up of 80 pediatric patients. *Bone Marrow Transplant.* May 1990;5(5):335-340.
34. Lipshultz SE, Colan SD, Gelber RD, Perez-Atayde AR, Sallan SE, Sanders SP. Late cardiac effects of doxorubicin therapy for acute lymphoblastic leukemia in childhood. *N Engl J Med.* Mar 21 1991;324(12):808-815.

35. Ogilvy-Stuart AL, Shalet SM, Gattamaneni HR. Thyroid function after treatment of brain tumors in children. *J Pediatr.* Nov 1991;119(5):733-737.

36. Sanders JE. Endocrine problems in children after bone marrow transplant for hematologic malignancies. The Long-term Follow-up Team. *Bone Marrow Transplant.* 1991;8 Suppl 1:2-4.

37. DeGroot LJ. Effects of irradiation on the thyroid gland. *Endocrinol Metab Clin North Am.* Sep 1993;22(3):607-615.

38. Hancock SL, Donaldson SS, Hoppe RT. Cardiac disease following treatment of Hodgkin's disease in children and adolescents. *J Clin Oncol.* Jul 1993;11(7):1208-1215.

39. Ali MK, Ewer MS, Gibbs HR, Swafford J, Graff KL. Late doxorubicin-associated cardiotoxicity in children. The possible role of intercurrent viral infection. *Cancer.* Jul 1 1994;74(1):182-188.

40. Boulad F, Bromley M, Black P, et al. Thyroid dysfunction following bone marrow transplantation using hyperfractionated radiation. *Bone Marrow Transplant.* Jan 1995; 15(1):71-76.

41. Lipshultz SE, Lipsitz SR, Mone SM, et al. Female sex and drug dose as risk factors for late cardiotoxic effects of doxorubicin therapy for childhood cancer. *N Engl J Med.* Jun 29 1995;332(26):1738-1743.

42. Fein DA, Hanlon AL, Corn BW, Curran WJ, Jr., Coia LR. The influence of lymphangiography on the development of hypothyroidism in patients irradiated for Hodgkin's disease. *Int J Radiat Oncol Biol Phys.* Aug 1 1996;36(1):13-18.

43. Chin D, Sklar C, Donahue B, et al. Thyroid dysfunction as a late effect in survivors of pediatric medulloblastoma/primitive neuroectodermal tumors: a comparison of hyperfractionated versus conventional radiotherapy. *Cancer.* Aug 15 1997;80(4):798-804.

44. Novakovic B, Fears TR, Horowitz ME, Tucker MA, Wexler LH. Late effects of therapy in survivors of Ewing's sarcoma family tumors. *J Pediatr Hematol Oncol.* May-Jun 1997;19(3):220-225.

45. Sorensen K, Levitt G, Bull C, Chessells J, Sullivan I. Anthracycline dose in childhood acute lymphoblastic leukemia: issues of early survival versus late cardiotoxicity. *J Clin Oncol.* Jan 1997;15(1):61-68.

46. Hudson MM, Poquette CA, Lee J, et al. Increased mortality after successful treatment for Hodgkin's disease. *J Clin Oncol.* Nov 1998;16(11):3592-3600.

47. Nysom K, Holm K, Lipsitz SR, et al. Relationship between cumulative anthracycline dose and late cardiotoxicity in childhood acute lymphoblastic leukemia. *J Clin Oncol.* Feb 1998;16(2):545-550.

48. Green DM, Hyland A, Chung CS, Zevon MA, Hall BC. Cancer and cardiac mortality among 15-year survivors of cancer diagnosed during childhood or adolescence. *J Clin Oncol.* Oct 1999;17(10):3207-3215.

49. Sklar C, Whitton J, Mertens A, et al. Abnormalities of the thyroid in survivors of Hodgkin's disease: data from the Childhood Cancer Survivor Study. *J Clin Endocrinol Metab.* Sep 2000;85(9):3227-3232.

50. Sklar CA, LaQuaglia MP. The long-term complications of chemotherapy in childhood genitourinary tumors. *Urol Clin North Am.* Aug 2000;27(3):563-568, x.

51. Green DM, Grigoriev YA, Nan B, et al. Congestive heart failure after treatment for Wilms' tumor: a report from the National Wilms' Tumor Study group. *J Clin Oncol.* Apr 1 2001;19(7):1926-1934.

52. Kadan-Lottick N, Marshall JA, Baron AE, Krebs NF, Hambidge KM, Albano E. Normal bone mineral density after treatment for childhood acute lymphoblastic leukemia diagnosed between 1991 and 1998. *J Pediatr.* Jun 2001;138(6):898-904.

53. Kremer LC, van Dalen EC, Offringa M, Ottenkamp J, Voute PA. Anthracycline-induced clinical heart failure in a cohort of 607 children: long-term follow-up study. *J Clin Oncol.* Jan 1 2001;19(1):191-196.

54. Oeffinger KC, Buchanan GR, Eshelman DA, et al. Cardiovascular risk factors in young adult survivors of childhood acute lymphoblastic leukemia. *J Pediatr Hematol Oncol.* Oct 2001;23(7):424-430.

55. Sklar C, Boulad F, Small T, Kernan N. Endocrine complications of pediatric stem cell transplantation. *Front Biosci.* Aug 1 2001;6:G17-22.

56. Keefe DL. Anthracycline-induced cardiomyopathy. *Semin Oncol.* Aug 2001;28(4 Suppl 12):2-7.

57. Lipshultz SE, Lipsitz SR, Sallan SE, et al. Long-term enalapril therapy for left ventricular dysfunction in doxorubicin-treated survivors of childhood cancer. *J Clin Oncol.* Dec 1 2002;20(23):4517-4522.

58. Mertens AC, Yasui Y, Liu Y, et al. Pulmonary complications in survivors of childhood and adolescent cancer. A report from the Childhood Cancer Survivor Study. *Cancer.* Dec 1 2002;95(11):2431-2441.

59. Adams MJ, Hardenbergh PH, Constine LS, Lipshultz SE. Radiation-associated cardiovascular disease. *Crit Rev Oncol Hematol.* Jan 2003;45(1):55-75.

60. Gurney JG, Kadan-Lottick NS, Packer RJ, et al. Endocrine and cardiovascular late effects among adult survivors of childhood brain tumors: Childhood Cancer Survivor Study. *Cancer.* Feb 1 2003;97(3):663-673.

61. Athanassiadou F, Kourti M, Papageorgiou T, Stamou M, Makedou A, Boufidou A. Severe hyperlipidemia in a child with acute lymphoblastic leukemia treated with L-asparaginase and prednisone. *Pediatr Int.* Dec 2004;46(6):743-744.

62. Huettemann E, Junker T, Chatzinikolaou KP, et al. The influence of anthracycline therapy on cardiac function during anesthesia. *Anesth Analg.* Apr 2004;98(4):941-947.

63. Metayer C, Lynch CF, Clarke EA, et al. Second cancers among long-term survivors of Hodgkin's disease diagnosed in childhood and adolescence. *J Clin Oncol.* Jun 2000; 18(12):2435-2443.

64. Swerdlow AJ, Barber JA, Hudson GV, et al. Risk of second malignancy after Hodgkin's disease in a collaborative British cohort: the relation to age at treatment. *J Clin Oncol.* Feb 2000;18(3):498-509.

65. Feig SA. Second malignant neoplasms after successful treatment of childhood cancers. *Blood Cells Mol Dis.* May-Jun 2001;27(3):662-666.

66. Neglia JP, Friedman DL, Yasui Y, et al. Second malignant neoplasms in five-year survivors of childhood cancer: childhood cancer survivor study. *J Natl Cancer Inst.* Apr 18 2001;93(8):618-629.

67. Bhatia S, Yasui Y, Robison LL, et al. High risk of subsequent neoplasms continues with extended follow-up of childhood Hodgkin's disease: report from the Late Effects Study Group. *J Clin Oncol.* Dec 1 2003;21(23):4386-4394.

68. Barnard DR, Woods WG. Treatment-related myelodysplastic syndrome/acute myeloid leukemia in survivors of childhood cancer—an update. *Leuk Lymphoma.* May 2005; 46(5):651-663.

69. Travis LB, Hill DA, Dores GM, et al. Breast cancer following radiotherapy and chemotherapy among young women with Hodgkin disease. *JAMA.* Jul 23 2003;290(4): 465-475.

70. Kenney LB, Yasui Y, Inskip PD, et al. Breast cancer after childhood cancer: a report from the Childhood Cancer Survivor Study. *Ann Intern Med.* Oct 19 2004;141(8): 590-597.

71. Lew SM, Morgan JN, Psaty E, Lefton DR, Allen JC, Abbott R. Cumulative incidence of radiation-induced cavernomas in long-term survivors of medulloblastoma. *J Neurosurg.* Feb 2006;104(2 Suppl):103-107.

72. Kourti M, Tragiannidis A, Makedou A, Papageorgiou T, Rousso I, Athanassiadou F. Metabolic syndrome in children and adolescents with acute lymphoblastic leukemia after the completion of chemotherapy. *J Pediatr Hematol Oncol.* Sep 2005;27(9):499-501.

73. Probert JC, Parker BR, Kaplan HS. Growth retardation in children after megavoltage irradiation of the spine. *Cancer.* Sep 1973;32(3):634-639.

74. Probert JC, Parker BR. The effects of radiation therapy on bone growth. *Radiology.* Jan 1975;114(1):155-162.

75. Noorda EM, Somers R, van Leeuwen FE, Vulsma T, Behrendt H. Adult height and age at menarche in childhood cancer survivors. *Eur J Cancer.* Mar 2001;37(5):605-612.

76. Gurney JG, Ness KK, Stovall M, et al. Final height and body mass index among adult survivors of childhood brain cancer: childhood cancer survivor study. *J Clin Endocrinol Metab.* Oct 2003;88(10):4731-4739.

77. Brownstein CM, Mertens AC, Mitby PA, et al. Factors that affect final height and change in height standard deviation scores in survivors of childhood cancer treated with growth hormone: a report from the childhood cancer survivor study. *J Clin Endocrinol Metab.* Sep 2004;89(9):4422-4427.

78. Goldsby RE, Taggart DR, Ablin AR. Surviving childhood cancer: the impact on life. *Paediatr Drugs.* 2006;8(2):71-84.

79. Oeffinger KC, Mertens AC, Sklar CA, et al. Obesity in adult survivors of childhood acute lymphoblastic leukemia: a report from the Childhood Cancer Survivor Study. *J Clin Oncol.* Apr 1 2003;21(7):1359-1365.

80. Sklar CA, Mertens AC, Walter A, et al. Changes in body mass index and prevalence of overweight in survivors of childhood acute lymphoblastic leukemia: role of cranial irradiation. *Med Pediatr Oncol.* Aug 2000;35(2):91-95.

81. Rogers PC, Meacham LR, Oeffinger KC, Henry DW, Lange BJ. Obesity in pediatric oncology. *Pediatr Blood Cancer.* Dec 2005;45(7):881-891.

82. Meacham LR, Gurney JG, Mertens AC, et al. Body mass index in long-term adult survivors of childhood cancer: a report of the Childhood Cancer Survivor Study. *Cancer.* Apr 15 2005;103(8):1730-1739.

83. Koocher GP, O'Malley JE. *The Damocles syndrome: psychosocial consequences of surviving childhood cancer.* New York: McGraw-Hill; 1981.

84. Schmale AH, Morrow GR, Schmitt MH, et al. Well-being of cancer survivors. *Psychosom Med.* May 1983;45(2):163-169.

85. Cella DF, Tross S. Psychological adjustment to survival from Hodgkin's disease. *J Consult Clin Psychol.* Oct 1986;54(5):616-622.

86. Mulhern RK, Wasserman AL, Kovnar EH, Williams JM, Ochs JJ. Serial neuropsychological studies of a child with acute lymphoblastic leukemia and subsequent glioblastoma multiforme. *Neurology.* Nov 1986;36(11):1534-1538.

87. Teta MJ, Del Po MC, Kasl SV, Meigs JW, Myers MH, Mulvihill JJ. Psychosocial consequences of childhood and adolescent cancer survival. *J Chronic Dis.* 1986; 39(9):751-759.

88. Williams JM, Ochs J, Davis KS, et al. The subacute effects of CNS prophylaxis for acute lymphoblastic leukemia on neuropsychological performance: a comparison of four protocols. *Arch Clin Neuropsychol.* 1986;1(2):183-192.

89. Mulhern RK, Wasserman AL, Friedman AG, Fairclough D. Social competence and behavioral adjustment of children who are long-term survivors of cancer. *Pediatrics.* Jan 1989;83(1):18-25.

90. Brown RT, Kaslow NJ, Hazzard AP, et al. Psychiatric and family functioning in children with leukemia and their parents. *J Am Acad Child Adolesc Psychiatry.* May 1992;31(3):495-502.

91. Gray RE, Doan BD, Shermer P, et al. Psychologic adaptation of survivors of childhood cancer. *Cancer.* Dec 1 1992;70(11):2713-2721.

92. Brown RT, Madan-Swain A. Cognitive, neuropsychological, and academic sequelae in children with leukemia. *J Learn Disabil.* Feb 1993;26(2):74-90.

93. Madan-Swain A, Brown RT, Sexson SB, Baldwin K, Pais R, Ragab A. Adolescent cancer survivors. Psychosocial and familial adaptation. *Psychosomatics.* Sep-Oct 1994; 35(5):453-459.

94. Chesler M, Zebrack B. *An Updated Report on Our Studies of Long-Term Survivorship of Childhood Cancer and a Brief Review of the Psychosocial Literature* Ann Arbor, MI: Center for research on Social Organization, University of Michigan; 1997.

95. Elkin TD, Phipps S, Mulhern RK, Fairclough D. Psychological functioning of adolescent and young adult survivors of pediatric malignancy. *Med Pediatr Oncol.* Dec 1997;29(6):582-588.

96. Kokkonen J, Vainionpaa L, Winqvist S, Lanning M. Physical and psychosocial outcome for young adults with treated malignancy. *Pediatr Hematol Oncol.* May-Jun 1997;14(3):223-232.

97. Pendley JS, Dahlquist LM, Dreyer Z. Body image and psychosocial adjustment in adolescent cancer survivors. *J Pediatr Psychol.* Feb 1997;22(1):29-43.

98. Zeltzer LK, Chen E, Weiss R, et al. Comparison of psychologic outcome in adult survivors of childhood acute lymphoblastic leukemia versus sibling controls: a cooperative Children's Cancer Group and National Institutes of Health study. *J Clin Oncol.* Feb 1997;15(2):547-556.

99. Richardson RC, Nelson MB, Meeske K. Young adult survivors of childhood cancer: attending to emerging medical and psychosocial needs. *J Pediatr Oncol Nurs.* Jul 1999;16(3):136-144.

100. Chen E, Zeltzer LK, Craske MG, Katz ER. Children's memories for painful cancer treatment procedures: implications for distress. *Child Dev.* Jul-Aug 2000;71(4):933-947.

101. Eiser C, Hill JJ, Vance YH. Examining the psychological consequences of surviving childhood cancer: systematic review as a research method in pediatric psychology. *J Pediatr Psychol.* Sep 2000;25(6):449-460.

102. Manne S, Nereo N, DuHamel K, et al. Anxiety and depression in mothers of children undergoing bone marrow transplant: symptom prevalence and use of the Beck depression and Beck anxiety inventories as screening instruments. *J Consult Clin Psychol.* Dec 2001;69(6):1037-1047.

103. Langer T, Martus P, Ottensmeier H, Hertzberg H, Beck JD, Meier W. CNS late-effects after ALL therapy in childhood. Part III: neuropsychological performance in long-term survivors of childhood ALL: impairments of concentration, attention, and memory. *Med Pediatr Oncol.* May 2002;38(5):320-328.

104. Alter CL, Pelcovitz D, Axelrod A, et al. Identification of PTSD in cancer survivors. *Psychosomatics.* Mar-Apr 1996;37(2):137-143.

105. Butler RW, Rizzi LP, Handwerger BA. Brief report: the assessment of posttraumatic stress disorder in pediatric cancer patients and survivors. *J Pediatr Psychol.* Aug 1996;21(4):499-504.

106. Stuber ML, Christakis DA, Houskamp B, Kazak AE. Posttrauma symptoms in childhood leukemia survivors and their parents. *Psychosomatics.* May-Jun 1996;37(3):254-261.

107. Barakat LP, Kazak AE, Meadows AT, Casey R, Meeske K, Stuber ML. Families surviving childhood cancer: a comparison of posttraumatic stress symptoms with families of healthy children. *J Pediatr Psychol.* Dec 1997;22(6):843-859.

108. Kazak AE, Barakat LP, Meeske K, et al. Posttraumatic stress, family functioning, and social support in survivors of childhood leukemia and their mothers and fathers. *J Consult Clin Psychol.* Feb 1997;65(1):120-129.

109. Stuber ML, Kazak AE, Meeske K, et al. Predictors of posttraumatic stress symptoms in childhood cancer survivors. *Pediatrics.* Dec 1997;100(6):958-964.

110. Kazak AE. Posttraumatic distress in childhood cancer survivors and their parents. *Med Pediatr Oncol.* 1998;Suppl 1:60-68.

111. Rourke MT, Stuber ML, Hobbie WL, Kazak AE. Posttraumatic stress disorder: understanding the psychosocial impact of surviving childhood cancer into young adulthood. *J Pediatr Oncol Nurs.* Jul 1999;16(3):126-135.

112. Hobbie WL, Stuber M, Meeske K, et al. Symptoms of posttraumatic stress in young adult survivors of childhood cancer. *J Clin Oncol.* Dec 15 2000;18(24):4060-4066.

113. Erickson SJ, Steiner H. Trauma spectrum adaptation: somatic symptoms in long-term pediatric cancer survivors. *Psychosomatics.* Jul-Aug 2000;41(4):339-346.

114. Manne S, DuHamel K, Nereo N, et al. Predictors of PTSD in mothers of children undergoing bone marrow transplantation: the role of cognitive and social processes. *J Pediatr Psychol.* Oct-Nov 2002;27(7):607-617.

115. Alderfer MA, Labay LE, Kazak AE. Brief report: does posttraumatic stress apply to siblings of childhood cancer survivors? *J Pediatr Psychol.* Jun 2003;28(4):281-286.

116. Brown RT, Madan-Swain A, Lambert R. Posttraumatic stress symptoms in adolescent survivors of childhood cancer and their mothers. *J Trauma Stress.* Aug 2003;16(4):309-318.

117. Kazak AE, Alderfer M, Rourke MT, Simms S, Streisand R, Grossman JR. Posttraumatic stress disorder (PTSD) and posttraumatic stress symptoms (PTSS) in families of adolescent childhood cancer survivors. *J Pediatr Psychol.* Apr-May 2004;29(3):211-219.

118. Kazak AE, Alderfer MA, Streisand R, et al. Treatment of posttraumatic stress symptoms in adolescent survivors of childhood cancer and their families: a randomized clinical trial. *J Fam Psychol.* Sep 2004;18(3):493-504.

119. Alderfer MA, Cnaan A, Annunziato RA, Kazak AE. Patterns of posttraumatic stress symptoms in parents of childhood cancer survivors. *J Fam Psychol.* Sep 2005; 19(3):430-440.

120. Barakat LP, Alderfer MA, Kazak AE. Posttraumatic growth in adolescent survivors of cancer and their mothers and fathers. *J Pediatr Psychol.* May 2006;31(4):413-419.

121. Stoppelbein LA, Greening L, Elkin TD. Risk of Posttraumatic Stress Symptoms: A Comparison of Child Survivors of Pediatric Cancer and Parental Bereavement. *J Pediatr Psychol.* 2006;31(4):367-376.

122. Mulhern RK, Ochs J, Fairclough D, Wasserman AL, Davis KS, Williams JM. Intellectual and academic achievement status after CNS relapse: a retrospective analysis of 40 children treated for acute lymphoblastic leukemia. *J Clin Oncol.* Jun 1987;5(6):933-940.

123. Mulhern RK, Wasserman AL, Fairclough D, Ochs J. Memory function in disease-free survivors of childhood acute lymphocytic leukemia given CNS prophylaxis with or without 1,800 cGy cranial irradiation. *J Clin Oncol.* Feb 1988;6(2):315-320.

124. Brown RT, Madan-Swain A, Pais R, et al. Cognitive status of children treated with central nervous system prophylactic chemotherapy for acute lymphocytic leukemia. *Arch Clin Neuropsychol.* Nov 1992;7(6):481-497.

125. Brown RT, Sawyer MB, Antoniou G, et al. A 3-year follow-up of the intellectual and academic functioning of children receiving central nervous system prophylactic chemotherapy for leukemia. *J Dev Behav Pediatr.* Dec 1996;17(6):392-398.

126. Brown RT, Madan-Swain A, Walco GA, et al. Cognitive and academic late effects among children previously treated for acute lymphocytic leukemia receiving chemotherapy as CNS prophylaxis. *J Pediatr Psychol.* Oct 1998;23(5):333-340.

127. Kazak AE, Simms S, Barakat L, et al. Surviving cancer competently intervention program (SCCIP): a cognitive-behavioral and family therapy intervention for adolescent survivors of childhood cancer and their families. *Fam Process.* Summer 1999;38(2):175-191.

128. Winqvist S, Vainionpaa L, Kokkonen J, Lanning M. Cognitive functions of young adults who survived childhood cancer. *Appl Neuropsychol.* 2001;8(4):224-233.

129. von der Weid N, Mosimann I, Hirt A, et al. Intellectual outcome in children and adolescents with acute lymphoblastic leukaemia treated with chemotherapy alone: age- and sex-related differences. *Eur J Cancer.* Feb 2003;39(3):359-365.

130. Buizer AI, de Sonneville LM, van den Heuvel-Eibrink MM, Veerman AJ. Behavioral and educational limitations after chemotherapy for childhood acute lymphoblastic leukemia or Wilms tumor. *Cancer.* Mar 27 2006;Prepublication release.

131. Beardslee C, Neff EJ. Body related concerns of children with cancer as compared with the concerns of other children. *Matern Child Nurs J.* Fall 1982;11(3):121-134.

132. Neff EJ, Beardslee CI. Body knowledge and concerns of children with cancer as compared with the knowledge and concerns of other children. *J Pediatr Nurs.* Jun 1990; 5(3):179-189.

133. Anholt U, Fritz G, Keener M. Self-concept in survivors of childhood and adolescent cancer. *J Psychosoc Oncol.* 1993;11(1):1-16.

134. Madan-Swain A, Brown RT, Foster MA, et al. Identity in adolescent survivors of childhood cancer. *J Pediatr Psychol.* Mar 2000;25(2):105-115.

135. Zebrack BJ, Chesler M. Health-related worries, self-image, and life outlooks of long-term survivors of childhood cancer. *Health Soc Work.* Nov 2001;26(4):245-256.

136. Landier W, Wallace WH, Hudson MM. Long-term follow-up of pediatric cancer survivors: education, surveillance, and screening. *Pediatr Blood Cancer.* Feb 2006;46(2):149-158.

137. Byrne J, Lewis S, Halamek L, Connelly RR, Mulvihill JJ. Childhood cancer survivors' knowledge of their diagnosis and treatment. *Ann Intern Med.* Mar 1 1989;110(5):400-403.

138. Kadan-Lottick NS, Robison LL, Gurney JG, et al. Childhood cancer survivors' knowledge about their past diagnosis and treatment: Childhood Cancer Survivor Study. *Jama.* Apr 10 2002;287(14):1832-1839.

139. Bashore L. Childhood and adolescent cancer survivors' knowledge of their disease and effects of treatment. *J Pediatr Oncol Nurs.* Mar-Apr 2004;21(2):98-102.

140. Caprino D, Wiley TJ, Massimo L. Childhood cancer survivors in the dark. *J Clin Oncol.* Jul 1 2004;22(13):2748-2750.

141. Zebrack BJ, Eshelman DA, Hudson MM, et al. Health care for childhood cancer survivors: insights and perspectives from a Delphi panel of young adult survivors of childhood cancer. *Cancer.* Feb 15 2004;100(4):843-850.

142. Mulhern RK, Tyc VL, Phipps S, et al. Health-related behaviors of survivors of childhood cancer. *Med Pediatr Oncol.* Sep 1995;25(3):159-165.

143. Hudson MM, Tyc VL, Srivastava DK, et al. Multi-component behavioral intervention to promote health protective behaviors in childhood cancer survivors: the protect study. *Med Pediatr Oncol.* Jul 2002;39(1):2-1; discussion 2.

144. Tyc VL, Hudson MM, Hinds P. Health promotion interventions for adolescent cancer survivors. *Cognitive and Behavioral Practice.* 1999;6:128-136.

145. Park EB, Emmons KM, Malloy NW, Seifer E. A qualitative exploration of health perceptions and behaviors among adult survivors of childhood cancers. *J Cancer Educ*. Winter 2002;17(4):211-215.

146. Cox CL, McLaughlin RA, Rai SN, Steen BD, Hudson MM. Adolescent survivors: A secondary analysis of a clinical trial targeting behavior change. *Pediatr Blood Cancer*. Mar 15 2005.

147. Demark-Wahnefried W, Werner C, Clipp EC, et al. Survivors of childhood cancer and their guardians. *Cancer*. May 15 2005;103(10):2171-2180.

148. Hollen PJ, Hobbie WL, Finley SM, Hiebert SM. The relationship of resiliency to decision making and risk behaviors of cancer-surviving adolescents. *J Pediatr Oncol Nurs*. Sep-Oct 2001;18(5):188-204.

149. Emmons K, Li FP, Whitton J, et al. Predictors of smoking initiation and cessation among childhood cancer survivors: a report from the childhood cancer survivor study. *J Clin Oncol*. Mar 15 2002;20(6):1608-1616.

150. Oeffinger KC, Mertens AC, Hudson MM, et al. Health care of young adult survivors of childhood cancer: a report from the Childhood Cancer Survivor Study. *Ann Fam Med*. Jan-Feb 2004;2(1):61-70.

151. Schidlow DV, Fiel SB. Life beyond pediatrics. Transition of chronically ill adolescents from pediatric to adult health care systems. *Med Clin North Am*. Sep 1990;74(5):1113-1120.

152. Rettig P, Athreya BH. Adolescents with chronic disease. Transition to adult health care. *Arthritis Care Res*. Dec 1991;4(4):174-180.

153. Blum RW, Garell D, Hodgman CH, et al. Transition from child-centered to adult health-care systems for adolescents with chronic conditions. A position paper of the Society for Adolescent Medicine. *J Adolesc Health*. Nov 1993;14(7):570-576.

154. Rosen DS. Transition to adult health care for adolescents and young adults with cancer. *Cancer*. May 15 1993;71(10 Suppl):3411-3414.

155. Betz CL. Facilitating the transition of adolescents with chronic conditions from pediatric to adult health care and community settings. *Issues Compr Pediatr Nurs*. Apr-Jun 1998;21(2):97-115.

156. Blum RW. Introduction. Improving transition for adolescents with special health care needs from pediatric to adult-centered health care. *Pediatrics*. Dec 2002;110(6 Pt 2):1301-1303.

157. Kelly AM, Kratz B, Bielski M, Rinehart PM. Implementing transitions for youth with complex chronic conditions using the medical home model. *Pediatrics*. Dec 2002;110(6 Pt 2):1322-1327.

158. Reiss J, Gibson R. Health care transition: destinations unknown. *Pediatrics*. Dec 2002;110(6 Pt 2):1307-1314.

159. Scal P. Transition for youth with chronic conditions: primary care physicians' approaches. *Pediatrics*. Dec 2002;110(6 Pt 2):1315-1321.

160. White PH. Access to health care: health insurance considerations for young adults with special health care needs/disabilities. *Pediatrics*. Dec 2002;110(6 Pt 2):1328-1335.

161. Merrick J, Kandel I. Adolescents with special needs and the transition from adolescent to adult health care. *Int J Adolesc Med Health*. Apr-Jun 2003;15(2):103.

162. Rosen DS, Blum RW, Britto M, Sawyer SM, Siegel DM. Transition to adult health care for adolescents and young adults with chronic conditions: position paper of the Society for Adolescent Medicine. *J Adolesc Health*. Oct 2003;33(4):309-311.

163. McDonagh JE. Growing up and moving on: transition from pediatric to adult care. *Pediatr Transplant*. Jun 2005;9(3):364-372.

164. Scal P, Ireland M. Addressing transition to adult health care for adolescents with special health care needs. *Pediatrics*. Jun 2005;115(6):1607-1612.

165. Ginsberg JP, Hobbie WL, Carlson CA, Meadows AT. Delivering long-term follow-up care to pediatric cancer survivors: transitional care issues. *Pediatr Blood Cancer.* Feb 2006;46(2):169-173.

166. Cunningham PJ, Kohn L. Health plan switching: choice or circumstance? *Health Aff (Millwood).* May-Jun 2000;19(3):158-164.

167. Smith MA, Bartell JM. Changes in usual source of care and perceptions of health care access, quality, and use. *Med Care.* Oct 2004;42(10):975-984.

168. Yarnall KS, Pollak KI, Ostbye T, Krause KM, Michener JL. Primary care: is there enough time for prevention? *Am J Public Health.* Apr 2003;93(4):635-641.

169. University of Minnesota Cancer Center. Surviving childhood cancer. November 1, 2002; http://www.cancer.umn.edu/ltfu. Accessed December 1, 2004.

170. Fordis M, Horowitz M, Landier W, et al. Investigation of the feasibility of developing an online decision support tool for healthcare providers managing the long-term follow-up of survivors of childhood cancer. Paper presented at: Society of Academic Continuing Medical Education (SACME)/Research in Continuing Medical Education (RICME); April 8, 2006; Key West, FL.

171. McKinley ED. Under Toad days: surviving the uncertainty of cancer recurrence. *Ann Intern Med.* Sep 19 2000;133(6):479-480.

172. Grant J, Cranston A, Horsman J, et al. Health status and health-related quality of life in adolescent survivors of cancer in childhood. *J Adolesc Health.* May 2006;38(5):504-510.

173. Mooney GA, Bligh JG. Computer-based learning materials for medical education: a model production. *Med Educ.* May 1997;31(3):197-201.

174. Landier W, Bhatia S, Eshelman DA, et al. Development of risk-based guidelines for pediatric cancer survivors: the Children's Oncology Group Long-Term Follow-Up Guidelines from the Children's Oncology Group Late Effects Committee and Nursing Discipline. *J Clin Oncol.* Dec 15 2004;22(24):4979-4990.

175. National Comprehensive Cancer Network. Categories of Consensus. 2006; http://www.nccn.org/professionals/physician_gls/categories_of_concensus.asp. Accessed April 19, 2006.

176. Lomas J, Anderson GM, Domnick-Pierre K, Vayda E, Enkin MW, Hannah WJ. Do practice guidelines guide practice? The effect of a consensus statement on the practice of physicians. *N Engl J Med.* Nov 9 1989;321(19):1306-1311.

177. Tunis SR, Hayward RS, Wilson MC, et al. Internists' attitudes about clinical practice guidelines. *Ann Intern Med.* Jun 1 1994;120(11):956-963.

178. Davis DA, Taylor-Vaisey A. Translating guidelines into practice. A systematic review of theoretic concepts, practical experience and research evidence in the adoption of clinical practice guidelines. *CMAJ.* Aug 15 1997;157(4):408-416.

179. Cabana MD, Rand CS, Powe NR, et al. Why don't physicians follow clinical practice guidelines? A framework for improvement. *JAMA.* Oct 20 1999;282(15):1458-1465.

180. Browman GP. Clinical practice guidelines and healthcare decisions: credibility gaps and unfulfilled promises? *Nat Clin Pract Oncol.* Oct 2005;2(10):480-481.

181. Feifer C, Fifield J, Ornstein S, et al. From research to daily clinical practice: what are the challenges in "translation"? *Jt Comm J Qual Saf.* May 2004;30(5):235-245.

182. Greenfield S, Kaplan S, Ware JE, Jr. Expanding patient involvement in care. Effects on patient outcomes. *Ann Intern Med.* Apr 1985;102(4):520-528.

183. Greenfield S, Kaplan SH, Ware JE, Jr., Yano EM, Frank HJ. Patients' participation in medical care: effects on blood sugar control and quality of life in diabetes. *J Gen Intern Med.* Sep-Oct 1988;3(5):448-457.

184. Von Korff M, Gruman J, Schaefer J, Curry SJ, Wagner EH. Collaborative management of chronic illness. *Ann Intern Med.* Dec 15 1997;127(12):1097-1102.

185. Stone EG, Morton SC, Hulscher ME, et al. Interventions that increase use of adult immunization and cancer screening services: a meta-analysis. *Ann Intern Med.* May 7 2002;136(9):641-651.

186. Shea S, DuMouchel W, Bahamonde L. A meta-analysis of 16 randomized controlled trials to evaluate computer-based clinical reminder systems for preventive care in the ambulatory setting. *J Am Med Inform Assoc.* Nov-Dec 1996;3(6):399-409.

187. Hunt DL, Haynes RB, Hanna SE, Smith K. Effects of computer-based clinical decision support systems on physician performance and patient outcomes: a systematic review. *JAMA.* Oct 21 1998;280(15):1339-1346.

188. Mitchell E, Sullivan F. A descriptive feast but an evaluative famine: systematic review of published articles on primary care computing during 1980-97. *BMJ.* Feb 3 2001; 322(7281):279-282.

189. Gandhi TK, Sequist TD, Poon EG, et al. Primary care clinician attitudes towards electronic clinical reminders and clinical practice guidelines. *AMIA Annu Symp Proc.* 2003:848.

190. Evans RS, Pestotnik SL, Classen DC, et al. A computer-assisted management program for antibiotics and other antiinfective agents. *N Engl J Med.* Jan 22 1998;338(4):232-238.

191. McCulloch DK, Price MJ, Hindmarsh M, Wagner EH. A population-based approach to diabetes management in a primary care setting: early results and lessons learned. *Eff Clin Pract.* Aug-Sep 1998;1(1):12-22.

192. Griffin S, Kinmonth AL. Systems for routine surveillance for people with diabetes mellitus. *Nurs Times.* Jul 5-11 2001;97(27):44.

193. Rundall TG, Shortell SM, Wang MC, et al. As good as it gets? Chronic care management in nine leading US physician organisations. *BMJ.* Oct 26 2002;325(7370):958-961.

194. Griffin SJ, Kinmonth AL, Veltman MW, Gillard S, Grant J, Stewart M. Effect on health-related outcomes of interventions to alter the interaction between patients and practitioners: a systematic review of trials. *Ann Fam Med.* Nov-Dec 2004;2(6):595-608.

195. Osheroff JA, Pifer EA, Teich JM, Sittig DF, Jenders RA. *Improving Outcomes with Clinical Decision Support: An Implementer's Guide.* Chicago, IL: Healthcare Information and Management Systems Society; 2005.

196. Teich JM, Osheroff JA, Pifer EA, Sittig DF, Jenders RA. Clinical decision support in electronic prescribing: recommendations and an action plan: report of the joint clinical decision support workgroup. *J Am Med Inform Assoc.* Jul-Aug 2005;12(4):365-376.

197. Connecting For Health Steering Group. The Connecting for Health Common Framework: Overview and Principles. April, 2006; http://www.connectingforhealth.org/commonframework/docs/Overview.pdf. Accessed May 24, 2006.

198. 104th U.S. Congress. Public Law 104-91—Health Insurance Portability and Accountability Act of 1996: An Act. August 21, 1996; http://aspe.hhs.gov/admnsimp/pl104191.htm. Accessed May 24, 2006.

Appendix D.4

Regional Approaches to Cancer Survivorship Care Planning

Tim Byers, MD, MPH

Professor, University of Colorado School of Medicine
Deputy Director, University of Colorado Cancer Center

Synopsis: State-level cancer control collaboratives could help to institute a widespread adoption of cancer survivorship planning, but most of the current collaboratives will first need to better engage health care providers.

Introduction

If cancer survivor plans are to constitute a standard in cancer care, many different organizations will need to collaborate to institute this new service as a medical care norm.[1] Regional organizations that currently collaborate in cancer control programs could be particularly helpful to broadly institute cancer survivor planning. The purpose of this paper is to examine this potential, and to critically assess both the capabilities and weaknesses of organizations engaged in regional cancer control activities.

Cancer Control as a Regional Issue

The term "regional" could define many different types of geopolitical units. In this review, "regional" will be considered mostly as statewide or as pertaining to subregions of a state, such as an urban area with its surrounding suburbs, or a defined rural area of a state with a regional identity. The term "regional" could also refer to areas of the country that include several states, such as the Southwest or the Midwest, but most multistate regional organizations, such as Department of Health and Human Services (DHHS) regions and American Cancer Society (ACS) Divisions, have been created principally for administrative convenience, and do not have functional collaborative programs. As most public health activity tends to be state-specific, and most cancer control programming is now at the state level, the term "regional" will mostly be used here as synonymous with "statewide."

State-based cancer organizations have been under development as a public health strategy over the past decade by the Centers for Disease Control and Prevention (CDC).[2] The CDC comprehensive cancer control strategy is to support public health departments to create state-wide collaborative organizations that join expertise from public health agencies, universities, nongovernmental voluntary cancer organizations, and health care providers. That CDC would designate state health departments as the conveners of statewide collaborative organizations derives from the historic relationship between CDC and state governments. States are the geopolitical units with primary responsibility for public health in the United States, and the historic role of CDC has been to support states in their public health efforts. CDC's cancer control strategy via states has been to build a program of comprehensive cancer control onto their earlier investments in chronic disease prevention and control, including state tobacco control programs, cancer registries, breast and cervical cancer screening, and behavioral risk factor surveillance systems.

The Current Status of State-Based Comprehensive Cancer Control

The CDC model for state-based comprehensive cancer control is to build programs in two stages: first planning, then implementation. The planning process can take from one to several years. Planning is a collaborative process in which the state health department cancer control program staff convene work groups to examine cancer trends and risk factors, then to examine existing resources and opportunities, and finally to create consensus objectives and strategies to reduce the state's cancer burden. At this time, 44 states have completed the cancer planning process, with publication of their state cancer plans.[3] The implementation stage then follows, a prolonged period with no definable ending, in which collaboratives in the state work to develop a comprehensive cancer control program and to accomplish the goals set out in the cancer plan. As the CDC budget for cancer control is not growing as rapidly as is the number of states entering into the implementation phase, the level of funding per state for implementation has been decreasing in recent years. Thus, comprehensive cancer control across the United states is progressing in terms of the numbers of states completing plans and moving into implementation, but it is at the same time regressing from the perspective of the availability of resources to implement plans within states.

The main strength of state-based cancer programs derives from their multiorganizational and multidisciplinary nature. State cancer coalitions (variously also called "alliances," or "partnerships") serve the function of communication and collaboration about various cancer control activities across many different sectors within states. These sectors include public health agencies, academic centers, nongovernmental voluntary health agencies, and health care providers. Most of the actual work of cancer control in the state cancer coalitions is conducted by the partner organizations. The purpose of the coalition is to motivate and coordinate the collective body of work done by partner organizations. Within the coalitions, most of the planning and communication occurs within work groups or task forces. The composition of these groups differs across states but usually includes disease-specific groups (e.g., breast cancer, colorectal cancer, prostate cancer, skin cancer), or groups focusing on specific issues that cut across cancer sites (e.g., surveillance, evaluation, health disparities).

There are two major weaknesses of state cancer control coalitions: insufficient funding and insufficient independence. CDC has provided funding for the development of cancer plans across states, but as states finish the planning process, there is insufficient funding to enact programs to achieve the lofty goals defined in the planning process. With the numbers of states entering into the implementation phase of comprehensive cancer control growing much more rapidly that the CDC budget for cancer control, the result has been lower budgets for states to effectively engage in implementation activities. A result, then, is that states can be proud of the glossy cancer plans on their shelves and empowered by the potentials of new partnerships formed in the planning process but can then have considerable difficulty maintaining that collaborative spirit as they try to implement lofty goals with insufficient resources.

Another weakness of state cancer programs is their lack of independence from their funding source. Comprehensive cancer programs are funded by CDC grants to state health departments, sometimes supplemented also by state monies, but in all cases the effort is managed by the state public health department. Although CDC properly envisions the role of the public health department as the convener of statewide collaboratives, and regards the strength of coalitions as coming from their multisectorial representation, the fact that cancer coalitions are convened and staffed by state public health department personnel means that coalition partners tend to regard the process as a state health department activity. As a result, many partners, especially health care providers, do not become as fully engaged as they otherwise might if the effort had a more independent identity. This problem is compounded, of course, by the problem of insufficient funding. Coalitions can often be hesitant to become fully engaged in issues that are politically sensitive, such as policy or legislative matters in which state employees (the conveners of coalitions) are disallowed from engagement due to their government employee status. Apart from these legal conflicts, the public health department identity of cancer coalitions also tends to distance the coalitions from health care providers because of the historic gap between public health departments and health care providers. Most public health workers who convene cancer coalitions have not been trained as health care providers and are much more fluent in public health skills such as mass marketing, health education, and surveillance, than in matters pertaining to clinical cancer care. One result of the low level of provider input into state cancer programs has been the low profile of goals and strategies to meet the many needs of cancer patients in treatment, rehabilitation, and survivorship.

Cancer Survivorship Content Within State Cancer Plans

There are 44 state cancer plans (Alaska, Idaho, Illinois, Mississippi, Montana, and Oklahoma are now drafting cancer plans).[3] State cancer plans are written in varying degrees of detail, and in many different formats. All plans include descriptions of cancer risk in the state and set specific targets for reducing cancer incidence and mortality as well as lowering the prevalence of cancer risk factors across the state. Nearly all plans are heavily weighted by objectives for cancer prevention and early detection. Most plans also include some mention of cancer survivorship issues by at least briefly acknowledging the importance of cancer survivorship. Many plans, for instance, simply define cancer survivorship by the National Cancer Institute (NCI) definition ("An individual is considered a cancer survivor from the time of diagnosis, through the balance of his or her life"), or state the many needs of survivors without defining specific objectives. Most plans cover pain control or end-of-life care as their principal cancer survivorship focus. The emphasis on pain control and end-of-life care are understandable as the evidence base in these areas is stronger than for most of the other issues in cancer survivorship. In fact, a recent Institute of Medicine (IOM) report that defined a set of measures for the State of Georgia (intended as a model set of quality measures for any state) included pain control and hospice utilization as the only cancer survivorship measures among 52 measures.[4] Many plans also make general reference to the need for better education of both cancer survivors and health care providers about cancer survivorship needs and support systems. Some plans specify more survivorship needs and objectives that could potentially be tied to cancer survivorship planning. Selected aspects of those more specific objectives are summarized in Table D.4-1.

Only two state plans specifically mention objectives that could be interpreted as promoting the specific idea of cancer survivorship plans (Minnesota and Oregon). In the Minnesota plan, objective #17 is to "Optimize

TABLE D.4-1 Specific Statements of Need and Objectives Related to Cancer Survivorship Support that Might Be Tied to Cancer Survivorship Plans in Selected State Cancer Plans

State (page in plan)	Need	Objective
Alabama (25)	Cancer support services are underutilized.	Increase knowledge of cancer support services by both providers and the public.
Arizona (127)	Cancer patients need better support services.	Promote patient navigator programs, help providers direct patients to supportive care, and monitor gaps in support services.
Colorado (62-66)	Rehabilitation after cancer treatment is lacking.	Support the development of navigation and rehabilitation services.
Connecticut (89-91)	Cancer patients find the survivorship process confusing.	Define "high-quality" care for cancer survivors.
Iowa (46-47)	Poor communication exists between providers and patients regarding cancer care.	Increase communication between providers and patients about cancer care, and also educate providers about the need to take care of themselves.
Indiana (47-49)	Cancer support services are underutilized.	Increase knowledge of cancer support services by both providers and the public.
Kansas (35-37)	Recovery and reintegration of cancer survivors into family, society and workplace is lacking.	A business standard of excellence is proposed for return to work, and an emphasis is placed also on preventive behaviors, including nutrition, among cancer patients.
Louisiana (71-74)	Rehabilitation after cancer treatment is needed.	Provide clearer information to both providers and patients about cancer rehab services.

continuity of care for cancer survivors during and beyond the initial course of treatment." That objective would be assessed by monitoring the proportion of primary care physicians who receive information about their patients' cancer treatment and follow-up recommendations from their patients' oncologists. Special surveys would be done to accomplish that assessment. In the Oregon plan, objective #3 is to "Increase the proportion of cancer patients who are informed and participate with their provider in their long-term follow-up care plan." That objective would be achieved

TABLE D.4-1 Continued

State (page in plan)	Need	Objective
Maine (61-62)	Rehabilitation and survivorship services are needed.	A "best practices" approach is suggested to define high-quality services statewide.
Maryland (92-94)	Need to develop survivorship awareness and services.	Several objectives are defined for education but also one for establishing cancer survivor clinics.
Minnesota (42-43)	Continuity of care is lacking.	Encourage oncologists to provide clear treatment summaries and care plans to primary care practitioners.
Nevada (18)	Develop a more comprehensive approach to long-term cancer survivorship.	The Nevada Cancer Institute is developing a cancer survivorship program that can be a model, made possible by LAF.
New York (30)	Employment and insurance issues are barriers for cancer survivors.	Employment and insurance will be addressed as statewide policy issues.
Oregon (73-77)	The transition from cancer care to survivorship is confusing.	Increase the proportion of cancer patients who are informed and participate with their provider in their long-term follow-up plan.
Texas (76-80)	Identifies many needs in information and access.	Increase knowledge of survivorship issues for the general public, cancer survivors, health care professionals, and policy makers.
Virginia (82)	Rehabilitation for cancer is insufficient.	Assure that cancer rehab services become available statewide.

using strategies that include increased communication with providers about follow-up guidelines and developing long-term follow-up plans as collaborative activities between providers and patients.

Survivorship planning is rarely pointed to in state cancer plans, probably because the idea of cancer survivorship plans is fairly new, and there is as yet little evidence basis for including it as a statewide objective. Many state cancer plans only generally acknowledge the many needs of cancer survivors, however, and many plans merely point to the general needs of health care providers as well as patients and family members for education about cancer survivorship. The fact that detailed objectives in most of the plans are much less common than the general rhetoric about the importance of survivorship may suggest that state cancer coalition members would be quite receptive to specific measurable objectives for cancer survivorship planning.

Cancer Survivorship as a Public Health Issue

The CDC has joined in a partnership effort with the Lance Armstrong Foundation (LAF) to better develop a public health role in cancer survivorship.[5] In their 2004 report entitled "A National Action Plan for Cancer Survivorship: Advancing Public Health Strategies", the CDC-LAF partnership defines four areas of traditional public health activity within which cancer survivorship can be relevant: (1) surveillance and applied research; (2) communication, education, and training; (3) programs, policies, and infrastructure; and (4) access to quality care and services.

Cancer surveillance might be the single most important area in which public health agencies could have an immediate impact on cancer survivorship. All states operate cancer registries. These registries were developed to monitor cancer incidence and survival. Outcomes apart from recurrence and survival have been assessed only as special studies tied to cancer registries. Over time, though, cancer registries have begun to also monitor the quality of cancer care.[6] In the near future, outcomes such as fatigue, pain, confusion, satisfaction with health care, and both the need for and utilization of community support services could become routinely measured as part of cancer surveillance systems in states. Communication, education, and training are traditional public health functions that fit well into the model of cancer coalition activities. These types of activities require far fewer resources than do the provision of services. Programs, policies, and infrastructure are more problematic for state comprehensive cancer control programs, both because of insufficient funding for programs and because of insufficient independence to affect policies. Access to quality care and services is also a challenge for public-health-dominated coalitions, as public health agencies provide very little cancer care, and health care access is now determined more by insurance and entitlement programs than by public health agencies.

Other State-Based Organizations Relevant to Cancer Survivorship

Many state-based organizations are active in cancer survivorship programs. In most states, these organizations are also active members of the state cancer coalition. These include comprehensive cancer centers, quality improvement organizations, health care professional organizations, health care provider systems, and nongovernmental cancer voluntary organizations.

Comprehensive Cancer Centers

NCI provides core support to 39 comprehensive cancer centers across the United States.[7] The principal mission of these centers is to conduct cancer research. In order to be designated as a comprehensive cancer center, centers must demonstrate their expertise in cancer control research and their connection to cancer control activities in the populations they serve. NCI funding does not directly support community outreach and cancer control service programs of cancer centers, but the requirement of community outreach as a criterion for the "comprehensive" designation is a strong incentive for cancer center researchers to collaborate in community-based programs such as state cancer coalitions. NCI provides core support for cancer centers to conduct research. Most of those resources support the basic science and clinical science core laboratories needed for research, but some cancer centers also use NCI resources to support community outreach and population sciences. Academic cancer center members who conduct community-based and population-based cancer research are frequently the faculty who become engaged in state cancer coalitions. In addition, cancer researchers with special interests in a particular type of cancer are often engaged in the work group or task force for that cancer type. With the recent drop in funding levels for cancer research by NCI, there has been a tightening of budgets not only for new research, but also for core support to cancer centers. Though new initiatives in cancer survivorship such as survivor planning will likely be supported by cancer centers, and though cancer centers would be excellent settings in which to conduct demonstration projects, it is unlikely that NCI will be a major source of new funding for this as a developmental project via cancer centers in the near future.

NCI does provide major support for clinical trials, however, both via cancer centers and via community-based trial organizations. It is in the realm of clinical trials where cancer survivor plans could emerge as a service project of cancer center investigators, blending service with research. All clinical trials now include at least some assessment of quality-of-life outcome measures. This happened as a mandated policy from the cooperative trial groups supported by NCI. NCI could, as a matter of policy, also mandate that that all patients exiting the first course of treatment in clinical trials be provided a full written treatment summary and follow-up plan, essentially a cancer survivorship plan. If such a policy were not accompanied by additional resources, it would be met with some resistance from clinicians, but clinical trial systems in both cancer centers and in the communities would be excellent places in which to support demonstration projects as addendums to ongoing trials.

Quality Improvement Organizations

The Center for Medicare and Medicaid Services (CMS) supports interventions to improve the quality of health care services principally through a system 53 of state and territory-based organizations called Quality Improvement Organizations (QIOs).[8] It is the mission of QIOs to conduct projects within each state to improve the quality of medical services provided to Medicare beneficiaries. These projects are often done in collaboration with other states as either national or multistate projects, under a general framework of themes and goals set by CMS. Important projects have been done to improve the quality and reach of proven interventions such as adult immunizations, the clinical management of diabetes, pneumonia, heart failure, and myocardial infarction. In the area of cancer quality improvement, projects have been done to increase mammography utilization and colorectal screening, but to date no projects have been done to improve the quality of cancer survivorship. As Medicare pays for a substantial proportion of cancer care in the United States, engaging the QIOs to implement and evaluate a cancer survivorship planning project might be a very effective way to develop, evaluate, and then, eventually, to implement cancer survivor plans. A widespread national quality improvement project on cancer survivorship planning would likely need to follow a stronger set of evidence for efficacy, but a small demonstration project could be done with CMS support. The advantage of this as a CMS QIO project is that such a project would be done in settings in which successful partnerships with hospital care systems have been done before, on statewide bases, with strong evaluations.

Health Care Professional Organizations

Health care professional societies such as the American Society of Clinical Oncology (ASCO), the American College of Surgeons (ACoS), and the Oncology Nursing Society (ONS) have been leaders in the development and implementation of guidelines to improve the standard of care. These professional organizations tend to impact problems of clinical care at a national level, but there are often viable local or state-level chapters, and many of the leaders in these organizations are also active members of state cancer coalitions. ASCO has been active in setting standards for cancer care, and cancer survivorship planning could eventually be added into quality cancer care standards. ACoS certifies hospitals across the United states according to their cancer treatment quality standards, so cancer survivorship planning could be added into other hospital-based quality standards. The ONS provides ongoing continuing education to nurses to improve the quality of nursing oncology practice, and nurses would likely play important roles in survivorship care planning and patient support. All three of these organizations, both via their national organizations and also via their local and state organizations, could be instrumental in developing and instituting cancer survivorship planning.

Health Care Systems

Health care systems and organizations are often organized with regional reach. Large HMOs, for instance, often capture a substantial proportion of patients in a region (e.g., Kaiser in the San Francisco Bay Area, or Group Health Cooperative in the Puget Sound area). Hospital systems can also have considerable influence on medical practice in an urban or rural region of a state. Health care systems such as these could therefore substantially influence practice norms in a region if they were to institute cancer survivorship plans as a matter of policy.

Nongovernmental Voluntary Organizations (NGOs)

There are many NGO cancer advocacy and support organizations across the United States that are active at regional or state levels. The ACS is now an approximately 1 billion dollar per year organization, with national local, regional, state, and local organizational features. ACS has a collaborative approach to cancer control and, in most states, is a key partner in cancer coalition activities. ACS is a provider of cancer patient support services but also is engaged in cancer control applied research, in policy formation, and in capacity development. ACS has partnered with CDC to institute state cancer control leadership development training. Teams of leaders representing the many sectors in cancer coalitions are trained together as teams to conduct both planning and programming in cancer control. Other NGO cancer voluntary organizations of importance in cancer coalitions include cancer site-specific organizations such as the Susan G. Komen Foundation and the Avon Foundation, and mission-specific organizations such as the LAF. The LAF has had mostly a national impact via successful publicity on cancer survivorship and rehabilitation tied to Lance Armstrong's personal story, but in addition it is now creating regional impact by creating LIVE**STRONG**™ Centers of Excellence in cancer survivorship at selected cancer centers across the United States (now in New York, Boston, Denver, Los Angeles, and Seattle).

Table D.4-2 summarizes the critical strengths and weaknesses of se-

lected organizations in terms of their potential to impact problems of cancer survivorship such as cancer survivorship planning.

How Might Cancer Survivorship Plans Be Regionally Instituted?

Cancer survivorship planning could most quickly have regional and
statewide impact if it were to be instituted as part of a state's comprehensive cancer control program. A successful process would need to engage
health care providers, however, much more than is currently the norm in
cancer control programs. Following a process to add specific objectives and
strategies into existing cancer plans could bring together cancer coalition
partners in states who have in the past expressed only general needs for
addressing the needs of cancer survivors, without specific measurable objectives. The initial objectives would likely not be statewide adoption of
cancer survivorship planning, but they could be phased objectives to first
implement demonstration projects, evaluate them, and then disseminate the
practice. The principal function of a planning (goal setting) phase might be
to engage regional partners to envision the possibilities of a set of demonstration projects in which cancer survivorship planning could be developed
and implemented in different ways, and evaluated in terms of patient and
provider satisfaction as well as other outcomes. Alternative ways can be
assessed to develop cancer survivorship plans, to deliver them to patients,
and to then navigate (or not) patients through recovery and long-term
survival. Outcomes can be assessed in many domains, including cost-effectiveness. The rudimentary coverage of cancer survivorship issues by most
state cancer plans is evidence for some preexisting dialogue between plan-
ners, public health-oriented professionals, and health cancer care providers.
Reconvening these partners around the specific proposal to conduct demonstration projects might be welcome in many states. A critical issue, of
course, will be the time and resources needed to conduct and evaluate
demonstration projects of this type. Those issues are discussed in the section that follows.

Recommendations

The IOM report *From Cancer Patient to Cancer Survivor: Lost in
Transition* makes important recommendations related to cancer survivorship planning:

• *Recommendation #1* calls for health care workers, patient advocates, and others to ". . . act to ensure the delivery of appropriate survivorship care."

TABLE D.4-2 A Summary of Selected Strengths, Weaknesses, and Opportunities Faced by Various Types of Organizations in Affecting the Uptake of Cancer Survivorship Planning in Regions

	Strengths	Weaknesses	Opportunities
State public health departments	Conveners of comprehensive cancer coalitions and programs	Only weakly linked to health care providers	Define objectives in cancer plans and increase surveillance coverage of cancer survivorship issues
Comprehensive cancer centers	Expertise in cancer control design and evaluation	Research focus is stronger than the service mission	Create and evaluate demonstration projects
Quality improvement organizations	Effective projects have been carried out for other chronic conditions	At this time, there is not a cancer survivorship mandate from CMS	Create and evaluate a demonstration quality improvement project in cancer survivorship planning
Health professional societies	Composed of the very individuals who would need to promote and carry out survivorship plans	Many competing issues for the health professions	High potential for education once models are developed
Health care systems	Provide direct services to regions, and have the ability to set practice norms	Many competing issues in terms of time and cost	Demonstration projects could assess outcomes including satisfaction with care
Nongovernmental cancer organizations	Driven largely by interests of cancer survivors	Tend to not be well connected to health care delivery	Could advocate for and fund demonstration projects

NOTE: CMS = Centers for Medicare & Medicaid Services.

• *Recommendation #2* deals specifically with survivorship planning: "Patients completing primary treatment should be provided with a comprehensive care summary and follow-up plan that is clearly and effectively explained. This Survivorship Care Plan should be written by the principal provider(s) who coordinated oncology treatment. This service should be reimbursed by third-party payors of health care."

• *Recommendation #5* calls for CMS, NCI, and others to ". . . support demonstration programs to test models of coordinated, interdisciplinary survivorship care. . . ."

• *Recommendation #6* states that "Congress should support the Centers for Disease Control and Prevention (CDC), other collaborating institutions, and the states in developing comprehensive cancer control plans that include consideration of survivorship care, and promoting the implementation, evaluation, and refinement of existing state cancer control plans."

Based on these recommendations, and in light of the regional organizations and opportunities reviewed above, the following specific recommendations are proposed:

1. Add cancer survivorship planning into to state cancer plans. Although the cancer planning process has been long for many states, and although most state plans target specific years for outcomes (e.g., 2010, etc.), states are able to add additional objectives to their plans at any time. Planning is, of course, not the same as action, but planning can serve to bring together sectors that otherwise seldom interact. In this instance, the planning process can energize the dialogue between professionals with public health skills in population science, behavioral science, and evaluation, with health care providers who are skilled in managing patients with cancer. Suggested objectives for the implementation of demonstration projects in cancer survivorship planning could be developed by an independent source, such as the CDC-LAF partnership, or they could be developed by some lead states, and then shared with other states. The planning process need not be lengthy. The critical need to move through planning and into implementation of demonstration projects will be to identify sufficient funding to support the work. Funding could come from various sources, but NGOs and foundations tied to health care systems might be well positioned to provide support for this type of work. With the engagement of state cancer coalitions in the demonstration phase of this work, state coalitions would then be ready to move toward statewide dissemination in the next step. Ongoing needs in state cancer coalitions are to close the gap between the public health and the clinical care sectors, and to create more independence from state departments of health. Cancer survivorship planning, if properly supported and independently funded, could serve to accomplish both of these needs.

2.   **Develop business models and support structures to provide widespread support for cancer survivorship planning should demonstration projects be successful.** If the demonstration projects show that the survivorship care plans provided to patients do, indeed, lead to reduced confusion, improved compliance with follow-up recommendations, and improved quality of life for long-term cancer survivors, then it will be important to develop mechanisms of widespread dissemination of this type of service. The providers who partner to demonstrate and evaluate this service will likely not be representative of all providers. A business model needs to also be developed to make cancer survivorship planning become as easy and as widespread as possible, with both time efficiency and cost efficiency in mind. Eventually, it is likely that plans could be developed in partnerships between providers and businesses, using web-based methods, and with standardized methods for patient communication and evaluation. This business model could be developed even during the demonstration phase of work, as a Small Business Innovation Research (SBIR) grant from NCI.

3.   **Include measures of cancer survivorship in current public health surveillance systems as well as in health care systems.** Cancer registries are already following patients for outcomes of recurrence and mortality, and special studies have shown that it is very feasible to also monitor quality-of-life outcomes after cancer treatment. Cancer registries could begin to systematically monitor cancer survivorship outcomes and needs such as fatigue, pain, the use of support systems, and satisfaction with care. This information would then inform statewide efforts and priorities in cancer survivorship systems. Through the support CDC provides for both comprehensive cancer control and state cancer registries, this type of outcome assessment could be supported first as special studies, then as core activities once cost-effective methods are determined. The Behavioral Risk Factor Surveillance System could also be used to monitor needs of long-term cancer survivors in each state. Either based on direct responses of cancer survivors who happen to be sampled, or (more likely) snowball sampling within families or acquaintances, the experiences and issues faced by cancer survivors in states could be systematically assessed.

Health care systems are increasingly conducting routine patient satisfaction surveys. Systematic surveys of cancer patients under care and of those who have been released from care could monitor performance of systems in meeting cancer survivors' needs. The IOM recommendation for the State of Georgia specifically calls for surveys of pain control, but in fact many other problems could be monitored in this way, including fatigue, confusion with recommendations, adherence with recommendations, and behavioral changes, as well as satisfaction with health care services.

REFERENCES

1. IOM (Institute of Medicine) 2006. From Cancer Patient to Cancer Survivor: Lost in Transition. Hewitt M, Greenfield S, Stovall E, eds. Washington, DC, The National Academies Press.
2. IOM (Institute of Medicine) 2003. Fulfilling the Potential of Cancer Prevention and Early Detection. Curry S, Byers T, and Hewitt M, eds. Washington, DC, The National Academies Press.
3. http://www.cancercontrolplanet.cancer.gov.
4. IOM (Institute of Medicine) 2005. Assessing the Quality of Cancer Care: An Approach to Measurement in Georgia. Eden J and Simone J, eds. Washington, DC, The National Academies Press.
5. CDC (Centers for Disease Control and Prevention) and LAF (Lance Armstrong Foundation) 2004. A National Action Plan for Cancer Survivorship: Advancing Public health Strategies. Atlanta, GA: CDC.
6. McDavid K, Schymura M, Armstrong L, Santilli L, Schmidt B, Byers T, et al. Rationale and design of the Breast, Colon, and Prostate Cancer Patterns of Care Study by the National Program of Cancer Registries. Cancer Causes and Control 2004;15:1057-66.
7. http://www3.cancer.gov/cancercenters.
8. Medicare Quality Improvement Organization Program Priorities. CMS, DHHS, January, 2006. Accessed via www.MedQIC.org.

Appendix D.5

Cancer Survivorship Care Planning: An Evaluation and Research Agenda

Craig C. Earle, MD, MSc

Harvard Medical School
Center for Outcomes and Policy Research
Dana-Farber Cancer Center

Introduction

The recent Institute of Medicine (IOM) report *From Cancer Patient to Cancer Survivor: Lost in Transition* recommended that "survivorship care plans" be created for patients as they complete primary therapy for cancer in order to ensure clarity for all involved about patients' diagnoses, treatment received, and plan for surveillance. The survivorship care plan should explicitly identify the providers responsible for each aspect of ongoing care and give information on resources available for psychosocial and other practical issues that may arise as a result of the prior cancer diagnosis. Creation of such a document would likely require a dedicated "off-treatment" or "transition" consultation in most cases. The IOM stated that such survivorship care plans "have strong face validity and can reasonably be assumed to improve care unless and until evidence accumulates to the contrary." This may be true, but it was an unusual step to make such a strong recommendation in the absence of much evidence. The logistics and resources required to implement survivorship care planning are nontrivial. If evidence eventually does not support their use, a lot of time, money and effort will have been wasted. Therefore, it is incumbent on the health services research community to quickly yet rigorously evaluate each element of the survivorship care plan and the effects, both good and bad, of its implementation.

The theory implicit in this focus on optimizing the transition from cancer patient to survivor is that if treatment summaries and survivorship care plans become part of standard practice and included in the medical record, they can facilitate communication among providers about the treatments patients have received and what the known toxicities have been, while also providing information as to the late effects they should be on the lookout for. Cancer care is often fragmented among many different specialists, and there has traditionally not been adequate communication back to primary care physicians (PCPs), for example, of such basic information as the specific diagnosis, stage, and treatment received. Moreover, the lack of clear practice guidelines for survivors creates uncertainty about what, if anything, nonspecialist providers should be doing to help follow cancer survivors. Survivorship care plans would provide clear direction about what should be done for a given patient and who should do it. Moreover, if standardized and available in electronically searchable formats, they may also assist broader efforts to monitor care patterns and evaluate the quality of care delivered.

Barriers to achieving the IOM's vision of survivorship care planning include: reaching consensus about what information these summaries should contain; making it feasible for busy oncologists to take the time to create them carefully; changing the oncology culture so that treatment summaries become part of expected practice; and educating patients about the potential benefits of such planning in order to maximize adherence to its content. Clearly, the summary described in Table D.5-1 would be a labor-intensive undertaking. On a larger scale, there are already manpower concerns in the oncology workforce brought about by the aging population, improved cancer therapeutics, and previous policy decisions limiting the training of specialist physicians. Spending more time on survivorship means there will be fewer available person-hours to care for patients with active cancer.

This review will not address the critical role of basic science research to elucidate such things as the mechanisms of long-term and late effects, and will not get into specific questions regarding surveillance for particular cancers. Rather it will focus on the general health services research questions around evaluating the implementation of various aspects and models of survivorship care planning at the point of transition from active cancer therapy.

Evaluation of Survivorship Care Plans

It is essential that we conduct rigorous systematic studies to see what works and what does not work in survivorship care planning. Table D.5-2 outlines key elements to be considered when envisioning such studies. Most study hypotheses or research questions related to survivorship care planning would be based to some extent on the notion that an element or elements of the care plan affect(s) one or more outcomes. The essentials of

TABLE D.5-1 The Institute of Medicine Survivorship Care Plan

Upon discharge from cancer treatment, including treatment of recurrences, every patient should be given a record of all care received and important disease characteristics. This should include, at a minimum:
1) Diagnostic tests performed and results.
2) Tumor characteristics (e.g., site(s), stage and grade, hormone receptor status, marker information).
3) Dates of treatment initiation and completion.
4) Surgery, chemotherapy, radiotherapy, transplant, hormonal therapy, or gene or other therapies provided, including agents used, treatment regimen, total dosage, identifying number and title of clinical trials (if any), indicators of treatment response, and toxicities experienced during treatment.
5) Psychosocial, nutritional, and other supportive services provided.
6) Full contact information on treating institutions and key individual providers.
7) Identification of a key point of contact and coordinator of continuing care.

Upon discharge from cancer treatment, every patient and his/her primary health care provider should receive a written follow-up care plan incorporating available evidence-based standards of care. This should include, at a minimum:
1) The likely course of recovery from acute treatment toxicities, as well as the need for ongoing health maintenance or adjuvant therapy.
2) A description of recommended cancer screening and other periodic testing and examinations, and the schedule on which they should be performed (and who should provide them).
3) Information on possible late and long-term effects of treatment and symptoms of such effects.
4) Information on possible signs of recurrence and second tumors.
5) Information on the possible effects of cancer on marital/partner relationship, sexual functioning, work, and parenting, and the potential future need for psychosocial support.
6) Information on the potential insurance, employment, and financial consequences of cancer and, as necessary, referral to counseling, legal aid, and financial assistance.
7) Specific recommendations for healthy behaviors (e.g., diet, exercise, healthy weight, sunscreen use, immunizations, smoking cessation, osteoporosis prevention). When appropriate, recommendations that first-degree relatives be informed about their increased risk and the need for cancer screening (e.g., breast cancer, colorectal cancer, prostate cancer).
8) As appropriate, information on genetic counseling and testing to identify high-risk individuals who could benefit from more comprehensive cancer surveillance, chemoprevention, or risk-reducing surgery.
9) As appropriate, information on known effective chemoprevention strategies for secondary prevention (e.g., tamoxifen in women at high risk for breast cancer; aspirin for colorectal cancer prevention).
10) Referrals to specific follow-up care providers (e.g., rehabilitation, fertility, psychology), support groups, and/or the patient's primary care provider.
11) A listing of cancer-related resources and information (e.g., Internet-based sources and telephone listings for major cancer support organizations).

SOURCE: IOM Report: *From Cancer Patient to Cancer Survivor: Lost in Transition*, Box 3-16, pp. 152-3, adapted from the President's Cancer Panel (2004).

TABLE D.5-2 Constructing Studies to Evaluate Survivorship Care Plans

Care plan element	Outcome	Population	Setting	Format of the Care Plan	Study Design

• Entire survivorship care plan
• Treatment summary
• Possible clinical course
• Surveillance plan
• Lifestyle recommendations
• Psychosocial issues and available resources
	Patient-level
	• Knowledge
	• Satisfaction
	• Symptoms
	  o Anxiety, depression
	  o Physical
	• Quality of life
	  o Functional status, perceived health, utility
	• Survival
	
	Systems-level
	• Communication/ coordination
	• Practice patterns
	• Processes/quality of care
	• Efficiency
	  o Resource utilization, time, cost
		• All survivors
		• Specific cancer types
		• Age groups
		• Racial/ethnic groups
		• Socioeconomic status
		• Geography
		• Family/caregiver effects
			• Oncology specialist
			• Nurse practitioner allied provider or other
			• Other specialists
			• Dedicated survivorship clinic
			
			• Other organizational characteristics (insurers, etc.)
				• Oral/informal
				• Written
				• Electronic
				
				• Standardized
				
				• Portable
					• Qualitative
					• Observational
					  o Cross-sectional surveys
					  o Medical record review
					  o Administrative data analysis
					• Interventional
					  o Prospective cohort
					  o Quasi-experimental
					  o Before/after
					  o Natural experiments
					  o Randomized controlled trials

the majority of research proposals could be summarized by describing the study design, population to be studied, the setting in which the care plan would be created and disseminated, and the format of the care plan or care plan element being evaluated. A hallmark of this research is its emphasis on understanding the integration and interaction of multidisciplinary domains. Based on these considerations and what is already known about the situation in question, an appropriate study design can then be chosen.

Care Plan Elements

The survivorship care plan as described by the IOM is a comprehensive proposal that was arrived at by expert opinion. One can take it for what it is and design evaluation exercises around implementation of the entire plan, or evaluate different parts of the plan in different settings. Some studies would be designed to ask focused questions about a particular element of care planning in a specific population and setting, while others could look at the overall effect of care planning on such outcomes as communication and coordination of care. Although the IOM provided guidance on the elements of the ideal survivorship care plan, there is still much content to be developed and many ways that the same information can be presented. Moreover, resource guides need to be created for issues such as employment and insurance in which medical providers are often not expert. What is outlined below is a discussion of the elements of study design that would contribute to the evidence base to support or refute the inclusion of individual components of the IOM's broad call to implement survivorship care planning as a standard of care in oncology practice.

Treatment Summary

While some specialists, by virtue of carrying out discrete treatments, routinely create summaries of their own therapies (e.g., operative notes or radiation completion summaries), there is usually not in common practice today an overall summary of cancer-related interventions and effects at the conclusion of primary cancer therapy. Whether the creation of such a document is beneficial is an open question, though. It would seem obvious that it would facilitate care; however, it could be that the treatment summary is superfluous for a straightforward clinical situation that is consistently managed in a very standard way. An example might be early-stage colon cancer treated with surgery alone: not much more needs to be known as even the histology is expected to be uniform and late effects uncommon. On the other hand, it can be crucial to understanding the risks faced by a patient with lymphoma who received multimodality therapy. The general utility of treatment summaries and their feasibility in terms of collation of information and the resources required for their creation need to be determined in specific clinical situations.

Possible Clinical Course

Several elements of the survivorship care plan can be summarized as being descriptions of the possible clinical course a patient will take. This includes estimating the time frame over which acute toxicities would be expected to subside, long-term effects that would not be expected to substantially improve, and/or late effects that could occur at some time in the distant future. It would also include advice about what signs and symptoms could portend a relapse and should prompt medical attention. Such information can be useful in alerting patients and providers to things that might not otherwise be recognized as being related to the antecedent cancer. Hopefully such recognition would lead to earlier intervention that could improve outcomes. On the other hand, they could also lead to increased anxiety and overinvestigation. Consequently, the optimal way to provide such information and the effects, both good and bad, of raising this awareness needs to be considered in a research program.

Surveillance Plan

Surveillance for recurrence: Recommendations for surveillance for cancer recurrence are unique to each type of cancer, stage, disease histology, and the presence of any suspected genetic predisposition. They are generally thought to be important because of an expectation that they can affect survival. However, they are often controversial. Surveillance of the primary tumor site can in some cases detect salvageable local recurrences, for example, in anal, rectal, and breast malignancies. For disease that has spread beyond the primary site, there are some cancers, like colon cancer, renal cell carcinoma, and some sarcomas in which a small proportion of patients who recur distantly with oligometastatic disease can undergo surgery for possible cure. In many situations, however, there is not even a plausible rationale to intensely monitor asymptomatic patients in order to find incurable distant metastases, as it has not been shown in most cancers that palliative chemotherapy in asymptomatic patients is advantageous.

Surveillance research presents several methodological challenges. Randomized trials are required because nonrandomized studies are susceptible to lead-time and length-time biases. Randomized trials are logistically difficult and expensive to carry out, however, because they have to be very large to detect usually small differences in survival. Furthermore, what is tested is generally a complex strategy, and so the chosen components, frequency, and the duration of surveillance are open to challenge. Moreover, differences in overall survival outcomes may be lessened by ever improving treatment for relapsed disease. In the absence of high-quality evidence, there is in most cases little agreement about surveillance recommendations among experts.[1] Consequently, further discussion of specific issues in surveillance for recurrence is beyond the scope of this manuscript.

Surveillance for late effects of treatment: Long-term effects are those that first occur during cancer treatment and persist after completion of primary therapy. An example would be scarring from surgery. Late effects, on the other hand, are toxicities that are not apparent during primary treatment but that manifest clinically some time later, such as second cancers from radiation or chemotherapy. Specific late effects vary greatly depending on the site of disease and treatment modalities involved. Surgery and radiotherapy are local treatments and so their long-term and late effects are mostly confined to the structures in and around the primary tumor, although there can also be systemic effects from removal or destruction of an endocrine gland or the spleen. On the contrary, the effects of systemic therapy are related to the specific drugs involved. The challenge when following cancer patients is to recognize potential problems related to their prior cancer treatment, but still to monitor and investigate symptoms judiciously. Cancer survivors, like the rest of us, are aging and will develop other comorbid conditions. It is important to understand whether survivorship care planning can help increase the likelihood of appropriate workup of symptoms that may portend cancer recurrence or treatment late effect while not causing overly aggressive investigation of vague unrelated symptoms.

Psychosocial Issues and Resources

The challenges of cancer survivorship go beyond physical issues. It can affect interpersonal relationships in many ways and raise concerns related to insurance, employment, and finances. The IOM report suggests that the survivorship care plan include information on these possible effects and recommends referrals for assistance where possible. It is reasonable to question how much of this need is currently going unfulfilled, and whether proactive identification of these problems is actually able to result in better resolution. For example, can we really improve their employment situation? Are the necessary services widely available, or is the recommendation for something that cannot practically be implemented in many settings? Is provision of cancer-related resources and information in the form of web addresses and telephone numbers enough? It seems likely that if we could ensure that survivors know their rights and put them in contact with available help, they will do better in these areas, but this is an empirical question.

Lifestyle Recommendations

The end of primary treatment for cancer has been called a "teachable moment."[2] This recognizes that with significant events in a patient's life, there is a greater opportunity than at other times to have an impact on health with programs that have been shown to help change risk behaviors. As a result, a comprehensive survivorship care plan should include specific recommendations about things that survivors can do to reduce the risk of cancer recurrence (chemoprevention), second primaries (e.g., diet, exercise, stopping smoking), or of developing other unrelated diseases (e.g., immunizations) now that their cancer is cured. Collecting data on how best to operationalize this recommendation and its effect on altering behavior is important to justify expending this effort at the already overwhelming time of transitioning from cancer treatment.

Outcomes

There are several outcomes on which survivorship care planning can have an impact. Most can be assessed using existing measures, but development and validation of instruments able to capture important constructs specific to the survivor population will likely be necessary as well. The challenge in designing research is to choose end points that are going to be responsive to the effects of survivorship care planning so that improvements will be feasibly detected, yet are still important enough to be worth the effort of care planning. It would be optimal for the health services research community to converge as much as possible on a set of consistent outcome measures so that separate research groups can assess different models of care and still produce results that can be compared across studies.

Knowledge and Communication

At the patient level, several elements of the care plan are designed to increase patients' awareness of their disease and the treatment they have received. Instruments to measure such knowledge can be developed and compared with situations in which there has and has not been a care plan implemented. Similarly, the availability of this information to practitioners is a practical measure of communication among providers. Other constructs like decisional conflict, which may be decreased when patients make decisions in the setting of enhanced knowledge about their situation, could also be evaluated.

Clarity around who will be delivering various aspects of care to cancer survivors is often missing. One study found that a third of cancer survivors were not sure which physician was in charge of their cancer follow-up.[3] Some patients are aware of this and are able to take responsibility for obtaining at least some of their necessary care. Others can be empowered if made aware of what the plan should be. There will always be a proportion of patients, however, who lack the knowledge or personality to advocate for themselves. As a result, one of the most valuable features of holding cancer providers responsible for a survivorship care plan may actually be in defining explicitly which providers will take responsibility for different aspects of a patient's care. Assessing whether the survivor and involved providers are aware of and agree on who will take on the various roles of cancer surveillance, screening for other cancers where appropriate, and noncancer and preventive care is an important end point to consider studying.

Acceptability and Satisfaction

As different methods of implementing survivorship care plans are developed and tested, the satisfaction with and acceptability of the format of care planning needs to be assessed. For example, will patients accept an off-treatment consult with a nurse practitioner in a survivorship clinic, and are they as satisfied with this as if their oncologist had done it? Will they interact with web-based applications or do they prefer written documents? There are several instruments designed to measure satisfaction that could be adapted to be relevant to questions related to survivorship care planning.

Survival

Quantity and quality of life are generally considered to be the primary outcomes of biomedical research. Survivorship care plans could affect overall survival by improving adherence to important surveillance recommendations, ensuring optimal noncancer care, and/or by causing positive lifestyle changes. It may be worthwhile to look for this in some studies, but as described above, it may be difficult to detect what would likely be relatively small survival differences in most cases, and follow-up would have to be very long.

Quality of Life

Quality of life may be affected more directly than survival by survivorship care planning. Having specific recommendations about what to do for follow-up may decrease patient anxiety and ameliorate depressive symptoms. Early identification of late effects with appropriate intervention may decrease physical symptoms and improve functional status. On the other hand, highlighting all of the long-term or late effects that are possible may actually increase distress. Perceived health and self-esteem may be improved for some patients while others may become overly focused on their previous cancer experience, have increased fear of recurrence, and have trouble moving on with their lives. Consequently, preferences for the health state resulting from implementation of survivorship care plans may be reflected in measurable differences in utility.

Processes and Quality of Care

While not enough is known about the efficacy of treatment summaries and survivorship care plans to establish the simple fact of their creation as indicators of quality cancer care, some of the processes embedded in the care plans do have sufficient evidence base to be evaluated as measures of quality. In this way, quality of care becomes an outcome by which different models of care can be evaluated. For example, it is widely accepted that colorectal cancer survivors should undergo regular endoscopic surveillance to detect recurrence, new primaries, and/or to remove premalignant polyps. Therefore, studies comparing different "best practice models" could be evaluated to see which one produced the most adherence to this recommendation.

Health Care Resource Utilization

On the systems level, efficiency is a very important outcome. Any form of care plan implementation is going to consume resources, especially provider time. On a larger scale, health care costs may be affected in uncertain ways. For example, formal plans could decrease patient anxiety and result in fewer interval visits to physicians. Clear information about the likely course of disease and surveillance plan may avert inappropriate workup of probably unrelated symptoms by providers who are less familiar with specific cancer situations. Alternatively, survivors may seek investigation for potential problems they have been made aware of by the survivorship care planning process and would not otherwise have pursued. Also, if successful, survivorship care plans may cause patients who currently are not receiving appropriate surveillance measures to receive them, thereby resulting in increased appropriate health care utilization and costs. Hopefully these latter interventions would also improve health outcomes, however, allowing evaluation of the cost-effectiveness of survivorship care plans. A consideration when studying the economics of this is that the analytic methodology of discounting generally makes interventions like survivorship care plans that have up-front costs but benefits that often do not accrue until many years in the future appear relatively unattractive.

Population

The next consideration when designing research is to define the population to be studied. The notion of survivorship care planning applies to all cancer survivors. However, certain elements are more important for some than for others. Patients with very early-stage cancers may not need a specific surveillance plan, as the risk of relapse is vanishingly small. Lifestyle recommendations are more important for a survivor of head and neck cancer, for example, smoking cessation, than they are for a lymphoma survivor. Psychological distress may be more likely in a patient who has undergone disfiguring surgery (mastectomy or colostomy) than one who has had little long-term effect from cancer treatment. The concerns of an adolescent or young adult cancer survivor may have little in common with those of a geriatric oncology patient. The emphasis of the survivorship care plan will have to be tailored to the situation of each survivor, and as such, studies focused on the specific concerns relevant to relatively homogeneous populations of survivors will usually be most informative.

Even a study focused on a narrowly defined clinical situation will have to consider the diversity of the survivor population, however. Investigators will need to decide whether they want to study a representative sample of all patients or to focus on the priority areas of a subgroup. For example, how does the information needs of Spanish-speaking Latino survivors differ from those of white English-speaking patients? Should surveillance recommendations be modified in the presence of significant comorbidity? Is a web-based application as helpful to elderly survivors as younger ones? How does socioeconomic status affect the importance of employment and insurance assistance? Are survivorship resources accessible to survivors in different geographic locations across the country and across the continuum of urban and rural settings? Should children and adolescents be included? The tradeoffs necessary when studying defined populations involve balancing the efficacy of a care planning intervention against effectiveness and generalizability, while also considering practical matters of ease of subject recruitment and statistical power.

Caregiver Burden

Cancer survivorship affects more than just the cancer patient. There is a growing literature on the burden of cancer treatment on caregivers, and the challenges cancer survivors face can similarly affect the health and quality of life of their loved ones. As a result, it is appropriate for investigators to design studies that inquire whether survivorship care planning could affect satisfaction and health-related quality of life outcomes for caregivers as well.

Setting

There is no single organizational model that must be adopted in order to deliver high-quality care to cancer survivors. Although the National Coalition for Cancer Survivorship (NCCS) articulated the proposal that "long-term survivors should have access to specialized follow-up clinics that focus on health promotion, disease prevention, rehabilitation, and identification of physiologic and psychological problems," in reality, whether follow-up is provided by oncologists, PCPs, or specialized survivor clinics is not the important issue. Rather, it is by ensuring that a named provider is responsible for each aspect of follow-up that the chances of quality care occurring will be maximized. In fact, the IOM's Committee on Health Care Quality in America affirmed that "care based on continuous healing relationships" is important. In other words, patients shouldn't necessarily be removed from the care of their treating PCPs and oncologists in order to receive specialized survivor care. In addition, other specialists may be involved, and/or a "shared care" model of cooperation between specialists and primary care physicians in the follow-up of the cancer survivors could be attempted. The logistics of implementing formal survivorship care planning would be quite different if it was envisioned to occur in an oncologist's office, primary care practice, or specialized survivorship clinic. Therefore, in most cases, possibly with the exception of patient-driven care planning formats discussed below, investigators will have to decide and clearly specify which model they will study.

Even within a setting there are questions to be addressed about the efficiency, acceptability, and quality of survivorship care planning when it is carried out by treating physicians, allied providers such as nurses or nurse practitioners familiar with the patient, or by providers specialized in survivorship care planning but not familiar with the individual patient, as would be encountered in a specialized survivorship clinic. Few dedicated survivorship clinics currently exist, and they are all quite different. Some only take over the mechanics of surveillance, while others focus on providing primary care, especially to disadvantaged populations. Still others take on a consultative role, looking for signs and symptoms of long-term and late effects and then making appropriate referrals, as well as assisting with the transition consultation and creating a survivorship care plan. In this way, specialized clinics could help with the workload barrier; however, patients and physicians may fear losing contact with each other and so the feasibility of such a model is a question requiring study. Consequently, the fifth recommendation of the IOM report calls for funding organizations to "support demonstration programs to test models of coordinated, interdisciplinary survivorship care in diverse communities and across systems of care."

Care Plan Format

If survivorship care planning is currently carried out at all, it is usually in the sense of informal discussions with patients near the end of treatment about what the plan will be going forward. The IOM report suggests that that should change and provides examples but does not give a specific prescription about what form the survivorship care plan should take. Simply having a consultation in which all the elements of the plan are discussed, leaving the patient responsible to write down or remember the salient points, would probably still be a large improvement over current transition practices. However, it is expected that some form of documentation of the process that can be shared with the patient and other providers would be even more successful. A written consultation note or letter will achieve some of the aims of the IOM, but because of a lack of standardization it is quite likely to miss some of the suggested elements.

Standardization of the survivorship care plan to some extent is probably desirable. Some clinics use a combination of general and tailored information to develop a plan for patients. For example, templates can have spaces for a provider to fill in the elements of a treatment summary and surveillance plan on forms preprinted with standard lifestyle recommendations and lists of available resources. There are several examples of this sort of program in individual pediatric oncology clinics, a larger province-wide program in the Canadian province of Ontario, and the patient-centered materials developed by the Lance Armstrong Foundation. Electronic and/or handwritten versions of the templates can be available as necessary and each evaluated scientifically.

Creating even a standardized survivorship care plan is time-consuming and difficult, however. Providers could attempt to create a document as they go along during the course of care, but realistically, busy oncologists are usually stretched to their limit dealing with the acute toxicities of treatment and are unable to also work consistently on posttreatment care planning. Templates could increase feasibility if nonphysician staff such as nurses or nurse practitioners could assemble much of the data. Automated systems can be envisioned in which drugs, cumulative doses of chemotherapy, and radiation sites and fractions could be pulled from pharmacy and other administrative records and fed into the evolving treatment summary. Even with standardization and automation, however, creation of a survivorship care plan will still require significant time and resources. Advocacy organizations like the American Cancer Society and Lance Armstrong Foundation have tried to support patient-directed models by providing information on survivorship issues for common cancer types and helping survivors summarize for themselves their medical treatment and plan for follow-up care. It may be that such an approach is more realistic than a physician-based model.

Another big challenge of survivor care is the mobile patient population. A wonderful care plan can be developed, but if the patient subsequently moves to a new area, changes insurers, or even just changes doctors, the information can become practically inaccessible to his/her new providers. Because of this, an important area in need of research is the evaluation of technologies that could create care plans that are truly portable and accessible from almost anywhere. Options include "smart cards" or other media that a patient could physically carry with a large amount of electronic data in a more portable form than a paper record. Another exciting possibility is web-based applications. Patients could control access to a web-based record through standard Internet security measures (e.g., passwords, USB keys). Physicians with limited electronic resources in their practices but with Internet access could contribute to and edit information for the treatment summary and care plan over the web. In this way, a patient's plan could have input from all relevant providers. If a provider did not have Internet access, it could still provide the information for the patient or another provider to input. If the patient does not have Internet access, the final product could be printed in a hard copy version, thereby getting around the problem of disparities in electronic resources among patients that currently exist. Such formats have been implemented in some controlled settings, but their utility as population-based interventions remains to be established.

Study Design

Qualitative Research

The evaluation of survivorship care plans can involve most types of health services research study designs. Because this is a new intervention, not actually in widespread use, there is a lot of qualitative work to be done to understand the current problems in, for example, coordination of follow-up, or what the most important barriers are to implementing survivorship care planning in practice. Focus groups or key informant interviews could be undertaken with different stakeholders (e.g., survivors, oncologists, PCPs) to explore these issues and inform the design of larger quantitative studies. Case reports can increase awareness of uncommon late effects or describe anecdotal situations in which survivors may find themselves related to work or insurance.

Observational Research

If the important questions are known, observational studies can be designed to attempt to quantify and prioritize the areas of need. Cross-sectional surveys can address current practices in the various aspects of survivorship care planning. They can be used to identify deficiencies in patients' knowledge of their disease and its treatment, the surveillance plan, possible late effects, and resources available to them. Surveys can also be used to document the amount of communication that has taken place between the various specialists and with PCPs. Lastly, surveys can assess satisfaction and acceptability of different models of survivorship care among diverse stakeholders.

Some aspects of care relevant to survivorship planning can be observed directly rather than relying on patient or physician report in surveys. Retrospective medical record review and examination of administrative claims data are examples of noninterventional study designs that can confirm practice patterns with respect to surveillance for recurrence and management of long-term and late effects. Studies employing such methods can provide important insight into actual care delivered.

Prospective Cohort Studies

Different settings and formats for the creation and implementation of survivorship care plans can be piloted in prospective cohort studies. Such studies would generally start with a baseline measure of the outcome of interest, say, knowledge or anxiety. The survivorship care plan would then be implemented and follow-up determinations of the change from baseline would indicate whether the program was considered a success or failure. Other cohort studies would evaluate a nonrandom mix of patients who did and did not receive various elements of a care plan, allowing assessment of outcomes for hypothesis generation.

Quasi-experimental studies, in which there are both intervention and control groups but without random allocation of subjects into these groups, can also provide evidence of the effectiveness of survivorship care plans. Such studies can take the form of before/after analyses of outcomes divided at the time of implementation of a survivorship care plan program. This type of research is susceptible to secular trends in outcome, however, which could result from increasing general awareness of cancer survivorship among patients and providers. Another quasi-experimental design could be to take advantage of a natural experiment in which some constituents of a care plan are implemented for one group of patients but not for another similar group. Comparison of outcomes between these groups could provide information about the effects of these parts of the care plan.

Randomized Controlled Trials

The most powerful study design is the randomized controlled trial. Randomization can be at the level of the patient, although this may lead to contamination as a provider may become generally more aware of the importance of planning for survivorship and bias the study toward the null by treating control patients more like the intervention patients than they otherwise would. The problem of contamination also precludes the use of crossover designs for most questions related to survivorship care planning. Alternative designs would be to randomize providers or practices, but then there may be an imbalance in characteristics of the providers in each group, or of the patients in these practices, that could affect the outcome of the study.

Given the IOM recommendation, investigators should be aware that institutional review boards may not consider it ethical to randomize patients to having no survivorship care planning and so a "usual care" intervention, rather than a placebo, may have to be devised. This could consist of tailored information rather than a formal consultation, for example. Unfortunately, providing an intervention to the control group will bias any study toward the null and necessitate a larger sample size.

Examples of Research Questions and Study Designs

• Question: What are the practical barriers to implementing survivorship care plans in oncology practice?

o Study Design: Focus groups with providers from a variety of settings (e.g., private practice versus academic centers, different specialties, managed care versus fee-for-service contractors). Questions could try to elicit ideas for ways to facilitate transition consultations and creation of survivorship care plans in real world settings. Key informant interviews with medical directors and practice managers may provide insight into the feasibility of programs that depend on additional investment in information technology. Estimating the resource burden of creating a survivorship care plan could inform policy decisions about reimbursement for survivorship transition consultations.

• Question: In what areas do patients currently need more information: their diagnosis, previous treatment, plan for surveillance and monitoring, possible late effects, resources available, and/or who to turn to for different problems?

o Study Design: Cross-sectional survey of survivors of all kinds to assess their current knowledge and desire for information in order to find which elements of the proposed survivorship care plan have the greatest gaps between desired and actual knowledge, and to identify subpopulations of patients in which certain needs are particularly prevalent.

- Question: Is there variation in surveillance practice?
  o   Study Design: Administrative data analysis of surveillance practices for patients with stage II and III colon cancer, analyzing practice patterns and outcomes by geography, provider and patient characteristics (e.g., age, sex, race, socioeconomic status), organizational and insurance structure, and whether disparities in the quality of follow-up care exist.
- Question: How much does a transition consultation for survivorship care planning increase patients' knowledge of their previous treatment and care plan?
  o   Study Design: Prospective cohort study in which there is a base-line assessment of stage I–III breast cancer survivors' knowledge of these areas just after completion of primary therapy via an interviewer-administered survey. All subjects would then have a transition consultation and be given a written survivorship care plan. Six months later another interviewer-administered survey would assess change in knowledge from baseline.

- Question: What are the effects of survivorship care planning on a survivor's family and caregivers?
  o   Study Design: Prospective cohort study in which prostate cancer caregivers' burden is evaluated over a 2-year period and related to whether the survivor received a survivorship care plan, adjusted for other explanatory variables.

- Question: Does survivorship care planning decrease anxiety and depression?
  o   Study Design: Before/after study in which anxiety and depression levels are measured in a cohort of patients finishing treatment for Hodgkin's disease in a major referral center. A transition consultation and survivorship care plan is then implemented at that institution and anxiety and depression levels are evaluated for patients completing treatment in the following year.

- Question: How does receipt of different parts of the survivorship care plan affect satisfaction with the transition from active cancer treatment?
  o   Study Design: Analysis of data from a natural experiment in which different practices have implemented different parts of the care plan. Patients in each practice can be surveyed to assess their levels of satisfaction and differences related to the part of the care plan they received.
- Question: Are transition consultations with a specialized survivorship nurse practitioner acceptable to patients?
  o   Study Design: Randomized controlled trial in which head and neck cancer patients are randomized between either having a survivorship

care plan created by a specialized nurse practitioner during a consultation in a survivorship clinic or during a routine visit with their medical oncologist near the end of primary therapy, comparing measures of satisfaction between the two groups.

• Question: Can specific interventions targeted to lifestyle changes to decrease risk behaviors be more successful in the context of survivorship care planning.
    o Study design: Randomized controlled trial in which breast cancer patients completing adjuvant chemotherapy all receive a transition consultation and survivorship care plan, but half are invited to take part in an intensive diet and exercise intervention immediately, while the other half receive the same intervention 6 months later. Acceptance, compliance, and measures of dietary and exercise improvement would be the outcomes.

• Question: Does survivorship care planning decrease unnecessary health care resource utilization?
    o Study Design: Practices are randomized between usual care: giving patients individually-tailored treatment summaries, informal discussion of surveillance plans, and standard information about available resources; and an intervention group in which the survivorship care plan explicitly lays out the plan for surveillance and which symptoms should prompt medical evaluation. Data collected will include the costs associated with creating the care plan, and enumeration of physician visits and investigations received. This study could also inform cost-effectiveness analyses should improvement in survival and/or quality of life be found to be attributable to institution of such plans.

• Question: Which format of survivorship care plan is most effective at increasing communication among providers?
    o Study Design: Practices are randomized between web-based and paper versions of the survivorship care plan (with copies sent to all involved physicians). Survivors' PCPs are later asked to answer basic questions about the survivor's cancer and its care, using records available in their office.

Conclusion

Over time, as studies evaluating the effects of survivorship care planning on relevant outcomes are carried out, they would serve as the basis for secondary data analyses such as systematic overviews and technology assessments. Surveillance practices have already been the subject of several meta-analyses and decision analyses but this is only one component of care planning. Rigorous efficacy and effectiveness data would lead to the development of evidence-based clinical practice guidelines for survivorship care planning (the IOM report's third recommendation), thereby creating standards of care. From such standards, quality indicators related to survivorship care (promulgated in the fourth recommendation of the IOM report) could be identified and validated. This would spawn a field of inquiry related to access to care and disparities for different survivor populations. The fifth recommendation in the IOM report calls for funded demonstration programs to test models of care, and the final recommendation advocates that public as well as private agencies such as insurance plans should increase their support of survivorship research and expand mechanisms for its conduct. This last recommendation is actually the first step in all of this, however, as establishing an evidence base for the creation and implementation of survivorship care plans through the type of research outlined herein is necessary to realize the IOM's vision in which attention to the transition from cancer survivor to cancer patient is accepted as a routine part of oncology practice.

REFERENCES

1. Johnson FE: Overview, in Johnson FE, Virgo KS (eds): Cancer Patient Follow-Up. St. Louis, Mosby, 1997, p. 4.
2. Ganz PA: A teachable moment for oncologists: cancer survivors, 10 million strong and growing! J Clin Oncol 23:5458-5460, 2005.
3. Miedema B, MacDonald I, Tatemichi S: Cancer follow-up care. Patients' perspectives. Can Fam Physician 49:890-895, 2003.

Appendix E

Template for
"Cancer Survivorship Care Plan"
Tested in
IOM Focus Groups and Interviews

Cancer Survivorship Care Plan

Name:_____   Date of
Preparation:_____

This Survivorship Care Plan summarizes information about your diagnosis, treatment, follow-up care, symptoms to watch for, and steps you can take to stay healthy.

The information in this care plan will be important for you to keep so that doctors and other health care providers that you see in the future will have information about your cancer, its treatment, and how best to work with you to monitor your health.

This Survivorship Care Plan has been sent to the following providers:

Health care provider	Address

In the future, your healthcare providers may need more details about your cancer and how you were treated. This Survivorship Care Plan may help you locate information related to your treatment.

Resources for cancer survivors are listed as part of the Survivorship Care Plan so that you may obtain additional information and identify support services immediately or in the future.

Date of note:

Provider
Name: **Affiliation:**   **Telephone number:**

Survivor
Name: **Date of birth:**

CANCER TREATMENT SUMMARY

Cancer Diagnosis:
Date of tissue diagnosis of cancer:
Stage of cancer:
Pathologic findings:

Diagnostic tests done: dates and results

Treatment history (attach relevant treatment summaries):

	Surgery	Chemotherapy	Radiation	Other
Date(s)				
Location(s)				
Provider name(s)				
Procedures				

Risk of cancer recurrence and second cancer:

Patient should report these signs and symptoms if persistent:

Recommended surveillance to detect recurrence/second cancer (specify frequency):

Potential late effects of treatment (e.g., cardiovascular, skeletal):

Surgery:

Radiation:

Chemo/Biotherapy:

Patient should report these signs and symptoms if persistent:

Recommended surveillance for late effects of treatment(s):

Preventive care recommendations (e.g., osteoporosis prevention, weight management, smoking cessation, diet):

Physician(s) who will monitor recurrence/second cancer, late effects, and preventive care:

Identified concerns:	**Referrals:**
☐Depression/anxiety:	☐Psychiatry
☐Fertility:	☐Psychology/social work
☐Marital/partner/family relationships:	☐Fertility/endocrinology
☐Sexuality:	☐Genetic counseling
☐Genetic risk:	☐Smoking cessation
☐Wellness (e.g., diet, exercise, smoking cessation)	☐Dietician/weight control
☐Employment, health insurance, finances:	☐Exercise program
☐Other:	☐Physical therapy/rehabilitation
	☐Counseling regarding employment, health insurance, finances
	☐Other:

Services to Think About (adapted from NCI's facing forward)

People who have had cancer agree that no one should have to go it alone after treatment. Your friends and family can help. Ask your doctor, nurse, social worker, or local cancer organization how to find services in your area like the ones listed below.

Service	How It Can Help You
Clergy-- Spiritual Counseling	Some members of the clergy are trained to help you deal with cancer concerns such as feeling alone, fear of death, searching for meaning, and doubts about faith.
Counseling	Trained mental health specialists help you deal with your feelings, such as anger, sadness, and concern for your future. Family support programs are available as are trained specialists who can help you address issues related to sex and intimacy.
Genetic Counseling	Trained specialists advise on whether to have gene testing for cancer and how to deal with the results. It can be helpful for you and for family members who have concerns for their own health. (See Genetic Counseling for ways to find genetic counselors.)
Home Care Services	State and local governments offer many services useful after cancer treatment. A nurse or physical therapist may be able to come to your home. You also may be able to get help with housework or cooking. The phone book has contact numbers under Social Services, Health Services, or Aging Services--both nonprofit and for-profit.
Long-Term Follow-up Clinics	All doctors can offer follow-up care, but there are a few clinics that specialize in long-term follow-up after cancer. These clinics most often see people who are no longer being treated by an oncologist and who are considered disease-free. You may want to ask your doctor if there are follow-up cancer clinics in your area.
Nutritionists/Dietitians	They can help you with gaining or losing weight and with healthy eating.
Occupational Therapists	They can help you regain, develop, and build skills that are important for independent living. They can help you relearn how to do daily activities such as bathing, dressing, or feeding yourself after cancer treatment.
Oncology Social Workers	These professionals are trained to counsel you about ways to cope with treatment issues and family problems related to your cancer. They can tell you about resources and connect you with services in your area.
Pain Clinics (also called Pain and Palliative Care Services)	These are centers with professionals from many different fields who are specially trained in helping people get relief from pain.
Physical Therapists	Physical therapists are trained in the way that the body parts interact and work. They can teach you about proper exercises and body motions that can help you gain strength and mobility after treatment. They can also advise you about proper postures that help prevent injuries.
Smoking Cessation Services	Research shows that the more support you have in quitting smoking, the greater your chance for success. Many communities have "quit smoking" programs. Ask your doctor, nurse, social worker, or local hospital about what is available, or call 1-800-4-CANCER (1-800-422-6237).

Speech Therapists	Speech therapists can evaluate and treat any speech, language, or swallowing problems you may have after treatment.
Stress Management Programs	These programs teach ways to help you relax and take more control over stress. Hospitals, clinics, or local cancer organizations may offer such programs and classes.
Support Groups for Survivors	In-person and online groups enable survivors to interact with others in similar situations.
Vocational Rehabilitation Specialists	If you have disabilities or other special needs after treatment, these services can help you find suitable jobs. Such services include counseling, education and skills training, and help in obtaining and using assistive technology and tools.

Here are a few national organizations that provide information and support and tell you about services in your local community

Organization	Website	Telephone number
American Cancer Society-provides resources online and in the community	www.cancer.org	To be added
CancerCare-provides resources online and by telephone	www.cancercare.org	
Lance Armstrong Foundation-provider resources online and in the community	www.livestrong.org	
National Cancer Institute-provides information online and by telephone. *Life After Cancer Treatment is a booklet available in English and Spanish*	*www.cancer.gov/cancertopics/life-after-treatment*	
National Coalition of Cancer survivorship provides the "Cancer Survival Toolbox: An Audio Resource Program"	www.cancersurvivaltoolbox.org/	
The Wellness Community provides information and services online and in the community	www.thewellnesscommunity.org	

Disclaimer

It is important to realize that many management questions have not been comprehensively addressed in randomized trials and guideline based recommendations cannot always account for individual variation among patients. These recommendations are not intended to supplant physician judgment with respect to particular patients or special clinical situations and cannot be considered inclusive of all proper methods of care or exclusive of other treatments reasonably directed at obtaining the same results Accordingly, we consider adherence to these recommendations to be voluntary, with the ultimate determination regarding their application to be made by the physician in light of each patient's individual circumstances.

Cancer Survivorship Care Plan
(completed using fictitious information)

Name:__John Smith_____ Date of
Preparation:___4/3/06_____

This Survivorship Care Plan summarizes information about your diagnosis, treatment, follow-up care, symptoms to watch for, and steps you can take to stay healthy.

The information in this care plan will be important for you to keep so that doctors and other health care providers that you see in the future will have information about your cancer, its treatment, and how best to work with you to monitor your health.

This Survivorship Care Plan has been sent to the following providers:

Health care provider	Address
Tony Adams, M.D. (Fam physician)	323 Locust St. Birmingham, AL
Susan Lyons. M.D. (GI physician)	525 Wine Ave. Birmingham, AL

In the future, your healthcare providers may need more details about your cancer and how you were treated. This Survivorship Care Plan may help you locate information related to your treatment.

Resources for cancer survivors are listed as part of the Survivorship Care Plan so that you may obtain additional information and identify support services immediately or in the future.

Date of note: 4/3/06
Provider
Name: Jo Ann Helms, M.D.   **Affiliation:** U Alabama   **Telephone number:** 519-336-5123
Survivor
Name: John Smith   **Date of birth: 5-25-59**
CANCER TREATMENT SUMMARY

Colorectal Cancer Diagnosis:
Date of tissue diagnosis of cancer: 7-15-05
Stage of cancer: III Lymph node involvement
Pathologic findings: high grade cancer arising in a large polyp, 3 of 10 nodes positive

Diagnostic tests done: dates and results
   Colonoscopy: 7-1-05, obstructing lesion at hepatic flexure
   CT scan Chest: no mets
   CT scan Abdomen: enlarged mass in right colon, no liver mets
   CT scan Pelvis; no abnormalities

Pre-operative and Post-operative serum CEA levels (dates and results): 7/5/05 10; 8/15/05 3.9
   Last CEA 2.0 on 3-10-06

Treatment history (attach relevant treatment summaries):

	Surgery	Chemotherapy	Radiation	Other
Date(s)	7-15-05	9-05 to 3-06	none	
Location(s)	U of Alabama	U of Alabama		
Provider name(s)	John Woods	Jo Ann Helms		
Procedures	Right hemicolectomy	Systemic chemo: 5 FU + Leucovorin +/- Oxaliplatin (FLOX)		

Risk of cancer recurrence and second cancer: Patient has high stage cancer with increased risk of recurrence.

Patient should report these signs and symptoms if persistent:
Blood in stool, abdominal pain, change in bowel habits, cough that doesn't go away, bone pain, new lumps, nausea, vomiting, loss of appetite, weight loss, fatigue

Recommended surveillance to detect recurrence/second cancer (specify frequency)**:**
- Clinical assessments:
  Every 3-6 months for the first three years after primary treatment, then every 6 months for years 4 and 5, and

  subsequently to be determined (ASCO, 2005)

- Tests:
  Serum CEA every 3 months for at least 3 years after diagnosis, if the patient is a candidate for surgery or systemic

  therapy (ASCO, 2005); data not sufficient to recommend other tests such as CBC, LFT"s, and stool for occult blood

  (ASCO, 2005)

- Imaging:
  -Annual CT of the chest and abdomen for 3 years after primary therapy (for patients who are at higher risk of recurrence and who could be candidates for surgery with curative intent).

- Other: -Colonoscopy at 3 years after operative treatment; if results normal, every 5 years thereafter (ASCO, 2005);
  -Genetic counseling for those who are high risk (colorectal cancer or polyps in a parent, sibling, or child younger than 60 or in two such relatives of any age or colorectal cancer syndromes in family) **This patient needs genetic testing due to young age and family history.**

Potential late effects of treatment (e.g., cardiovascular, skeletal)**:**
Surgery: Bowel problems, such as diarrhea, fecal leakage/incontinence, constipation, bowel obstruction, hernia, pain, psychological distress

Chemo/Biotherapy: fatigue, peripheral neuropathy

Patient should report these signs and symptoms if persistent:
Diarrhea, constipation, pain with urination, erectile dysfunction, painful intercourse, infertility, numbness or tingling in hands or feet

Recommended surveillance for late effects of treatment(s): monitor for recovery of peripheral neuropathy

Preventive care recommendations (e.g., osteoporosis prevention, weight management, smoking cessation, diet)**: This patient needs counseling about smoking cessation and weight loss.**

Physician(s) who will monitor recurrence/second cancer, late effects, and preventive care:

Dr. Adams will monitor for late effects and preventive care recommendations. Dr. Adams will monitor CEA and do endoscopy and imaging studies at prescribed intervals.

Identified concerns:	Referrals:
xDepression/anxiety:	☐Psychiatry
☐Fertility:	xPsychology/social work

□Marital/partner/family relationships: □Sexuality: xGenetic risk: xWellness (e.g., diet, exercise, smoking cessation) □Employment, health insurance, finances: □Other:	□Fertility/endocrinology xGenetic counseling xSmoking cessation xDietician/weight control □Exercise program □Physical therapy/rehabilitation □Counseling regarding employment, health insurance, finances □Other:

Services to Think About (adapted from NCI's facing forward)

People who have had cancer agree that no one should have to go it alone after treatment. Your friends and family can help. Ask your doctor, nurse, social worker, or local cancer organization how to find services in your area like the ones listed below.

Service	How It Can Help You
Clergy-- Spiritual Counseling	Some members of the clergy are trained to help you deal with cancer concerns such as feeling alone, fear of death, searching for meaning, and doubts about faith.
Counseling	Trained mental health specialists help you deal with your feelings, such as anger, sadness, and concern for your future. Family support programs are available as are trained specialists who can help you address issues related to sex and intimacy.
Genetic Counseling	Trained specialists advise on whether to have gene testing for cancer and how to deal with the results. It can be helpful for you and for family members who have concerns for their own health. (See Genetic Counseling for ways to find genetic counselors.)
Home Care Services	State and local governments offer many services useful after cancer treatment. A nurse or physical therapist may be able to come to your home. You also may be able to get help with housework or cooking. The phone book has contact numbers under Social Services, Health Services, or Aging Services--both nonprofit and for-profit.
Long-Term Follow-up Clinics	All doctors can offer follow-up care, but there are a few clinics that specialize in long-term follow-up after cancer. These clinics most often see people who are no longer being treated by an oncologist and who are considered disease-free. You may want to ask your doctor if there are follow-up cancer clinics in your area.
Nutritionists/Dietitians	They can help you with gaining or losing weight and with healthy eating.
Occupational Therapists	They can help you regain, develop, and build skills that are important for independent living. They can help you relearn how to do daily activities such as bathing, dressing, or feeding yourself after cancer treatment.
Oncology Social Workers	These professionals are trained to counsel you about ways to cope with treatment issues and family problems related to your cancer. They can tell you about resources and connect you with services in your area.
Pain Clinics (also called Pain and Palliative Care Services)	These are centers with professionals from many different fields who are specially trained in helping people get relief from pain.

Physical Therapists	Physical therapists are trained in the way that the body parts interact and work. They can teach you about proper exercises and body motions that can help you gain strength and mobility after treatment. They can also advise you about proper postures that help prevent injuries.
Smoking Cessation Services	Research shows that the more support you have in quitting smoking, the greater your chance for success. Many communities have "quit smoking" programs. Ask your doctor, nurse, social worker, or local hospital about what is available, or call 1-800-4-CANCER (1-800-422-6237).
Speech Therapists	Speech therapists can evaluate and treat any speech, language, or swallowing problems you may have after treatment.
Stress Management Programs	These programs teach ways to help you relax and take more control over stress. Hospitals, clinics, or local cancer organizations may offer such programs and classes.
Support Groups for Survivors	In-person and online groups enable survivors to interact with others in similar situations.
Vocational Rehabilitation Specialists	If you have disabilities or other special needs after treatment, these services can help you find suitable jobs. Such services include counseling, education and skills training, and help in obtaining and using assistive technology and tools.

Here are a few national organizations that provide information and support and tell you about services in your local community

Organization	Website	Telephone number
American Cancer Society-provides resources online and in the community	www.cancer.org	To be added
CancerCare-provides resources online and by telephone	www.cancercare.org	
Lance Armstrong Foundation-provider resources online and in the community	www.livestrong.org	
National Cancer Institute-provides information online and by telephone. *Life After Cancer Treatment is a booklet available in English and Spanish*	*www.cancer.gov/cancertopics/life-after-treatment*	
National Coalition of Cancer survivorship provides the "Cancer Survival Toolbox: An Audio Resource Program"	www.cancersurvivaltoolbox.org/	
The Wellness Community provides information and services online and in the community	www.thewellnesscommunity.org	

Disclaimer

It is important to realize that many management questions have not been comprehensively addressed in randomized trials and guideline based recommendations cannot always account for individual variation among patients. These recommendations are not intended to supplant physician judgment with respect to particular patients or special clinical situations and cannot be considered inclusive of all proper methods of care or exclusive of other treatments reasonably directed at obtaining the same results Accordingly, we consider adherence to these recommendations to be voluntary, with the ultimate determination regarding their application to be made by the physician in light of each patient's individual circumstances.

Appendix F

Treatment Summary Forms
Developed by the
Children's Oncology Group (COG)

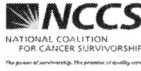 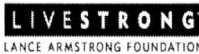 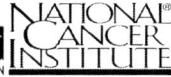

May 8, 2006

Dear Colleagues,

On behalf of the Children's Oncology Group (COG) Nursing Discipline and Late Effects Committees, Smita Bhatia and Wendy Landier have provided the attached treatment summary forms. These forms were developed through multidisciplinary collaboration within the COG and are designed to interface with COG's *Long-Term Follow-Up Guidelines for Survivors of Childhood, Adolescent, and Young Adult Cancers.*

Although a comprehensive summary is certainly preferred in the clinical setting - it is not always possible to obtain all the details of each patient's treatment, particularly when therapy was completed many years ago. Therefore, an abbreviated version of the therapeutic summary form was also developed.

The one-page abbreviated version includes only those elements required to generate patient-specific, exposure-related, long-term follow-up guidelines using *COG's Long-Term Follow-Up Guidelines for Survivors of Childhood, Adolescent, and Young Adult Cancers.* The two-page comprehensive version of the therapeutic summary form includes the required elements but also allows for a more detailed summary of the patient's medical history and cancer therapy. It is accompanied by a "Key" to assist in form completion (this is actually the list of the "drop-down menus" available for completing the computerized version of this form).

Both versions will eventually be accessible via a web-based interface that will allow for computerized generation of therapeutic summaries and accompanying patient-specific long-term follow-up guidelines. This web-based interface, known as "*Passport for Care,*" is a collaborative effort of Texas Children's Cancer Center, Baylor College of Medicine's Center for Collaborative and Interactive Technologies, and the Children's Oncology Group, and will provide clinicians with access to efficient, patient-specific application of the *COG's Long-Term Follow-Up Guidelines for Survivors of Childhood, Adolescent, and Young Adult Cancers.*

CureSearch
Children's Oncology Group

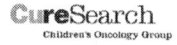

SUMMARY OF CANCER TREATMENT
(Abbreviated)

DEMOGRAPHICS

Name:	Sex:	Date of Birth:

CANCER DIAGNOSIS

Diagnosis:	Date of Diagnosis:	Date Therapy Completed:

CHEMOTHERAPY: ☐ Yes ☐ No *If yes, complete chart below*

Drug Name	Route	Additional Information*

* Anthracyclines: Include cumulative dose in mg/m^2; Carboplatin: Indicate if dose was myeloablative;
 IV Methotrexate and Cytarabine: Indicate if any single dose was $\geq$1000 mg/m^2.
 Note: Cumulative doses, if known, should be recorded for all agents, particularly for alkylators and bleomycin.

RADIATION ☐ Yes ☐ No *If yes, complete chart below*

Site/Field	Total Dose (cGy)	Boost Site	Boost Dose (cGy)	Total Dose with Boost (cGy)

HEMATOPOIETIC CELL TRANSPLANT ☐ Yes ☐ No *If yes, answer question below*

Was this patient ever diagnosed with **chronic** graft-versus-host disease (cGVHD)? ☐ Yes ☐ No

SURGERY ☐ Yes ☐ No *If yes, complete chart below*

Procedure	Site (if applicable)	Laterality (if applicable)

OTHER THERAPEUTIC MODALITIES ☐ Yes ☐ No *If yes, answer questions below*

Did this patient receive radioiodine therapy (I-131 thyroid ablation)?	☐ Yes ☐ No
Did this patient receive systemic MIBG (in therapeutic doses)?	☐ Yes ☐ No
Did this patient receive bioimmunotherapy?	☐ Yes ☐ No

Summary prepared by: | Date prepared:

CureSearch
Children's Oncology Group

SUMMARY OF CANCER TREATMENT
(Comprehensive)

DEMOGRAPHICS

Name: (last, first, middle)		Sex: (M/F)	Date of Birth:	COG Reg #:
Address: (number, street, city, state/province, postal code, country)				
Phone:	SS#		Race/Ethnicity: (see list #1)	
Alternate contact:		Relationship:		Phone:

CANCER DIAGNOSIS

Diagnosis: (see list #2)

Date of Diagnosis:	Age at Diagnosis:	Date Therapy Completed:
Sites involved/stage/diagnostic details:	Laterality: (Right/Left/NA)	

Hereditary/congenital history: (see list #3)

Pertinent past medical history:

Treatment Center:	Medical Record #:

MD/APN Contact Information:

RELAPSE(S) ☐ Yes ☐ No *If yes, provide information below*

Date:	Site(s):	Laterality: (Right/Left/NA)	Date Therapy Completed:

SUBSEQUENT MALIGNANT NEOPLASM(S) ☐ Yes ☐ No *If yes, provide information below*

Date:	Type: (see list #4)	
Stage/Site(s):		Date Therapy Completed:

CANCER TREATMENT SUMMARY

PROTOCOL(S) ☐ Yes ☐ No *If yes, provide information below*

Acronym/Number	Title/Description	Initiated	Completed	On-Study

CHEMOTHERAPY ☐ Yes ☐ No *If yes, complete chart below*

Drug Name (see list # 5)	Route (see list #6)	Additional Information (see list #7)

* Anthracyclines: Include cumulative dose in mg/m^2; Carboplatin: Indicate if dose was myeloablative;
IV Methotrexate and Cytarabine: Indicate if any single dose was $\geq$1000 mg/m^2.
Note: Cumulative doses, if known, should be recorded for all agents, particularly for alkylators and bleomycin.

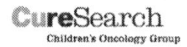

SUMMARY OF CANCER TREATMENT (continued)

RADIATION ☐ Yes ☐ No *If yes, complete chart below*

Site/Field	Laterality	Start Date	Stop Date	Fractions	Dose per Fraction (cGy)	Total Dose (cGy)	Boost Site	Boost Dose (cGy)	Total Dose with Boost (cGy)	Type
(see list #8)							(see list #9)			(see list #10)

Radiation oncologist: | **Institution:**

HEMATOPOIETIC CELL TRANSPLANT ☐ Yes ☐ No *If yes, complete chart below*

Type	Source	Date of Infusion	Conditioning Regimen	Institution/Treating MD
(see list #11) Tandem? **Yes/No**	(see list #12)		(see list #13)	

GVHD prophylaxis/treatment (For transplant patients only) ☐ Yes ☐ No *If yes, complete chart below*

Type	First Dose	Last Dose
(see list #14)		

Was this patient ever diagnosed with **chronic** graft-versus-host disease (cGVHD)? ☐ Yes ☐ No

---

SURGERY ☐ Yes ☐ No *If yes, complete chart below*

Date	Procedure	Site (if applicable)	Laterality (if applicable)	Surgeon/Institution
	(see list #15)			

OTHER THERAPEUTIC MODALITIES ☐ Yes ☐ No *If yes, complete chart below*

Therapy	Route	Cumulative Dose (if known)
(see list # 16)	(see list #6)	(see list #7)

COMPLICATIONS/LATE EFFECTS ☐ Yes ☐ No *If yes, complete chart below*

Problem	Date onset	Date resolved	Status
(see list #17)			(Active/Resolved)
			(Active/Resolved)
			(Active/Resolved)
			(Active/Resolved)
			(Active/Resolved)
			(Active/Resolved)

Adverse Drug Reactions/Allergies ☐ Yes ☐ No *If yes, complete chart below*

Drug	Reaction	Date	Status
			(Active/Resolved)
			(Active/Resolved)

Additional Information/Comments ☐ Yes ☐ No *If yes, provide information below*

Summary prepared by: (name/title/institution) | **Date prepared:**

Summary updated by: (name/title/institution) | **Date updated:**

CureSearch
Children's Oncology Group

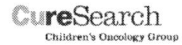

**Key for Completing
Summary of Cancer Treatment
(Comprehensive Version)**

#1: Race/Ethnicity

Asian
Black
Caucasian (non-Hispanic)
Hispanic
Native American/Alaskan Native
Native Hawaiian/Pacific Islander
Multi-racial/multi-ethnic
Other (specify):

#2: Cancer Diagnosis

Central Nervous System Tumor
Astrocytoma
Cerebellar astrocytoma
Supratentorial astrocytoma
Brainstem glioma
Choroid plexus neoplasm
Craniopharyngioma
Ependymoma
Germ cell tumor, intracranial, specify type:_____
Optic glioma
Pineal tumor
PNET
Cerebellar (medulloblastoma)
Supratentorial PNET
Spinal cord tumor, intramedullary
CNS tumor, other, specify:_____
Endocrine tumor
Adrenal tumor (non-neuroblastoma)
Thyroid tumor
Parathyroid tumor
Gastroenteropancreatic tumor
Multiple endocrine neoplasia syndrome
Endocrine tumor, other, specify:_____
Germ cell tumor (extracranial)
Seminoma
Germinoma
Dysgerminoma
Non-seminomas
Yolk sac tumor
Embryonal carcinoma
Choriocarcinoma
Teratoma
Mature
Immature
With malignant transformation
Germ cell tumor, other, specify:_____

CureSearch
Children's Oncology Group

#2: Cancer Diagnosis (continued)

Leukemia
Acute lymphoblastic leukemia
Acute myeloid leukemia
Chronic myeloid leukemia
Myelodysplastic syndrome
Myeloproliferative disorder
Leukemia, other, specify:_____
Liver tumor
Hepatoblastoma
Hepatocellular carcinoma
Liver tumor, other, specify: _____
Lymphoma
Hodgkin lymphoma
Non-Hodgkin lymphoma
Lymphoblastic lymphoma
Burkitt's lymphoma
Large cell lymphoma
Anaplastic large cell lymphoma
Diffuse large B-cell lymphoma
Lymphoma, other, specify:_____
Nasopharyngeal carcinoma
Neuroblastoma
Ganglioneuroblastoma
Renal tumor
Wilms tumor
Clear cell sarcoma
Renal cell carcinoma
Renal tumor, other:
Retinoblastoma
Sarcoma
Ewing's sarcoma/peripheral PNET
Osteogenic sarcoma
Rhabdomyosarcoma
Soft tissue sarcoma (nonrhabdomyosarcomatous)
Alveolar soft part sarcoma
Fibrosarcoma
Leiomyosarcoma
Liposarcoma
Malignant fibrous histiocytoma
Malignant peripheral nerve sheath tumor
Neurofibrosarcoma
Synovial sarcoma
Undifferentiated sarcoma
Sarcoma, other, specify: _____
Skin cancer
Basal cell carcinoma
Malignant melanoma
Squamous cell carcinoma
Skin cancer, other, specify:_____
Malignancy, other, specify:
Langerhans cell histiocytosis
Diagnosis, other, specify:
Unknown

CureSearch
Children's Oncology Group

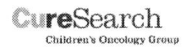

#3: Hereditary/Congenital History

Congenital heart disease
Congenital disease, other, specify:
Hemihypertrophy
Neurofibromatosis
Type I
Type II
Down syndrome
Syndrome, other, specify:
Hereditary condition, other, specify:
None
Unknown

#4: Subsequent Malignancy Diagnosis

Leukemia
Acute lymphoblastic leukemia
Acute myeloid leukemia
Chronic myeloid leukemia
Myelodysplastic syndrome
Myeloproliferative disorder
Leukemia, other, specify:
Lymphoma
Hodgkin lymphoma
Non-Hodgkin lymphoma
Lymphoblastic lymphoma
Burkitt's lymphoma
Large cell lymphoma, specify type:_____
Post-transplant lymphoproliferative disorder (PTLD)
Lymphoma, other, specify:
Sarcoma
Ewing's sarcoma/peripheral PNET
Osteosarcoma
Rhabdomyosarcoma
Nonrhabdomyosarcomatous soft tissue sarcoma, specify type:
Undifferentiated sarcoma
Other sarcoma, specify:
Thyroid cancer
Skin cancer
Basal cell carcinoma
Malignant melanoma
Squamous cell carcinoma
Breast cancer
Central nervous system tumor
Malignant, specify type and location:
Meningioma, specify location:
Other CNS tumor, specify type:
Gastrointestinal cancer
Esophageal cancer
Stomach cancer
Colorectal cancer
Hepatocellular carcinoma
Pancreatic cancer
Other GI cancer, specify:

CureSearch
Children's Oncology Group

#4: Subsequent Malignancy Diagnosis (continued)

Lung cancer
Bladder cancer
Renal cancer
Renal cell carcinoma
Clear cell sarcoma
Other renal cancer, specify:_____
Cervical cancer
Peripheral nerve sheath tumor/Schwannoma
Malignancy, other, specify:
None
Unknown

#5: Chemotherapy

Asparaginase
Bleomycin
Busulfan
Carboplatin
Myeloablative dose? Yes/No
Carmustine (BCNU)
Chlorambucil
Cisplatin
Cladribine
Clofarabine
Cyclophosphamide
Cytarabine
If IV: Any single dose $\geq$1000 mg/m^2? Yes/No
Dacarbazine (DTIC)
Dactinomycin
Daunorubicin
Dexamethasone
Docetaxel
Doxorubicin
Epirubicin
Etoposide (VP-16)
Fludarabine
Fluorouracil
Gemcitabine
Hydrocortisone
Hydroxyurea
Idarubicin
Ifosfamide
Imatinib Mesylate
Irinotecan
Lomustine (CCNU)
Mechlorethamine
Melphalan
Mercaptopurine
Methotrexate
If IV: Any single dose $\geq$1000 mg/m^2? Yes/No
Mitoxantrone
Oxaliplatin
Paclitaxel
Prednisone

#5: Chemotherapy (continued)

Procarbazine
Temozolomide
Teniposide (VM-26)
Thioguanine (6-TG)
Thiotepa
Topotecan
Trimetrexate
Vinorelbine
Vinblastine
Vincristine
Other, specify:
None
Unknown

#6: Route

PO
IM
IV
SQ
IT
IO
Other, specify:
Unknown

#7: Cumulative Dose *(Note: this is a required field for anthracyclines and optional but suggested for all others)*

mg/m^2
$units/m^2$
mg/kg *(Note: computer will multiply mg by 30 and display as mg/m^2)*
Not available
Not applicable
Other, specify:
Unknown

#8: Radiation Site/Field

Head/brain
Cranial
Craniospinal *(Note: if selected, computer will prompt user to enter data for both cranial <u>and</u> spinal fields]*
Orbital/eye, specify: Right, left, bilateral
Ear/infratemporal, specify: Right, left, bilateral
Nasopharyngeal
Oropharyngeal
Waldeyer's Ring
Other head/brain radiation, specify:_____
Neck
Cervical (neck), specify: Right, left, bilateral
Supraclavicular, specify: Right, left, bilateral
Spine
Spine - cervical
Spine - thoracic
Spine - lumbar
Spine - sacral

#8: Radiation Site/Field (continued)

Chest (thorax)
Lung (whole), specify: Right, left, bilateral
Mantle
Mini-Mantle
Extended Mantle
Mediastinal
Hilar
Axilla, specify: Right, left, bilateral
Chest, other, specify: _____
Abdomen
Whole abdomen
Upper abdomen, specify field(s) if applicable:
Hepatic
Hemiabdomen/flank, specify: Right, left
Upper quadrant, specify: Right, left, bilateral
Renal bed, specify: Right, left, bilateral
Spleen, specify: partial, entire
Splenic pedicle
Inverted Y
Paraaortic
Pelvis
Pelvic
Vagina
Prostate
Bladder
Iliac
Inguinal
Femoral
Inverted Y
Testicular, specify: Right, left, bilateral
Skeletal
Extremity
Upper, specify: Right, left, bilateral; specify: proximal, distal, entire
Lower, specify: Right, left, bilateral; specify: proximal, distal, entire
Bone, specify:
Other, specify:
Total Body Irradiation (TBI)
Total Lymphoid Irradiation (TLI)
Subtotal Lymphoid Irradiation (STLI)
Other, specify:
Add comment:
None
Unknown

#9: Radiation Boost

Tumor bed, specify location:
Other location, specify:
None
Unknown
Add comment:

#10: Radiation Type

Brachytherapy
Conformal
External beam (conventional)
IMRT
Stereotactic
Other, specify:
None
Unknown

#11: Hematopoietic Cell Transplant - Type

Autologous
Matched related
Mismatched related
Haploidentical related
Syngeneic
Matched unrelated
Other, specify:
None
Unknown

#12: Hematopoietic Cell Transplant - Source

Bone marrow
Peripheral blood stem cells
Cord blood
Other, specify:
None
Unknown

#13: Hematopoietic Cell Transplant - Conditioning Regimen

ATG
Busulfan
Carmustine (BCNU)
Cyclophosphamide
Etoposide
Fludarabine
Melphalan
Thiotepa
TBI
Other, specify:
None
Unknown

#14: GVHD Prophylaxis/Treatment

ATG
Cyclosporine
Methotrexate
MMF (mycophenolate mofetil)
Prednisone
PUVA
Sirolimus
Tacrolimus
Other, specify:
None
Unknown

CureSearch
Children's Oncology Group

#15: Surgery

Amputation, specify: Right, left, bilateral; specify site:
Central venous catheter
Cystectomy
Enucleation specify: Right, left, bilateral
Laparotomy
Limb sparing procedure, specify: Right, left, bilateral; specify site:
Nephrectomy, specify: Right, left, bilateral
Neurosurgery - brain
Craniotomy
Ventriculoperitoneal shunt
Other, specify:
Neurosurgery - spinal
Laminectomy
Other, specify:
Orchiectomy, specify: Right, left, bilateral
Pelvic surgery
Hysterectomy
Oophoropexy
Oophorectomy, specify: Right, left, bilateral
Pelvic surgery, other, specify:
Pulmonary lobectomy, specify site:
Pulmonary wedge resection, specify site:
Pulmonary metastasectomy, specify site:
Splenectomy
Thyroidectomy
Other, specify:
None
Unknown

#16: Other Therapeutic Modalities

Systemic Radiation
Radioiodine therapy (I-131 thyroid ablation)
Systemic MIBG (in therapeutic doses)
Other, specify:
Bioimmunotherapy
Hematopoietic growth factors:
G-CSF
Erythropoietin
Thrombopoietin
Interferon:
Alpha interferon
Gamma interferon
Interleukin:
IL-2
IL-11
Other, specify:
Monoclonal antibody, specify type:
Retinoic acid, specify type:
Other, specify:
Other therapeutic modality, specify:
None
Unknown

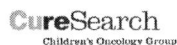

#17: Complications/Late Effects (by system)

Psychosocial
Behavioral problems/behavioral change
Educational problems
Fatigue
Limitations in healthcare access and/or insurance
Psychosocial disability due to pain
Anxiety
Depression
Post-traumatic stress
Psychosocial disability due to pain
Social withdrawal
Risky behaviors
Tobacco use
Alcohol abuse
Substance abuse
Other, specify:
Psychosocial maladjustment
Impaired quality of life
Psychosocial complication, other, specify:
Ocular
Cataract
Enophthalmos
Orbital hypoplasia
Glaucoma
Keratitis
Xerophthalmia (keratoconjunctivitis sicca)
Lacrimal duct atrophy
Optic chiasm neuropathy
Retinopathy
Telangiectasia
Maculopathy
Papillopathy
Chronic painful eye
Visual impairment (uncorrectable)
Ocular nerve palsy
Gaze paresis
Nystagmus
Papilledema
Optic atrophy
Ocular complication, other, specify:
Auditory
Eustachian tube dysfunction
Hearing loss (requires hearing aids? - Yes/No)
Sensorineural hearing loss
Conductive hearing loss
Otosclerosis
Tinnitus
Tympanosclerosis
Vertigo
Auditory complication, other, specify:
Dental
Dental abnormalities
Enamel dysplasia
Root thinning/shortening

CureSearch
Children's Oncology Group

Tooth/root agenesis	
Microdontia	
Periodontal disease	
Tooth decay	
Malocclusion	
Xerostomia (salivary gland dysfunction)	
Osteoradionecrosis	
Temporomandibular joint dysfunction	
Dental complication, other, specify:	
Cardiovascular	
Arrhythmia	
Atherosclerotic heart disease	
Cardiomyopathy	
Congestive heart failure	
Myocardial infarction	
Pericardial fibrosis	
Pericarditis	
Subclinical left ventricular dysfunction	
Valvular disease	
Carotid artery disease	
Subclavian artery disease	
Thrombosis/vascular insufficiency (related to central line)	
Vasospastic attacks (Raynaud's phenomenon)	
Cardiovascular complication, other, specify:	
Pulmonary	
Bronchiolitis obliterans	
Interstitial pneumonitis	
Pulmonary fibrosis	
Pulmonary dysfunction	
Acute respiratory distress syndrome (ARDS)	
Obstructive lung disease	
Restrictive lung disease	
Chronic bronchitis	
Bronchiectasis	
Pulmonary complication, other, specify:	
Gastrointestinal/Hepatic	
Abdominal adhesions	
Bowel obstruction	
Bowel strictures	
Fecal incontinence	
Cholelithiasis	
Cholecystitis	
Chronic enterocolitis	
Esophageal stricture	
Fistula	
Malabsorption	
Nutritional deficiency	
Vitamin B12, folate or carotene deficiency	
Cirrhosis	
Hepatic fibrosis	
Hepatic dysfunction	
Chronic hepatitis (non-infectious)	
Iron overload	
Venocclusive disease (VOD) of the liver	
Gastrointestinal/hepatic complication, other, specify:	

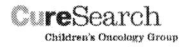

Endocrine/Metabolic
Hypothyroidism
Primary hypothyroidism (thyroid gland failure)
Secondary (central) hypothyroidism (TR/TSH deficiency)
Hyperthyroidism
Thyroid nodule
Precocious puberty
Gonadal dysfunction/failure
Gonadotropin deficiency (LH/FSH deficiency) [central gonadal failure]
Gonadal dysfunction – testicular: See Reproductive (male)
Gonadal dysfunction – ovarian: See Reproductive (female)
Metabolic syndrome
Overweight (Age 2-20 yrs: BMI for age $\geq$85 - <95%ile; Age >20 yrs: BMI 25 to 29.9)
Obesity (Age 2-20 yrs: BMI for age $\geq$95%ile; Age >20 yrs, BMI $\geq$30)
Underweight (FTT)
Insulin resistance
Impaired glucose tolerance
Diabetes mellitus
Type I
Type II
Gestational
Dyslipidemia
Adrenal insufficiency
Primary adrenal insufficiency (adrenal gland failure)
Secondary (central) adrenal insufficiency (ACTH deficiency)
Hyperprolactinemia
Growth deceleration
Growth hormone deficiency
Short stature (<5th percentile)
Endocrine/metabolic complication, other, specify:
Musculoskeletal
Amputation, specify type and site:
Osteonecrosis (avascular necrosis – AVN), specify site:
Craniofacial abnormalities
Impaired cosmesis
Contractures
Functional and activity limitation, specify:
Hypoplasia, specify site:
Kyphosis
Limb length discrepancy
Limb salvage, specify type and site:
Osteopenia
Osteoporosis
Phantom pain
Prosthesis, malfunction (poor fit, loosening, non-union, fracture)
Prosthesis, revision required due to growth
Residual limb integrity problems
Fracture (radiation-induced)
Increased energy expenditure (related to amputation/limb salvage)
Fibrosis (musculoskeletal)
Scoliosis
Short stature
Shortened trunk height
Reduced/uneven growth
Musculoskeletal complication, other, specify:

CureSearch
Children's Oncology Group

Central Nervous System (CNS)
Clinical leukoencephalopathy
With imaging abnormalities
Without imaging abnormalities
Learning disorder/disability
Math
Reading
Other, specify:
Motor deficit
Neurocognitive deficit, specify:
Diminished IQ
Executive function (planning/organization)
Sustained attention
Memory
Processing speed
Visual-motor integration
Moyamoya
Ataxia
Movement disorder
Neurogenic bladder
Neurogenic bowel
Paralysis
Occlusive cerebral vasculopathy
Seizures
Stroke
CNS complication, other, specify:
Peripheral Nervous System (PNS)
Peripheral sensory neuropathy
Peripheral motor neuropathy
PNS complication, other, specify:
Urinary
Hydronephrosis, specify: Right, left, bilateral
Hypertension
Mononephric
Renal insufficiency
Renal glomerular disorder
Hyperfiltration
Renal tubular disorder
Hypophosphatemic rickets
Renal Fanconi syndrome (dyselecrolytemia)
Renal tubular acidosis
Vesicoureteral reflux
Bladder fibrosis
Urinary incontinence
Reservoir calculi
Dysfunctional voiding
Hemorrhagic cystitis
Proteinuria
Chronic UTI
Neobladder perforation
Urinary tract obstruction (due to retroperitoneal fibrosis)
Stricture, urinary tract, specify:
Urinary complication, other, specify:

Reproductive - Female
Breast tissue hypoplasia
Uterine vascular insufficiency
Adverse pregnancy outcome
Pregnancy complications
Delivery complications
Fetal malposition
Low birthweight infant
Spontaneous abortion
Premature labor
Neonatal death
Gonadal dysfunction - ovarian
Primary ovarian failure
Delayed/arrested puberty
Premature menopause
Infertility
Inability to conceive (despite normal ovarian function)
Dyspareunia
Symptomatic ovarian cysts
Pelvic adhesions
Sexual dysfunction
Vaginal stenosis/fibrosis

Reproductive - Male
Gonadal dysfunction - testicular
Germ cell failure
Azoospermia
Oligospermia
Infertility
Leydig cell failure
Hypogonadism (testosterone deficiency)
Delayed/arrested puberty
Sexual dysfunction - male
Erectile dysfunction
Anejaculation
Retrograde ejaculation
Hydrocele

Dermatologic
Alopecia (permanent)
Dysplastic nevi
Altered skin pigmentation
Skin fibrosis
Nail dysplasia
Scleroderma
Telangiectasia
Vitiligo

Immune
Asplenia
Functional asplenia
Surgical asplenia
History of life-threatening infection (OPSI) related to asplenia
Chronic sinusitis
Chronic graft versus host disease (GVHD)
Chronic Hepatitis B
Chronic Hepatitis C

CureSearch
Children's Oncology Group

Chronic infection, specify:	
Human immunodeficiency virus (HIV) infection	
Hypogammaglobulinemia	
Secretory IgA deficiency	
Pain, chronic	
Musculoskeletal	
Neuropathic	
Other, specify:	
Other, specify	
No late effects identified	
Unknown	

Appendix G

Memorial Sloan-Kettering Cancer Center Treatment Summary and Follow-Up Plan

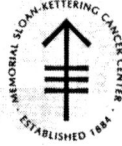

Mary S. McCabe
Director
Survivorship Program

To: Maria Hewitt,
             Senior Program Officer, Institute of Medicine

From: Mary S. McCabe, RN, MA
             Director, Survivorship Program

Date: May 10, 2006

Subject: Patient Treatment Summary

Attached is the draft Patient Treatment Summary that is being used and evaluated in the adult survivor clinics at Memorial Sloan-Kettering with individuals who have been treated for prostate cancer, thoracic malignancies and lymphoma. Both the patient and the primary care provider receive a copy of the summary.

The current draft has online pull down menus to make it simpler to complete since the clinics are busy and include a large number of patients. In our discussions with local primary care providers, we were asked to keep the form to one page so that it would be useful for physicians in busy practices.

As the next step in development, we are putting together a listing of relevant long term and late effects for inclusion in the summary.

Memorial Sloan-Kettering Cancer Center
1275 York Avenue, New York, New York 10021
Telephone 212.639.2581 • FAX 212.717.3414
E-mail: mccabem@mskcc.org

NCI-designated Comprehensive Cancer Center

Memorial Sloan Kettering Cancer Center
Summary of Cancer Treatment and Follow-up Plan
Date of preparation: _____

Name:	**Date of Birth:**
Cancer Diagnosis:	**Date of Diagnosis:**
Date Completed Therapy:	**Relapse:**

Cancer Treatment

Surgery

Date:	**Procedure:**
Surgeon/phone:	**Pathology:**

Radiation Therapy

Radiation Oncologist/phone:

Date start	Date Stop	Field	Dose (cGy)

Chemo/Biotherapy

Medical Oncologist/phone:

Drug Name	Cumulative Dose (units or mg/m^2)

Follow-up Plan

Visit Schedule	Testing

Screening Recommendations	
Colonoscopy	
Prostate specific antigen (PSA)	
Mammogram	
Other	
	NP: